LIBRARY
POST GRADUATE
KETTERING GENE

D1797273

WITHDRAWN

K D L I S

018464

COLOR ATLAS OF
GLAUCOMA

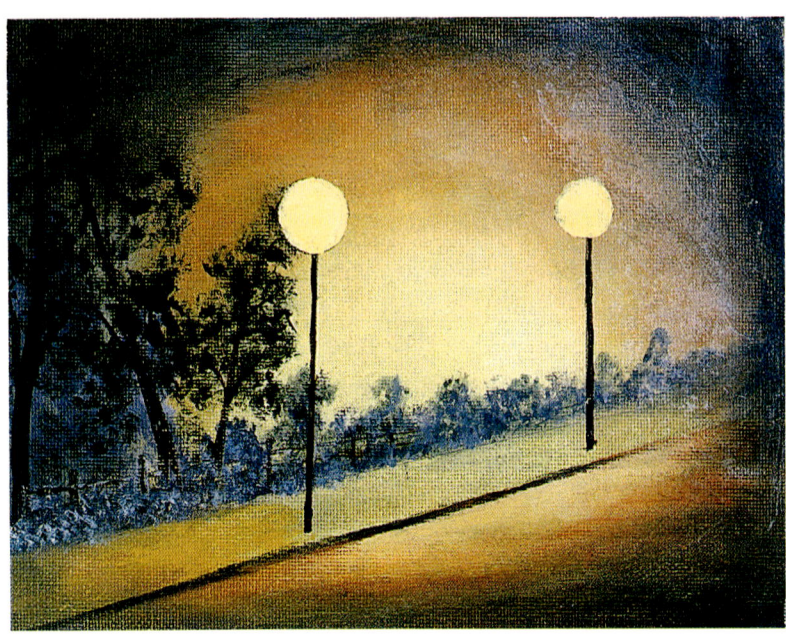

"Let There be Light"

By Robert L. Bimm

Mr. Bimm, a glaucoma patient, painted this picture as a farewell gift upon my departure from Duke. His gratitude and joy in sight are the ultimate rewards for those who labor to prevent the blindness of glaucoma.

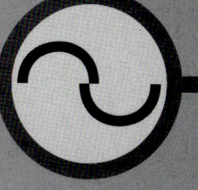

COLOR ATLAS OF
GLAUCOMA

M. Bruce Shields, M.D.

Sears Professor and Chairman
Department of Ophthalmology and Visual Science
Yale University School of Medicine
and
Chief of Ophthalmology
Yale-New Haven Hospital

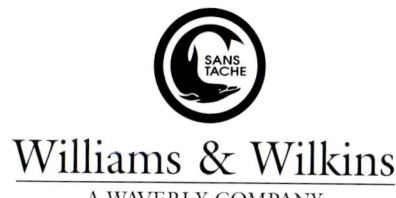

Williams & Wilkins
A WAVERLY COMPANY

BALTIMORE • PHILADELPHIA • LONDON • PARIS • BANGKOK
HONG KONG • MUNICH • SYDNEY • TOKYO • WROCLAW

PG-
WN 290 SH 1
KUA

Editor: Darlene Barela Cooke
Managing Editor: Frances M. Klass
Marketing Manager: Diane M. Harnish
Production Coordinator: Peter J. Carley
Book Project Editor: Thomas Lehr
Designer: Susan Blaker
Illustration Planner: Peter J. Carley
Cover Designer: Maria Karkucinski
Typesetter: Bi-Comp, Incorporated
Printer: Everbest Printing Co. Ltd.
Digitized Illustrations: All Systems Color, Inc.
Binder: Everbest Printing Co. Ltd.

Copyright © 1998 Williams & Wilkins

351 West Camden Street
Baltimore, Maryland 21201-2436 USA

Rose Tree Corporate Center
1400 North Providence Road
Building II, Suite 5025
Media, Pennsylvania 19063-2043 USA

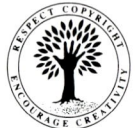

All rights reserved. This book is protected by copyright. No part of this book may be reproduced in any form or by any means, including photocopying, or utilized by any information storage and retrieval system without written permission from the copyright owner.

Accurate indications, adverse reactions and dosage schedules for drugs are provided in this book, but it is possible that they may change. The reader is urged to review the package information data of the manufacturers of the medications mentioned.

Printed in Hong Kong

Library of Congress Cataloging-in-Publication Data

Shields, M. Bruce.
    Color atlas of glaucoma / M. Bruce Shields.
      p. cm.
    Companion v. to: Textbook of glaucoma / M. Bruce Shields. 4th ed.
    Includes index.
    ISBN 0-683-07696-5
    1. Glaucoma—Atlases. I. Shields, M. Bruce. Textbook of
glaucoma. II. Title.
    [DNLM: 1. Glaucoma—atlases. WW 17 S554c 1997]
  RE871.S447 1997 Suppl.
  616.7'41—dc21
  DNLM/DLC
  for Library of Congress   96-48757
                                          CIP

The publishers have made every effort to trace the copyright holders for borrowed material. If they have inadvertently overlooked any, they will be pleased to make the necessary arrangements at the first opportunity.

To purchase additional copies of this book, call our customer service department at **(800) 638-0672** or fax orders to **(800) 447-8438.** For other book services, including chapter reprints and large quantity sales, ask for the Special Sales department.

Canadian customers should call **(800) 665-1148**, or fax **(800) 665-0103.** For all other calls originating outside of the United States, please call **(410) 528-4223** or fax us at **(410) 528-8550.**

Visit Williams & Wilkins on the Internet: http://www.wwilkins.com or contact our customer service department at **custserv@wwilkins.com.** Williams & Wilkins customer service representatives are available from 8:30 am to 6:00 pm, EST, Monday through Friday, for telephone access.

97 98 99 00
1 2 3 4 5 6 7 8 9 10

PREFACE

This *Color Atlas of Glaucoma* has been prepared as a companion to the *Fourth Edition of the Textbook of Glaucoma*. The diagnosis and management of ocular disease is a visual science from the standpoint of both the patient's health and the physician's practice. In no other discipline of medicine are the physical findings more readily available to the physician's visual inspection than in ophthalmology. It is hoped, therefore, that these color illustrations will enhance the understanding of the discussions in the textbook.

Each color plate is accompanied by legends on the facing page. This legend text is brief because the pictures, as we all know, are "worth a thousand words." More detailed information, related to each figure, can be found in the textbook. Cross-referencing is provided in both volumes to facilitate comparisons of pictures and text.

I am grateful for the assistance of my longtime secretary and friend, Ms. Robin Goodwin, who typed the text for the atlas and served as the model for many of the illustrations. Most of the pictures in the atlas are from my personal collection, amassed over the past 20 years. For those photographs, I am indebted to our award-winning ophthalmic photographer, Ms. Ruth Shirmer, and her outstanding staff of Ms. Teresa Jackson, Mr. Jeffrey Napoli, and Ms. Kim Salmon. I am also very grateful to many thoughtful friends who shared their slides with me to fill in the gaps in my collection and whose names are listed on the next page.

M. Bruce Shields, M.D.

ACKNOWLEDGMENTS

My sincere thanks to the following colleagues who were kind enough to share their slides for use in this atlas.

R Rand Allingham, MD

A Robert Bellows, MD

John F Bigger, MD

Theodore A Boutacoff

David G Campbell, MD

Carl B Camras, MD

L Frank Cashwell, Jr, MD

D Jackson Coleman, MD

Karim F Damji, MD

David Donaldson, MD

Jonathan J Dutton, MD, PhD

Gary N Foulks, MD

Jeffrey Freedman, MD, PhD

Sharon F Freedman, MD

Douglas E Gaasterland, MD

Barrett G Haik, MD

Eve J Higginbothan, MD

Roger A Hitchings, FRCS

H Dunbar Hoskins, MD

Andrew G Iwach, MD

Theodore Krupin, MD

William E Layden, MD

Charles M Lederer, MD

William A MacIlwaine, IV, MD

Wayne F March, MD

Brooks W McCuen, II, MD

Donald S Minckler, MD

Timothy O'Brien, PhD

Irvin P Pollack, MD

John W Reed, MD

Robert Ritch, MD

George O Rosenwasser, MD

Ruth Schirmer

Joel S Schuman, MD

Jerry A Shields, MD

Paul R Singer, MD

George L Spaeth, MD

H Saul Sugar, MD

Ramesch C Tripathi, MD, PhD

Martin Uram, MD

Rohit Varma, MD

David S Walton, MD

George O Waring, III, MD

CONTENTS

Section II

THE CLINICAL FORMS OF GLAUCOMA   57

Section III

THE MANAGEMENT OF GLAUCOMA

CROSS REFERENCES

to M. B. Shields: Textbook of Glaucoma,
Fourth Edition
Baltimore: Williams & Wilkins, 1998

Section I

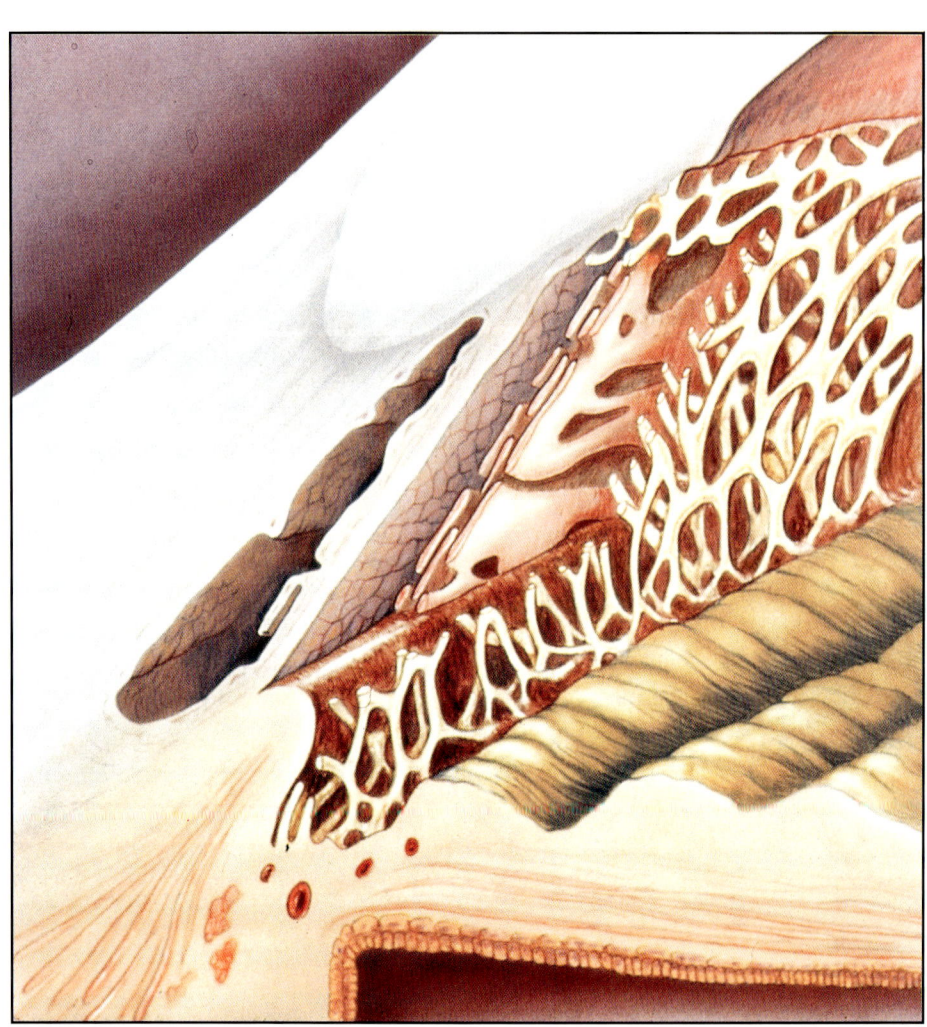

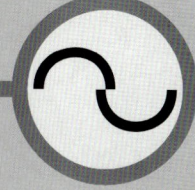

THE BASIC ASPECTS OF
GLAUCOMA

AQUEOUS HUMOR DYNAMICS

The Ciliary Body

12a. A human autopsy eye has been cut at the equator and photographed from the posterior side to show the full 360° of the ciliary body. The pars plicata is the innermost part of the ciliary body and is identified by the lighter, radial ridges of the ciliary processes, of which approximately 70 major processes are visible (*small arrow*). The pars plana is the broader, more posterior portion of the ciliary body, which joins the choroid at the ora serrata (*large arrow*). The iris has been removed in this specimen.

12b. The side view of a human autopsy eye, in which the iris has been removed, shows the relationship of the ciliary body to the aqueous humor outflow structures in the anterior chamber angle. The brown band (*arrow*) is the trabecular meshwork. Just below the meshwork is a thin, white line (the scleral spur) and below that is a light brown region (the ciliary body band). The row of ciliary processes is seen just below the ciliary body band, with the wider pars plana posterior to the processes and terminating at the ora serrata.

12c. Higher magnification of this human autopsy eye shows more detail of the ciliary processes. The iris in this specimen has been left intact and is seen just above the processes. Approximately 17 major ciliary processes and at least one minor or intermediate ciliary process (*arrow*) are visible in this view. The pars plana is the remaining brown portion posterior to the radial ridges of the ciliary processes.

12d. A cross-section view shows that the ciliary body has the shape of a right triangle, in which the ciliary processes occupy the innermost and anteriormost portion (*large arrow*). The lighter colored portion of the triangle represents ciliary muscle, which includes circular fibers in the wider anterior portion and longitudinal fibers, which insert into the scleral spur (*small arrow*) and extend posteriorly through the narrower pars plana. Note that the iris inserts into the anterior side of the ciliary body.

12e. Light microscopy of a human autopsy eye shows the relationship of the ciliary body (CB), anterior chamber angle (AC) structures, iris (I), and lens (L). The darker-staining, triangular-shaped portion of the ciliary body represents the ciliary muscle, which inserts anteriorly into the scleral spur just behind the trabecular meshwork and Schlemm's canal (*small arrow*), and tapers posteriorly through the pars plana. The ciliary processes are the fingerlike projections from the innermost, anteriormost portion of the ciliary body (*large arrow*). Note that the iris inserts into the anterior side of the ciliary body.

12f. Higher magnification shows further details of the ciliary processes, which are lined by two layers of epithelium, an outer layer of pigmented epithelium and an inner layer of nonpigmented epithelium. The innermost, anteriormost portion of the ciliary muscle is seen in the upper righthand corner, and the peripheral iris is seen to the left as it enters the ciliary body.

(Figures 12a, 12b and 12d were provided courtesy of David G. Campbell, M.D.)

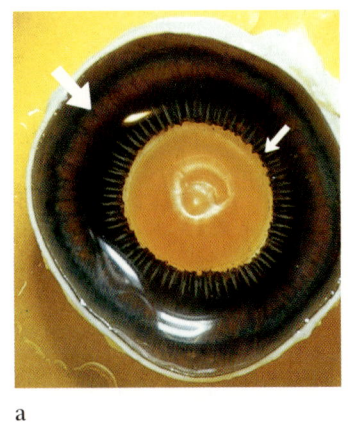

a

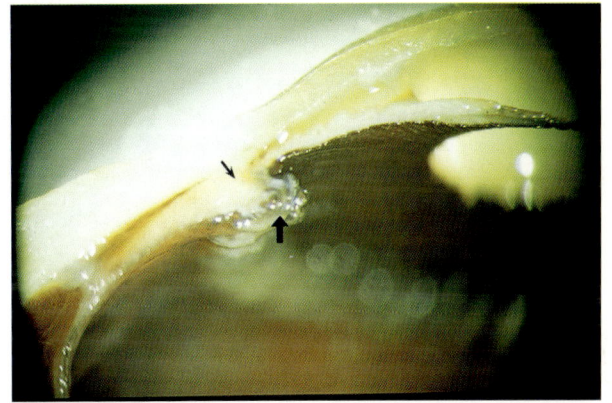

b

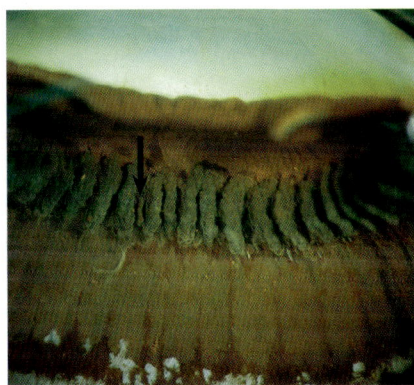

c

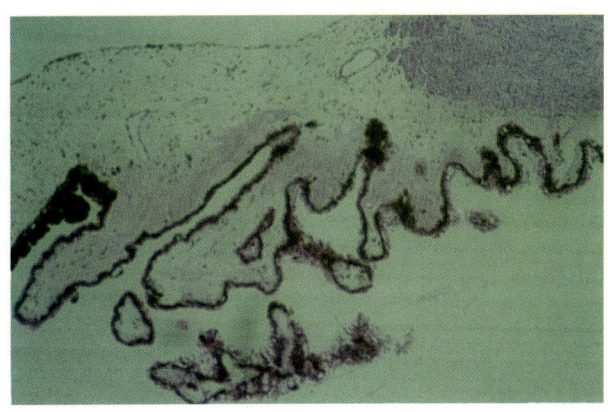

d

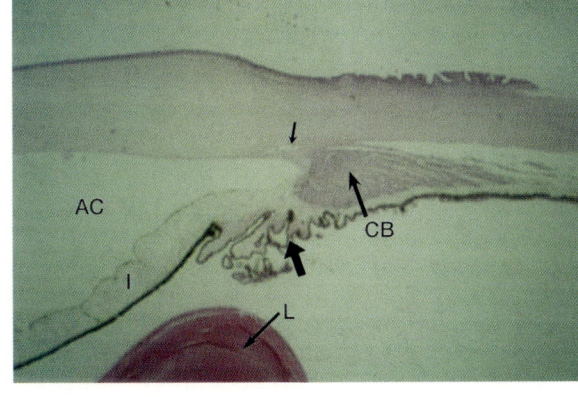

e

f

AQUEOUS HUMOR DYNAMICS

The Aqueous Humor Outflow Structures

13a.   Light microscopic view of human autopsy eye shows the anterior chamber angle (AC), with the relationship of the aqueous humor outflow structures to the anterior portion of the ciliary body. The longitudinal ciliary muscle inserts into the scleral spur, which is the lip of sclera just behind Schlemm's canal (*large arrow*). The trabecular meshwork (*small arrow*) extends anteriorly from the scleral spur to Schwalbe's line (SL), converting the scleral sulcus into the elongated Schlemm's canal.

13b.   Higher magnification shows details of trabecular meshwork and Schlemm's canal. The meshwork (*large arrow*) is seen as several lamellae of tissue, which consist of a connective tissue core, surrounded by endothelium, and are separated by intertrabecular spaces, through which the aqueous humor passes. The innermost lamellae (adjacent to the anterior chamber) constitute the uveal meshwork, which extends from the iris root and ciliary body to the peripheral cornea. The corneoscleral meshwork is the next several layers of lamellae, which extend from the scleral spur to the anterior wall of the scleral sulcus. The outermost portion of the meshwork (adjacent to Schlemm's canal) is the juxtacanalicular tissue. Note that the inner and outer walls of Schlemm's canal are connected by a tissue bridge (*small arrow*) in this section.

13c.   This histologic specimen of a normal human autopsy eye shows cystlike vacuoles along the inner wall of Schlemm's canal (*arrow*). These structures have been referred to as giant vacuoles and are believed to represent part of the transcellular pathway of aqueous humor from the trabecular meshwork to Schlemm's canal.

13d.   This light microscopic section of a human autopsy eye also shows the trabecular meshwork and Schlemm's canal in the lower half of the figure, but also shows an intrascleral channel (*arrow*), the aqueous vein of Ascher, which connects Schlemm's canal to episcleral and conjunctival veins.

13e.   Slit-lamp view of a normal eye shows episcleral veins (*arrows*), which begin as small tapered vessels near the limbus and become larger as they extend posteriorly. The more prominent vessels are anterior ciliary arteries, which are easily recognized by their tortuous configuration and abrupt termination behind the limbus.

13f.   This human autopsy eye is being perfused with India ink into the anterior chamber (note metal fitting in cornea). The ink can be seen filling veins in the small portion of remaining conjunctiva (*small arrow*) and in the episclera (*large arrow*). This demonstrates the routes that aqueous humor takes in returning to the venous system. The episcleral veins drain into the cavernous sinus by way of anterior ciliary and superior ophthalmic veins, while the conjunctival veins drain into the superior ophthalmic or facial veins via the palpebral and angular veins.

(Figure 13c was provided courtesy of R. Rand Allingham, M.D.)

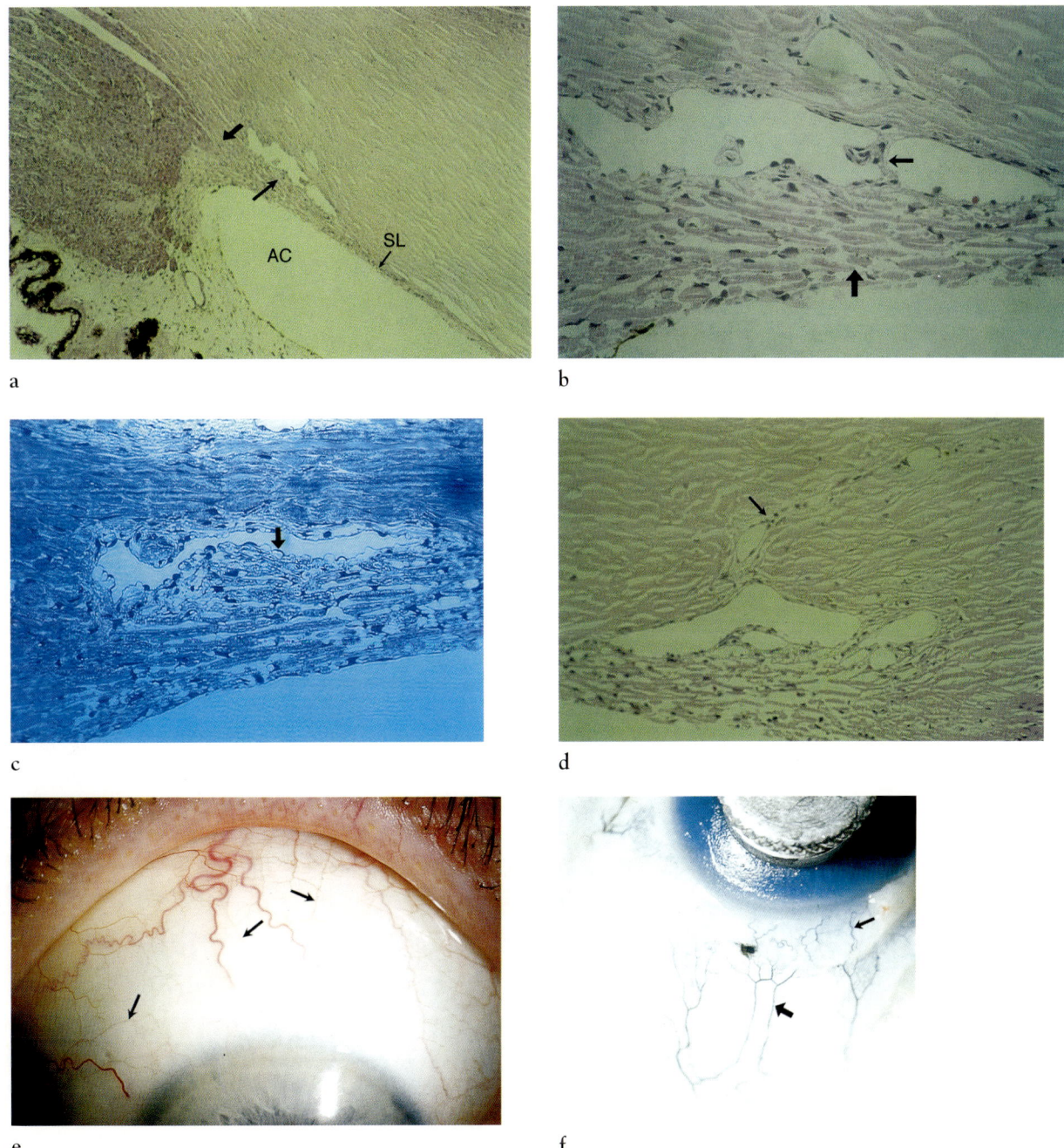

AC   SL

a   b   c   d   e   f

AQUEOUS HUMOR DYNAMICS

Indirect Gonioscopy

14a.   This grouping of instruments shows some of the gonioprisms and goniolenses that are available for evaluation of the anterior chamber angle. Gonioprisms are used for indirect gonioscopy, in which light rays are reflected by a mirror in the contact lens. The Goldmann three-mirror lens (the two black instruments) has two mirrors for examination of the fundus and one for the anterior chamber angle. The Posner lens (in center of grouping with handle) is a modification of the Zeiss four-mirror lens, in which all four mirrors are tilted to allow evaluation of the anterior chamber angle. The Koeppe lens (three lenses in foreground) is used for direct gonioscopy, which is discussed on the next page.

14b.   Goldmann three-mirror lens in use. The dome-shaped mirror, which is used for gonioscopy, is at the 12 o'clock position, allowing visualization of the angle at the 6 o'clock position. The lens must be rotated 360° to allow visualization of all quadrants of the anterior chamber angle.

14c.   Closer detail of the Posner lens shows the four gonioscopic mirrors permanently attached to a holding rod. The original Zeiss four-mirror lens is mounted on a detachable holding fork (Unger holder).

14d.   Posner lens in use. Because all four mirrors are angled for gonioscopy, it is not necessary to rotate the lens. In addition, unlike the Goldmann-type lenses, in which a viscous material must be used to fill the gap between the cornea and lens, the posterior curvature of the four-mirror lenses is similar to that of the cornea, allowing the patient's own tears to be used as the fluid bridge.

14e.   The Sussman lens is another modification of the Zeiss four-mirror lens and differs primarily from the others in that the lens is held directly, without the use of a holding rod or fork.

14f.   Sussman lens in use. As with the other four-mirror lenses, all quadrants of the anterior chamber angle can be seen without rotating the lens. The Sussman lens, however, is somewhat easier to rotate a few degrees in either direction to better see portions of the angle that might otherwise not be seen between two mirrors.

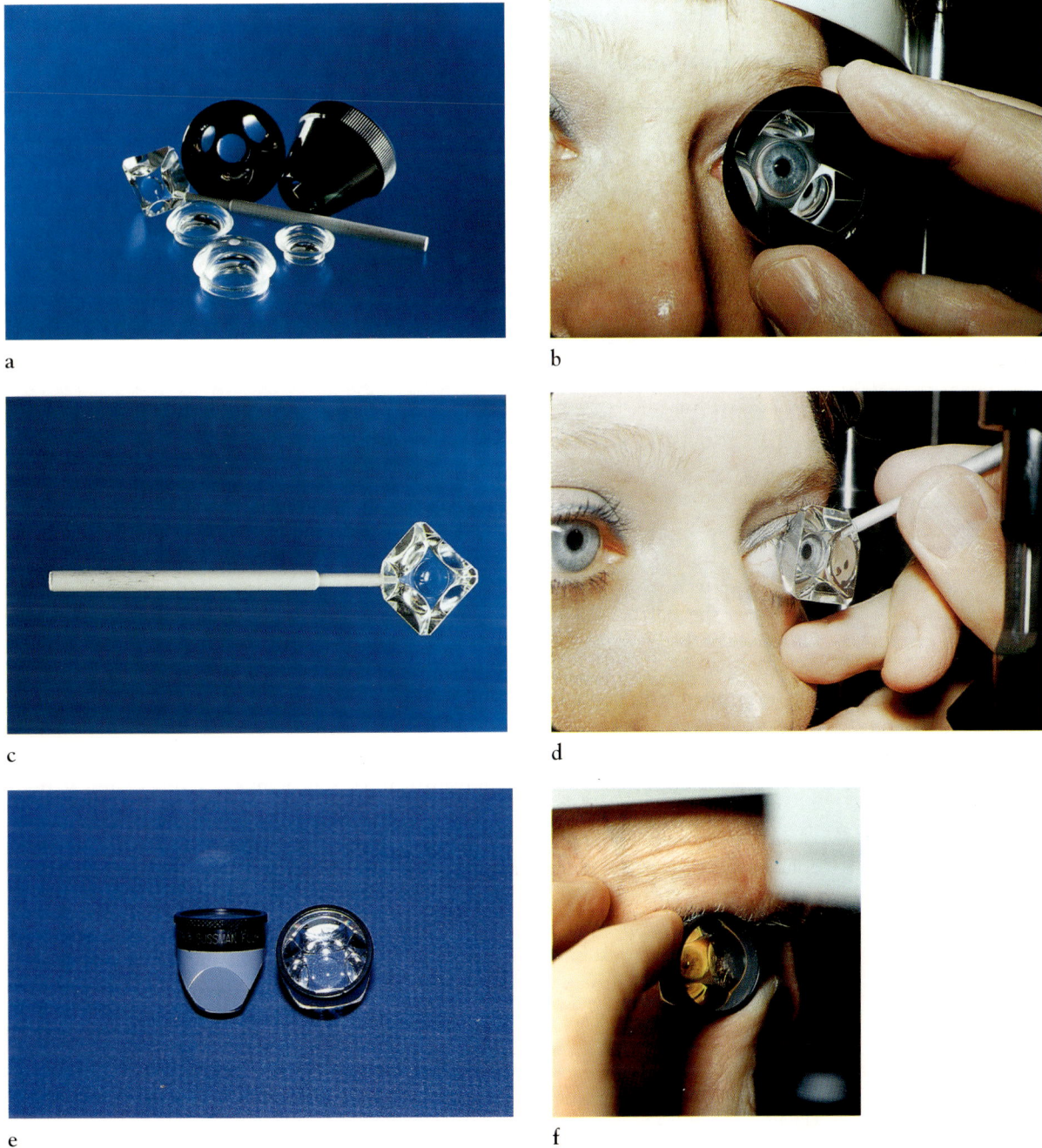

a

b

c

d

e

f

AQUEOUS HUMOR DYNAMICS

Gonioscopy: Normal Anterior Chamber Angle

16a.   Going from the iris (I) to the cornea (C), the structures normally seen by gonioscopy in the open, adult anterior chamber angle are the ciliary body band (CBB), scleral spur (SS) and the functional portion of the trabecular meshwork (TM).

16b.   In this normal anterior chamber angle, the ciliary body band is wider and more prominent than in the previous picture, while the trabecular meshwork is lightly pigmented. In addition, the faint, gray line above the meshwork represents Schwalbe's line (*small arrow*), which is the junction between the anterior chamber angle structures and the cornea. Notice also the loops of blood vessels that obscure part of the ciliary body band centrally (*large arrow*). These vessels are derived from the major arteriolar circle and are seen in some normal eyes.

16c.   While the ciliary body band may have a dark brown appearance in some eyes, as in the two examples above, it may be seen in other eyes as a slate gray band, as seen in this photo just above the iris root. The other feature of note in this picture is the numerous iris processes, which typically extend across the ciliary body band and scleral spur to the trabecular meshwork, which in this eye has a medium brown appearance.

16d.   In this eye, the ciliary body band also has a light gray appearance. The trabecular meshwork is heavily pigmented. The thinner, pigmented line above the meshwork (*arrow*) is Schwalbe's line, which is more easily seen in some eyes because of the buildup of pigment along the ridge, especially in the inferior quadrant.

16e.   In some cases, angle pigmentation is so heavy that the normal structures are difficult to identify. This is seen most commonly in the inferior quadrant, as in this picture in which the heavy pigment obscures portions of the ciliary body band and scleral spur.

16f.   In the same eye as I6e, the gonioprism has been rotated 90° to the temporal quadrant, where the reduced amount of pigment allows visualization of the scleral spur. This maneuver of rotating the gonioprism to identify angle structures is especially useful when performing laser trabeculoplasty, in which accurate identification of the trabecular meshwork is critical.

16g.   In other cases, the trabecular meshwork is difficult to identify because of light pigmentation. This can sometimes lead to the incorrect impression that the angle is closed. In this eye, the clues that the angle is open are the several iris processes that extend up to the faintly visible meshwork (*arrows*).

16h.   Another clue that is sometimes helpful in identifying the location of a lightly pigmented trabecular meshwork is blood reflux in Schlemm's canal (*arrow*).

(Figure I6c was provided courtesy of Ruth Schirmer.)

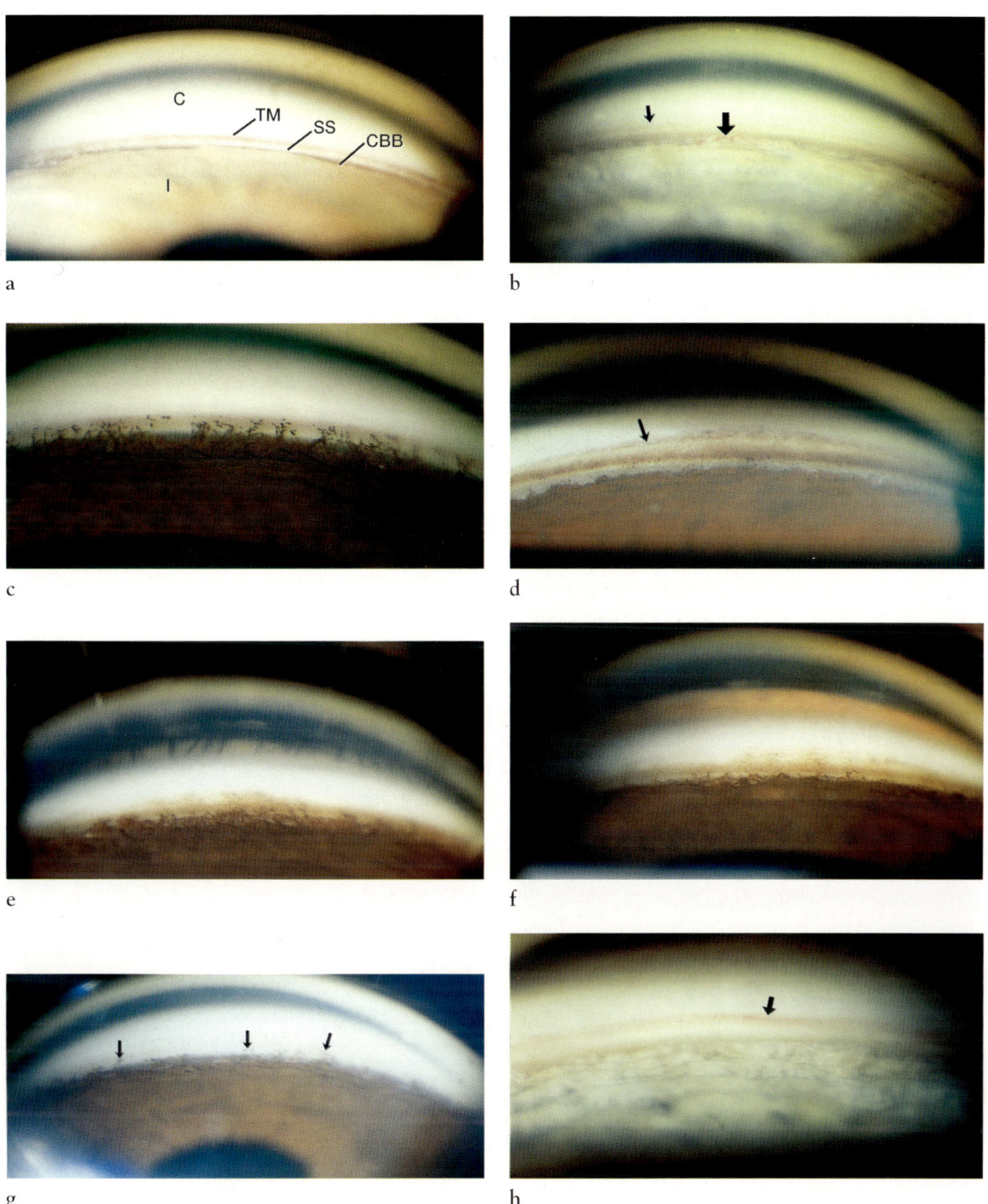

INTRAOCULAR PRESSURE

Indentation and Applanation Tonometry

I7a.   Schiøtz indentation tonometer, which shows footplate (F), plunger (P), weight (W), needle (N), and scale (S).

I7b.   Schiøtz tonometer in use. The footplate rests on the anesthetized cornea and must be kept perpendicular so the plunger will move freely within the shaft of the footplate. The extent of corneal indentation by the plunger and weight, which is inversely proportional to the intraocular pressure, is indicated by the needle on the scale. The pressure is derived from a conversion table, using the scale reading and plunger weight.

I7c.   Goldmann applanation tonometer. Plastic biprism (B) is attached by a rod to the housing (H) of the tonometer, which is attached to the slit lamp. The housing contains a coil spring and series of levers, which are adjusted by the knurled knob (K) to control the force of the biprism against the cornea.

I7d.   Technique of applanation tonometery with Goldmann tonometer. With patient seated at slit lamp and looking straight ahead, the biprism is brought into contact with the anesthetized cornea. The force is then adjusted until the inner margins of two semicircular mires overlap, at which point the intraocular pressure is read from the scale on the housing knob.

I7e.   Perkins applanation tonometer. This is a hand-held Goldmann-type applanation tonometer, which uses the same biprism (B) as the Goldmann tonometer. The light source (L) is powered by a battery, and the force is varied manually by a knurled knob (K).

I7f.   Technique of Perkins applanation tonometry. The platform is rested on the forehead, and the biprism is brought into contact with the anesthetized cornea. As with the Goldmann tonometer, the force is adjusted until the inner margins of the semicircular mires overlap, at which time the pressure is read directly from the scale beside the knob. A counter-balance in the tonometer makes it possible to use the instrument in either the vertical or horizontal position.

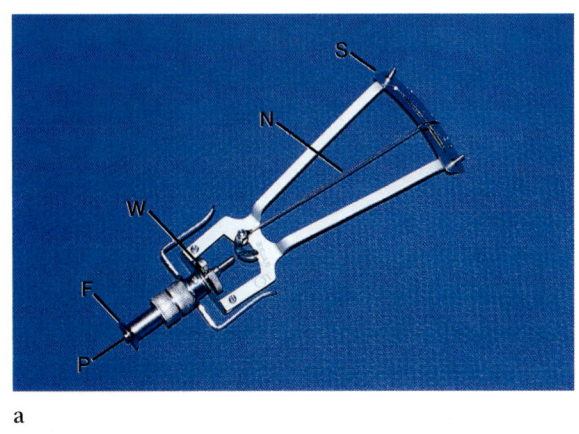

a

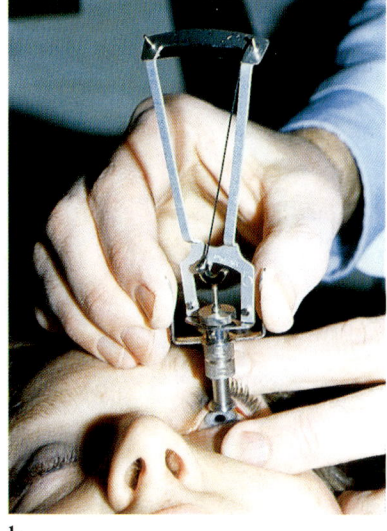

b

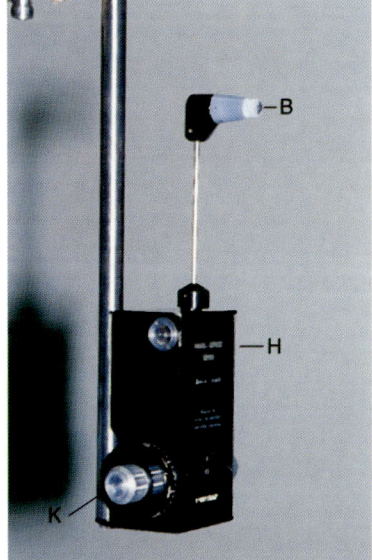

c

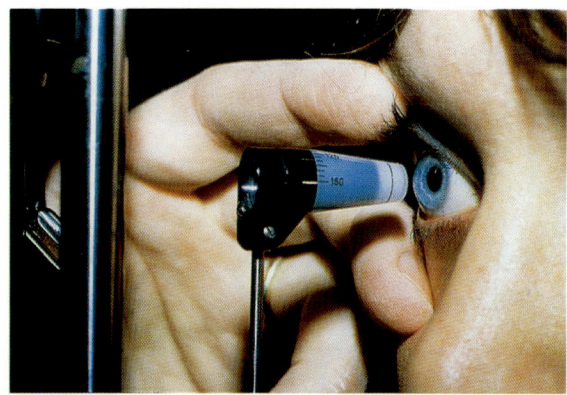

d

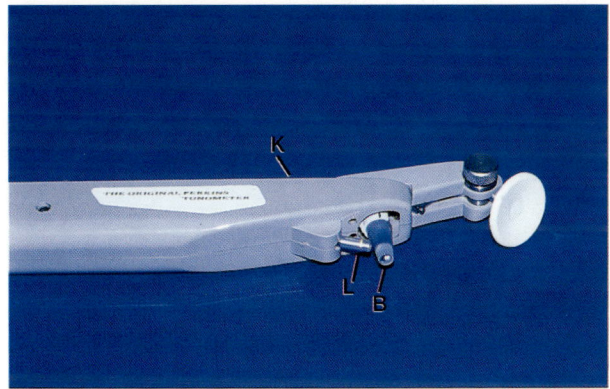

e

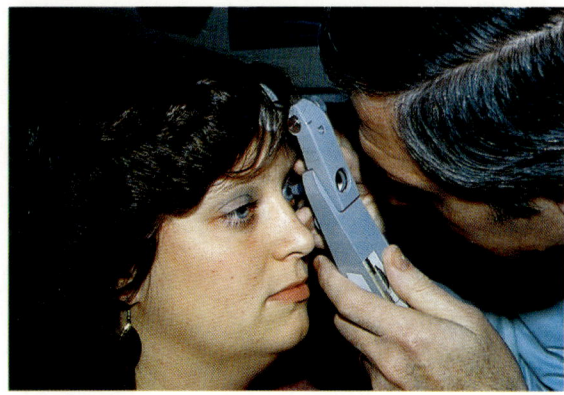

f

INTRAOCULAR PRESSURE

Electronic Tonometers

18a.   Pneumotonometer, showing the end of the pencil-like holder, which contains a sensing nozzle (*arrow*) covered with a silastic diaphragm. Air pressure in the central chamber is dependent on resistance to exhaust at the face of the nozzle, which is influenced by contact of the silastic diaphragm with the cornea.

18b.   The main body of the pneumotonometer contains a pneumatic-to-electronic transducer, which converts air pressure to intraocular pressures and provides them on a paper strip and in a digital window.

18c.   Pneumotonometer in use. With the patient either sitting or supine, the lids are gently separated and the hand-held unit is gently applied to the anesthetized cornea. A beeping sound indicates when the recordings have begun and ended. The instrument takes a series of readings, which are recorded on the paper strip and provided as an average on both the strip and the digital read-out.

18d.   An earlier version of the pneumotonometer shows the placement of the hand-held unit, with the conversion and recording unit in the background.

18e.   The Tono-Pen uses the McKay-Marg principle, in which an electronically controlled plunger is kept flush with a surrounding footplate as the tip is brought in contact with the cornea. The amount of force required to keep the plunger flush against the pressure of corneal deformation is electronically recorded and provided digitally as the intraocular pressure.

18f.   The Tono-Pen in use. The intraocular pressure is measured with a momentary touch to the cornea, and a microprocessor averages four to 10 readings to give a final digital read-out.

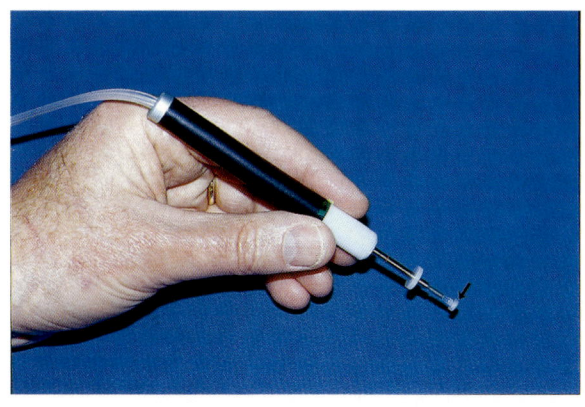

a

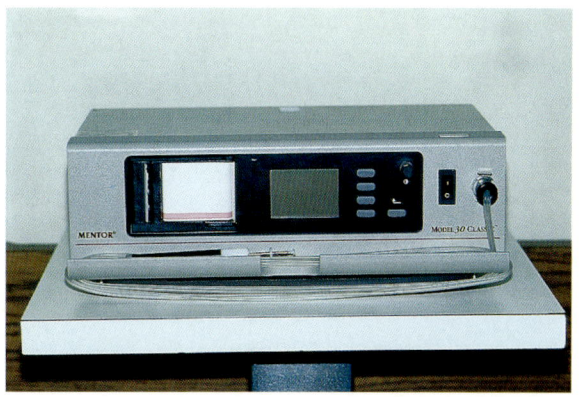

b

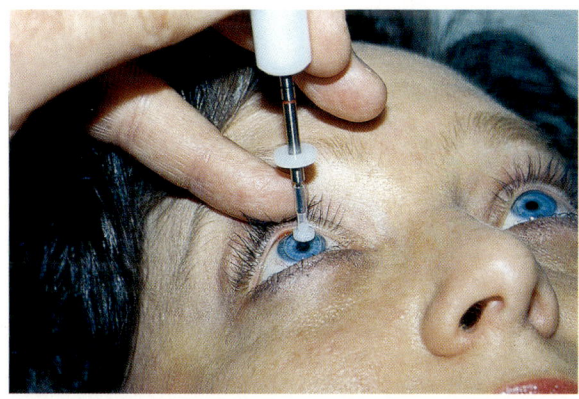

c

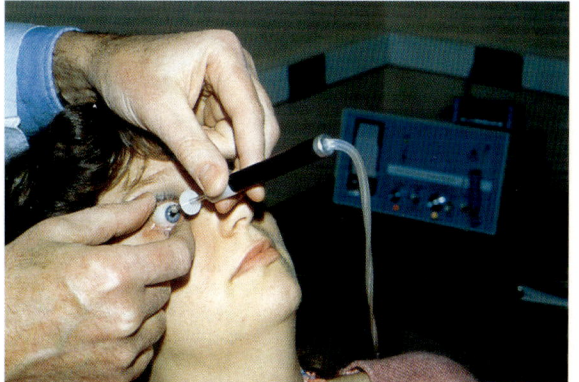

d

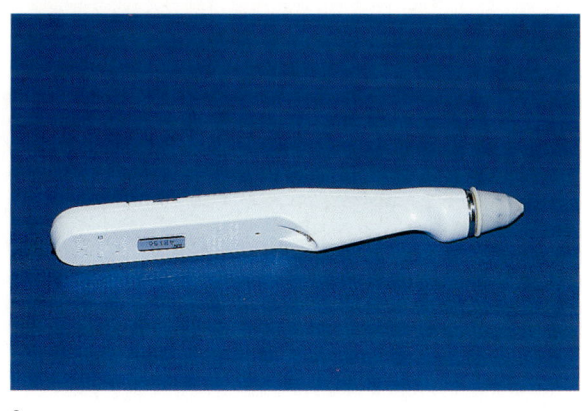

e

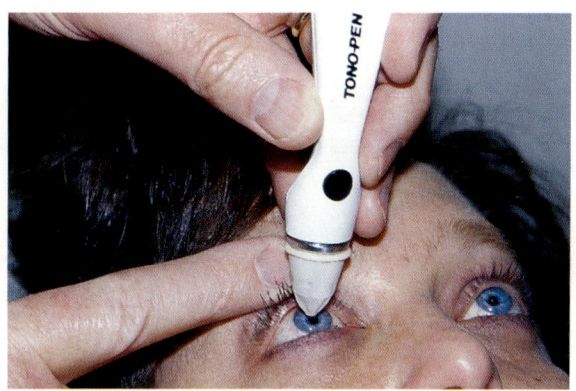

f

INTRAOCULAR PRESSURE

Air Puff and Home Tonometers

19a.   The X-Pert non-contact tonometer is a modified version of the original non-contact tonometer, in which a puff of room air creates a force that momentarily deforms the cornea. The extent of corneal deformation, which is influenced by the intraocular pressure, is determined by an opto-electronic system that receives and detects the amount of light reflected from the cornea. The force of air required to achieve peak light detection is converted to intraocular pressure and provided in the digital read-out.

19b.   The X-Pert non-contact tonometer is shown from the patient's side. The patient fixes on an internal light source. Unlike all other tonometers, nothing touches the eye except the puff of air.

19c.   The X-Pert non-contact tonometer is seen from the operator's side. After the eye is properly aligned, the air puff is automatically triggered and the intraocular pressure is displayed on the digital read-out.

19d.   An earlier model of the non-contact tonometer is shown, in which the operator manually triggered the air puff when alignment criteria were judged to be satisfied. This instrument also differed in that time to the moment of applanation, rather than force, was used to estimate the intraocular pressure.

19e.   The Zeimer Home Tonometer uses the McKay-Marg principle. It is designed so that patients can take it home and measure their own pressure around-the-clock for several days.

I9f.   The Home Tonometer in use. The patient rests her head against the instrument, fixes on an internal light source, and triggers the instrument to acquire the pressure reading. The readings are stored on a computer disk that can be read by the physician on a personal computer.

(Figures I9e and I9f were provided courtesy of Joseph A. Khawly, M.D.)

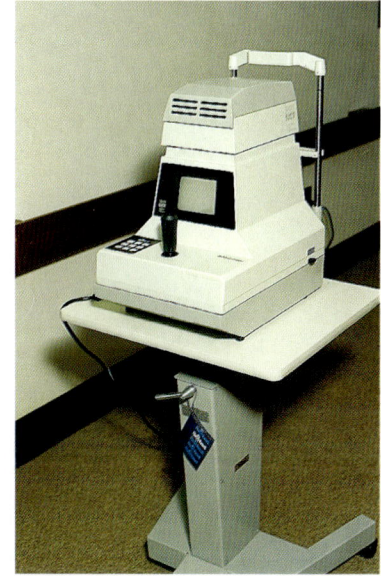

a

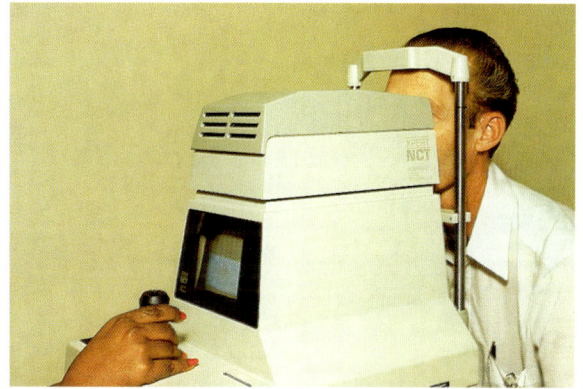

b

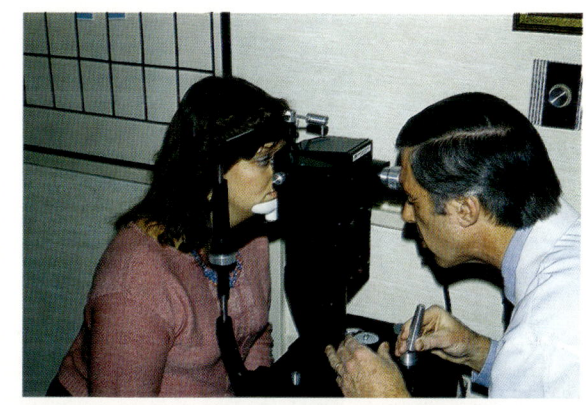

c

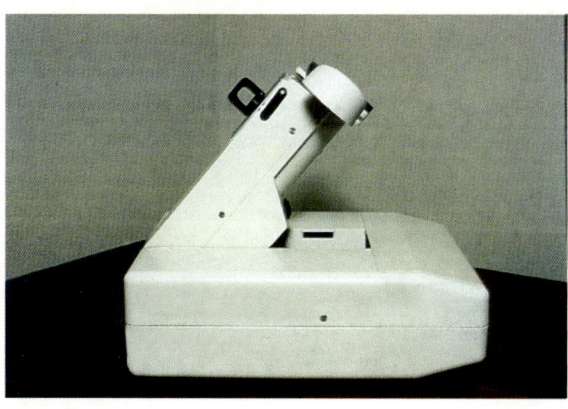

d

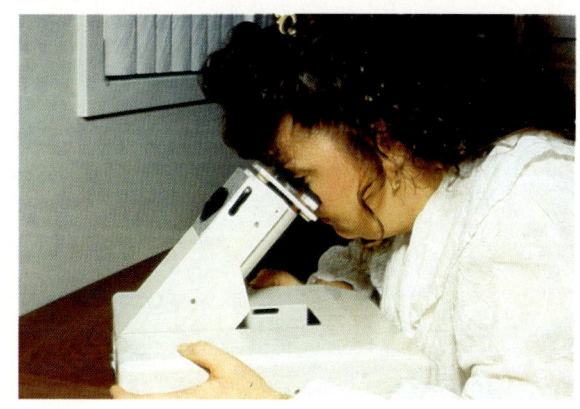

e

f

OPTIC NERVE HEAD

Normal Histology and Morphology

I10a. Light microscopic view shows the normal optic nerve head (*large arrow*), which has an average diameter of 1.5mm and enlarges to approximately 3mm just behind the sclera (*small arrow*), where the neurons acquire a myelin sheath.

I10b. Higher magnification of the optic nerve head and peripapillary structures shows the surface nerve fiber layer (1), prelaminar region (2), lamina cribrosa region (3), and the retrolaminar region (4). The peripapillary structures include the retina (R), choroid (C), and sclera (S). A portion of the meningeal sheaths (MS) is also seen surrounding the optic nerve.

I10c. The morphologic appearance of the normal optic nerve head consists of the central, pale depression or cup, which is surrounded by the orange neural rim. One characteristic of the normal optic nerve head is an even width of the neural rim in all quadrants. A slight variation, however, often occurs in the width of the physiologic neural rim. In this photograph, the neural rim is typically broadest in the inferior quadrant, followed by the superior and then nasal quadrants, with the temporal rim being the thinnest. Another characteristic of the physiologic neural rim is a sharp border between cup and rim supero-temporally, compared with a more sloping infero-temporal neural rim (this is seen best in the photo by observing the deviation of the major vessels in those two quadrants).

It is also important to recognize several structures that may surround the normal optic nerve head. The retinal nerve fiber layer can be seen faintly in this photo as fine striations, arching out from the infero-temporal portions of the disc in the peripapillary retina. Three zones of pigmentary variation also may surround a portion of the normal disc, all of which can be seen in this photo: the scleral lip (S), which appears as a thin, even white rim adjacent to the disc; zone beta (B), which is a broader, more irregular zone of depigmentation just peripheral to the scleral lip; and zone alpha (A), which is a crescent of increased pigmentation peripheral to zone beta.

I10d–f. The size of the physiologic cup may vary considerably, as shown in these three pictures. A rough method of recording the relative size of the cup in either the physiologic or glaucomatous state is to estimate the ratio between the size of the cup and the disc. For example, in these three photographs, the cup/disc ratio might be estimated at 0.4 in I10d, 0.5 in I10e, and 0.7 in I10f. It should be emphasized, however, that the size of the cup does not distinguish between the physiologic and glaucomatous state, and that it is more important to observe and record additional features of the optic nerve head, as will be discussed in the following pages.

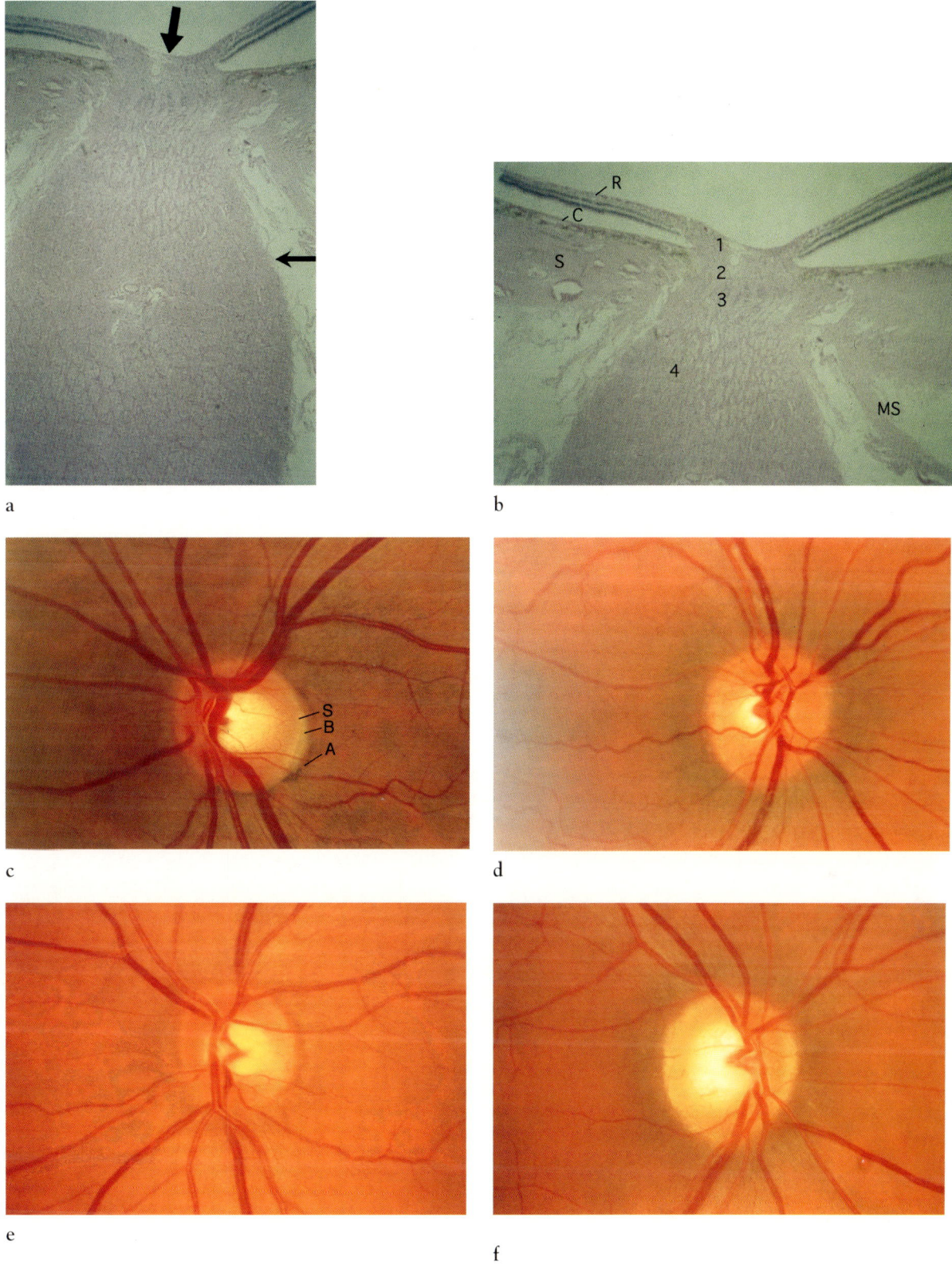

a

b

c

d

e

f

OPTIC NERVE HEAD

Large Physiologic Cups

I11a–b. A second important feature in distinguishing the physiologic from the glaucomatous state (in addition to evenness of the neural rim) is symmetry between the size of the cup in the two eyes. In this set of photos, we see the right and left eye of a patient with large physiologic cups. Note that the cups are of the same size in both eyes and that the neural rim is even in all quadrants of both eyes.

I11c–d. These photographs also show the right and left eyes of a patient with large physiologic cupping. The infero-temporal sloping of the neural rim is sometimes difficult to distinguish from the early saucerization of glaucoma. It is helpful in such cases, however, to look carefully at the nerve fiber layer, which is intact in the physiologic state.

I11e–f. Another feature that can be seen in the physiologic optic nerve head is the gray crescent in the optic nerve head. This thin crescent is seen just inside the scleral lip in the temporal quadrant of the right eye and the infero-temporal quadrant of the left eye. The importance of recognizing this feature is that it might otherwise be interpreted as a parapapillary pigmented crescent, which would cause the neural rim to appear unusually narrow in that quadrant. This can be especially significant when a patient has large physiologic cups, as in these photographs, in which case they might be misinterpreted as glaucomatous.

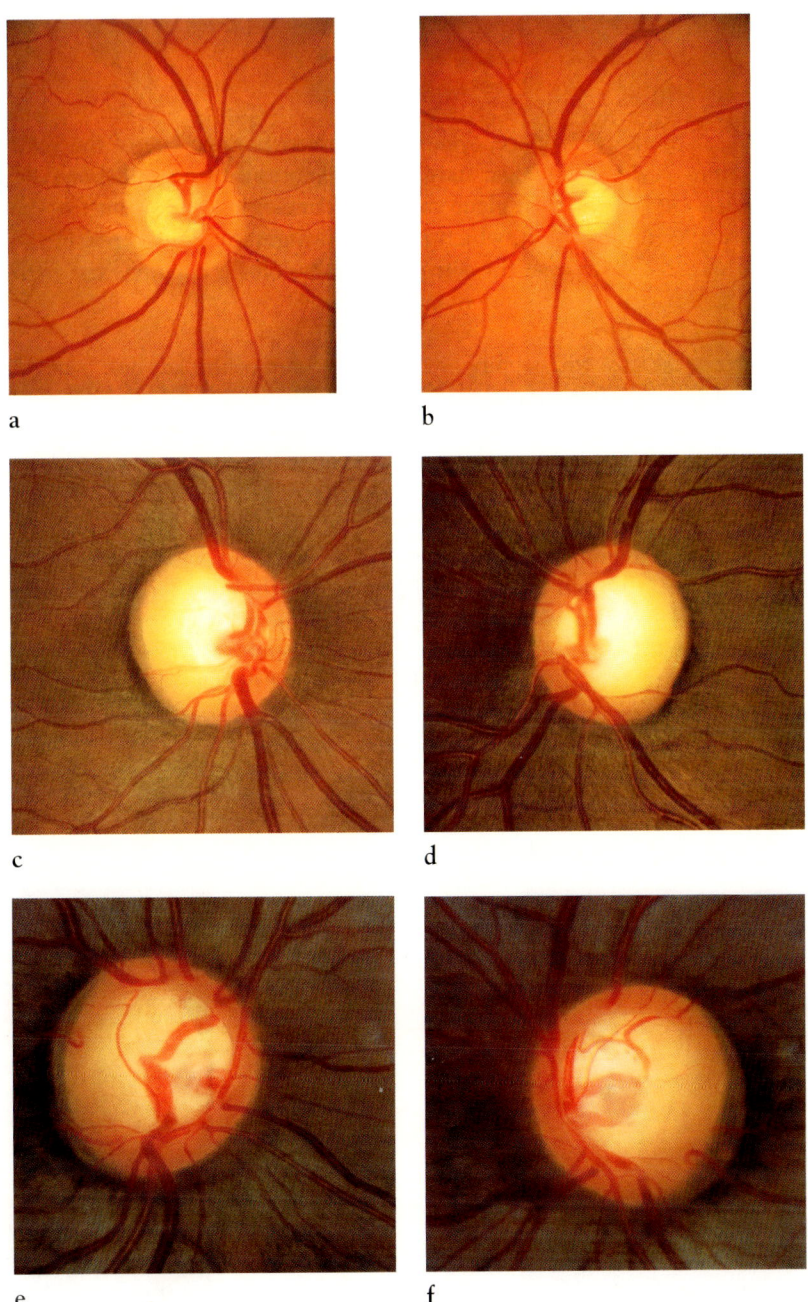

a

b

c

d

e

f

OPTIC NERVE HEAD

Focal Atrophy of the Neural Rim

I13a–b.   As the natural course of glaucomatous optic atrophy progresses, the most typical pattern is a focal loss of neural rim tissue, which is seen most commonly in the supero-temporal and the infero-temporal quadrants. This is seen first as a shallow cupping of the neural rim in that quadrant with retention of color, which has been referred to as focal saucerization. This can be seen in the infero-temporal quadrant of the right eye. As the process continues the color is lost, and both cupping and pallor extend to the margin of the disc, often with an undermining of the margin in that quadrant, as is seen in the inferior quadrant of the left eye.

I13c.   In this patient, the infero-temporal cupping and pallor have extended to involve a broad width of the infero-temporal quadrant, leaving only a thin nasal and superior neural rim.

I13d.   In this photo (the left eye of the patient in I13c), an example of what has been called vertical cupping can be seen. This is a situation in which the cupping and pallor have extended in both the superior and inferior directions, resulting in a cup shape that is more vertically oval than the shape of the disc, with retention of neural rim in the nasal and temporal quadrants.

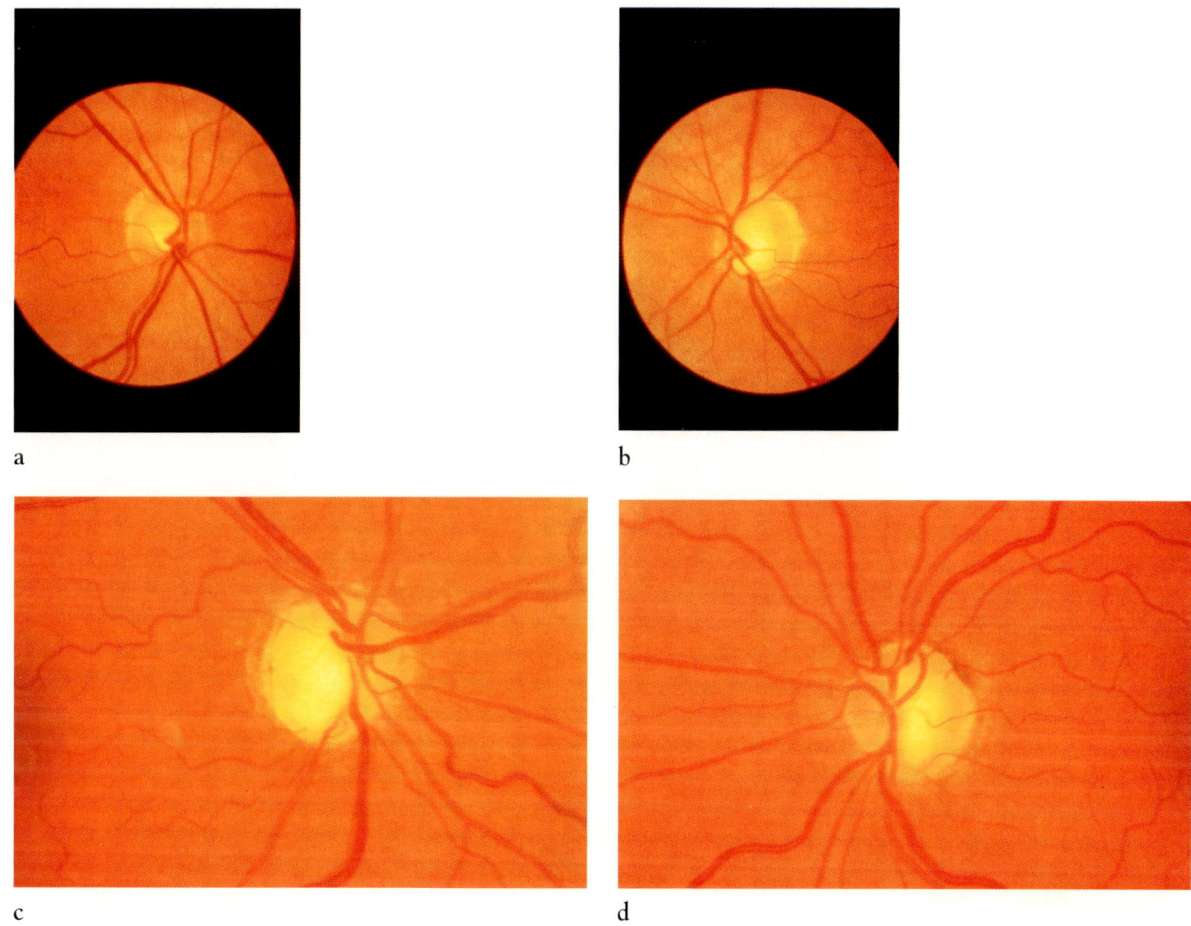

a

b

c

d

OPTIC NERVE HEAD

Optic Disc Hemorrhages

I14a–b.   In this patient, at least two signs of glaucomatous damage are visible. The first is an asymmetry of the cup size, in which the cup of the left eye is larger than that of the right eye. The right eye, however, contains a small hemorrhage on the disc margin in the supero-temporal quadrant (*arrow*), which is another sign that is highly suggestive, although not pathognomonic, of glaucomatous optic atrophy.

I14c–d.   Optic disc hemorrhages, also called flame hemorrhages or splinter hemorrhages, typically resolve, but often reappear in either the same area or in a different area of that or the fellow eye. In this rather unusual case, the patient had simultaneous, bilateral hemorrhages, with a flame hemorrhage in the supero-temporal quadrant of the right eye and the infero-temporal quadrant of the left eye.

I14e–f.   The significance of a flame hemorrhage is the indication of active glaucomatous damage in the zone of the hemorrhage. For example, in this patient we see a small flame hemorrhage in the infero-temporal quadrant of the left eye (*arrow, I14e*). In I14f, we see the same disc three years later, in which a notch of cupping and pallor in the infero-temporal quadrant are now present at the previous site of the flame hemorrhage (*arrow*).

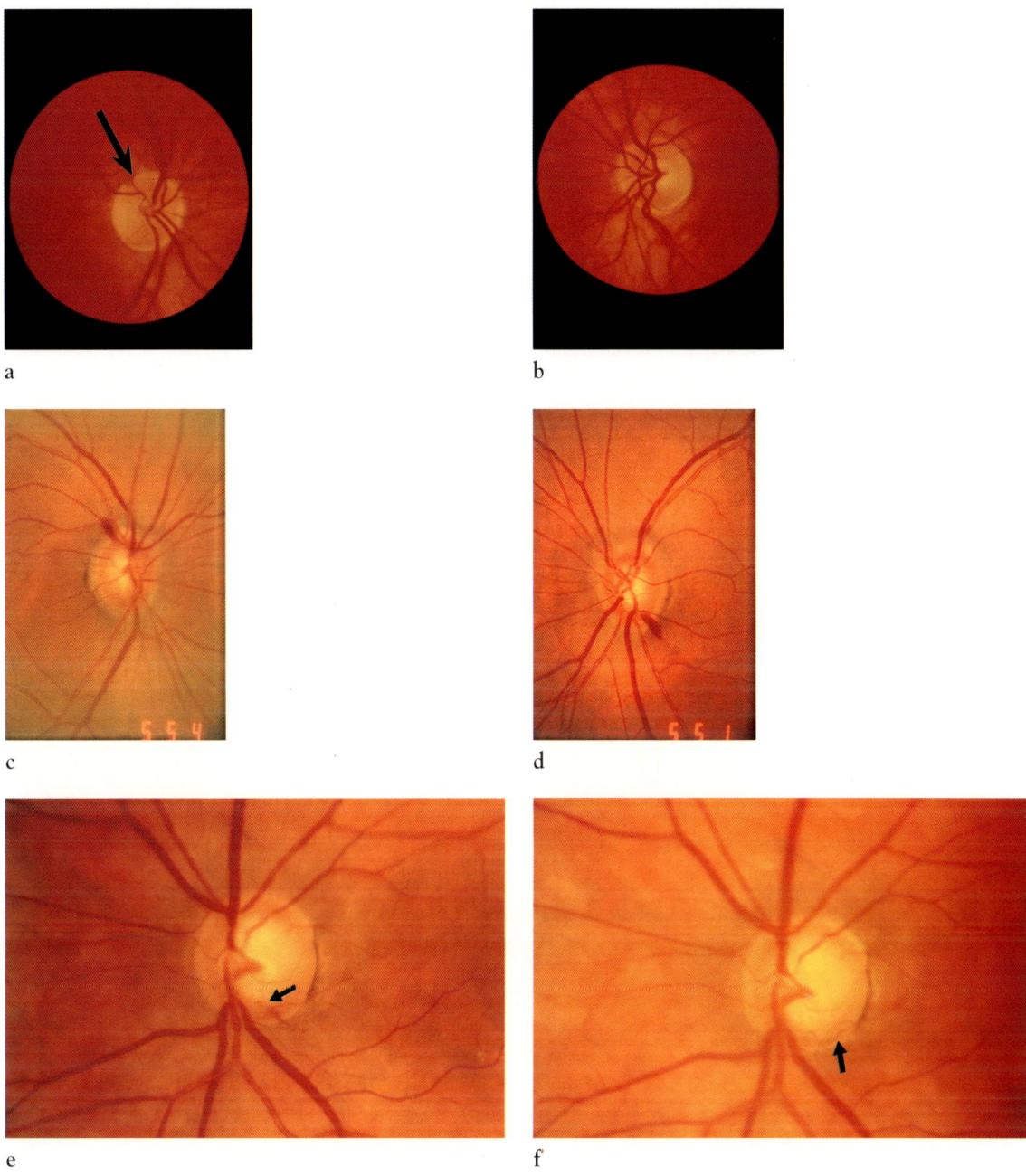

a

b

c

d

e

f

OPTIC NERVE HEAD

Flame Hemorrhages and Pseudo-Hemorrhages

I15a–b.   In some cases the flame hemorrhage of the optic disc can be rather obvious, as in these two patients, both of whom have a large flame hemorrhage crossing the neural rim in the infero-temporal quadrant of their right eye.

I15c.   In some cases, however, the flame hemorrhage may be subtle, as in this photograph in which a thin splinter hemorrhage in the infero-temporal quadrant (*arrow*) could have been easily misinterpreted as a blood vessel.

I15d.   In other cases, what might appear to be an obvious flame hemorrhage may have another explanation. For example, in this photograph, we see a vascular anomaly of tortuous vessels in the infero-nasal quadrant of the left eye.

I15e–f.   Another feature that may mimic a flame hemorrhage is the development of shunt vessels. For example, we see no apparent abnormality in this patient's left eye in I15e. The photograph I15f was taken six years later, following a branch retinal vein occlusion, in which tortuous shunt vessels have now developed in the inferior quadrant, which could have been misinterpreted as flame hemorrhages. It is important to remember, however, that retinal vessel occlusions and shunt vessels are more common in eyes with glaucoma.

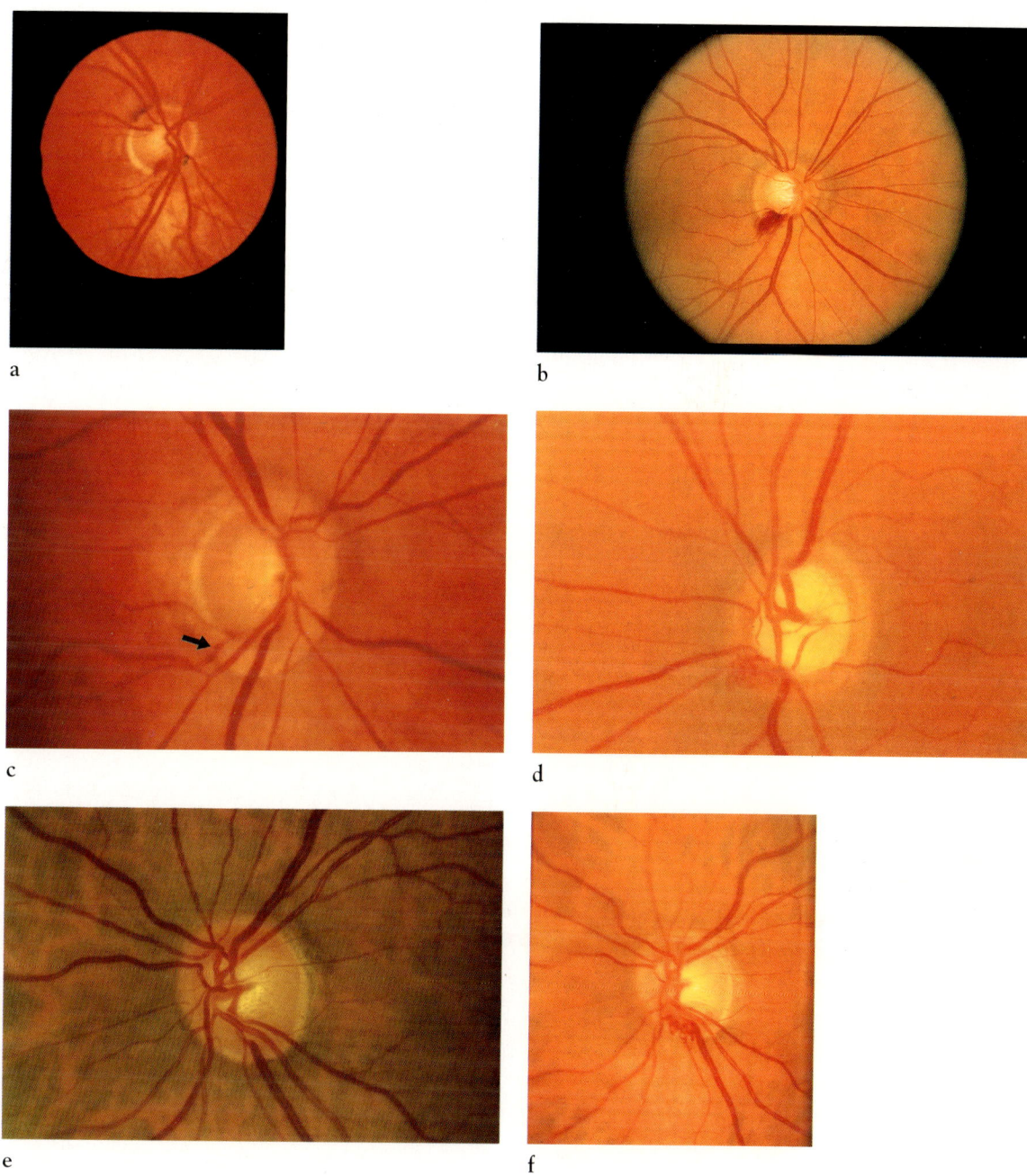

a

b

c

d

e

f

OPTIC NERVE HEAD

Other Vascular Signs of Glaucomatous Optic Atrophy

116a–b. This patient has several features of glaucomatous optic atrophy. Obvious asymmetry of the cupping is present, as well as a thinning of the inferior neural rim in the left eye. In addition, both eyes have a sign that has been referred to as baring of the circumlinear vessel. A circumlinear vessel is one that runs along the margin between the cup and neural rim for a short distance before crossing the neural rim to the peripapillary retina. These are most commonly seen in the supero-temporal and infero-temporal quadrants. As the neural rim becomes thinner as the result of glaucomatous optic atrophy, the rim separates from the circumlinear vessel, leaving an area of pallor between the remaining neural rim and the circumlinear vessel. This can be seen in the superior quadrants of both eyes (*arrows*), although it is more prominent in the left eye, which has the more advanced glaucomatous damage.

116c–d. Another vascular sign of glaucomatous damage is proximal constriction of the retinal arteries near the optic nerve head. This can be seen in both the superior and inferior quadrants of both eyes of this patient (*arrows*).

116e–f. Yet another vascular change that is associated with glaucomatous atrophy is shunt vessels of the optic disc, which are shown in the right eye of these two patients. As demonstrated on the previous page, shunt vessels can occur in association with retinal vascular occlusive disorders. In other cases, however, they may be seen with advanced glaucomatous optic atrophy, apparently because of obstruction of venous flow through the distorted lamina cribrosa.

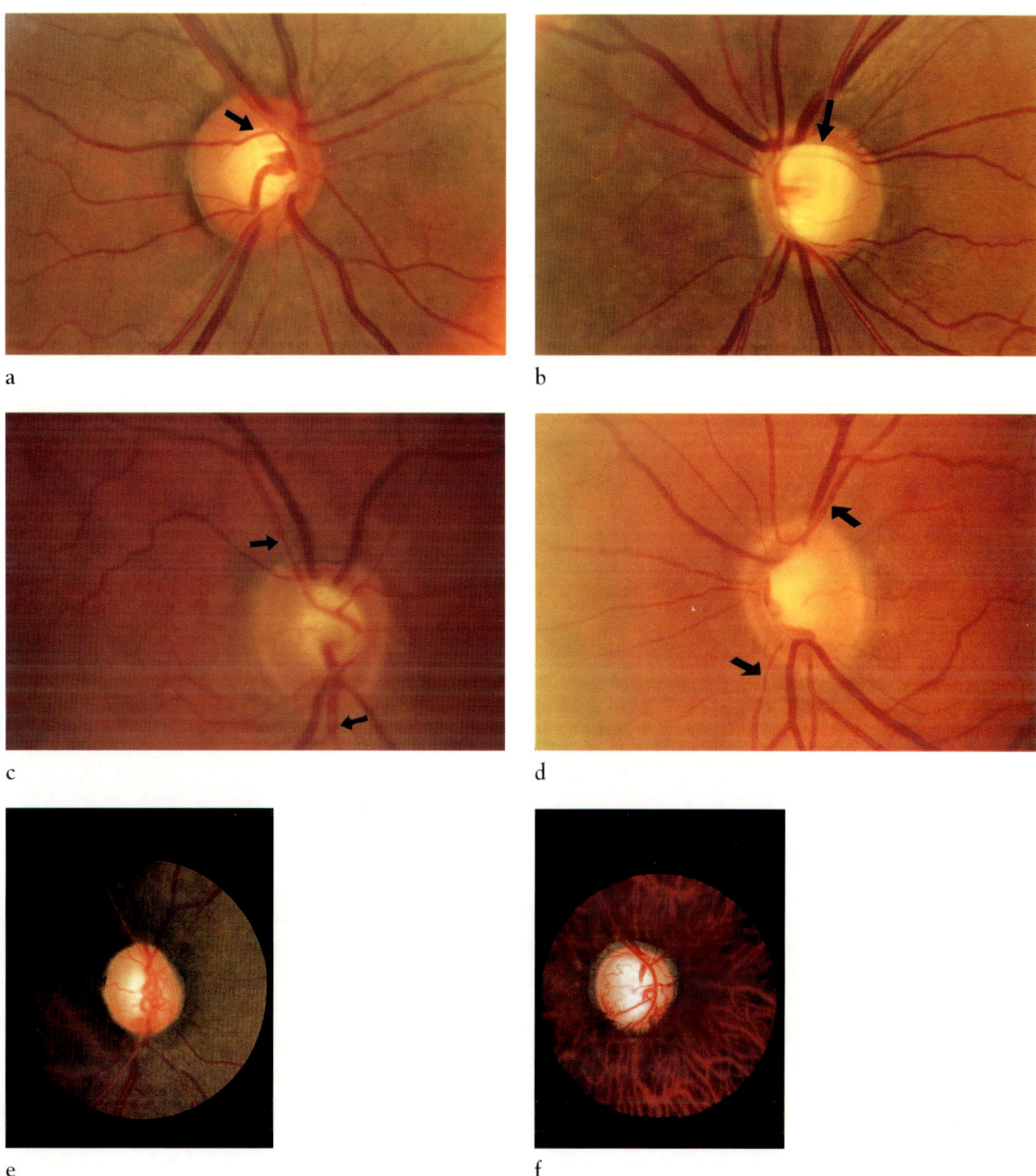

a

b

c

d

e

f

OPTIC NERVE HEAD

Peripapillary Changes with Glaucomatous Optic Atrophy

I17a. As discussed previously, the normal optic nerve head may be surrounded by several zones of variation in pigmentation. Zone alpha and beta tend to occur more frequently in eyes with glaucomatous optic atrophy. In this photo, we see the depigmented zone beta extending clockwise from nearly the 12 o'clock position around to the 8 o'clock position, with a thinner rim of pigmented zone alpha peripheral to the depigmented zone.

I17b. Not only do the zones of parapapillary atrophy occur more frequently in eyes with glaucoma, but they also tend to occur more frequently in the quadrant of neural rim atrophy. In this patient, for example, in which focal saucerization of the infero-temporal quadrant occurs, an area of zones alpha and beta are also in the same quadrant.

I17c–d. This patient with early glaucomatous damage has a prominent zone beta in the infero-temporal quadrant of the right eye and a zone beta extending from the 12 o'clock to the 6 o'clock position of the left eye with a very thin zone alpha.

I17e–f. A more significant peripapillary change associated with glaucomatous optic atrophy is the nerve fiber bundle defect. This represents the loss of axonal bundles in the peripapillary retina and is best seen in the supero-temporal and infero-temporal quadrants. In this patient, a broad, dense nerve fiber defect is seen in the infero-temporal quadrant of the right eye, corresponding to loss of neural rim tissue in the same quadrant.

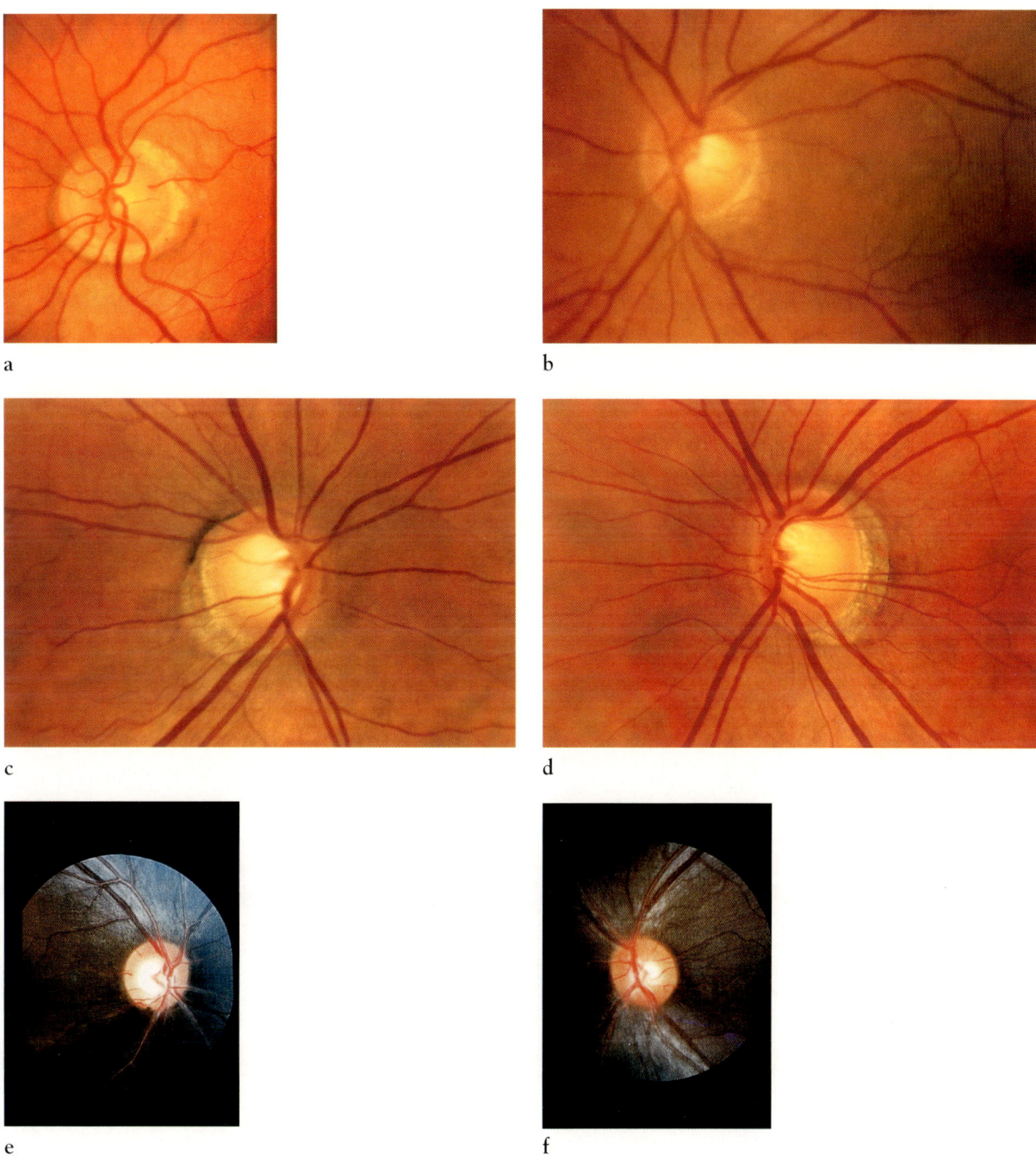

a

b

c

d

e

f

OPTIC NERVE HEAD

Advanced Glaucomatous Optic Atrophy

I18a–b.   If the process of glaucoma optic atrophy is allowed to progress, it will eventually lead to total cupping and pallor of the optic nerve head. This often leads to a deep cup with undermining of the disc margins, which has been referred to as bean-pot cupping. In some cases, however, this diagnosis may not be immediately apparent, if a halo surrounding the disc might be misinterpreted as neural rim. An example of this is seen in the right eye in these photos, in which total cupping and pallor with an even peripapillary halo occur. In the left eye, retention of neural rim color is seen in the superior and infero-temporal margins of the disc, which is surrounded by the peripapillary halo.

I18c–d.   This patient has total cupping of both optic nerve heads except for a thin nasal rim in the right eye, with retention of color in the periphery of the cup temporally in both eyes.

I18e–f.   This patient also has nearly total cupping except for a thin rim of nasal neural rim, which is wider in the right eye than the left. This patient also has an example of the gray crescent in the optic nerve head, which is seen in the temporal quadrants of both eyes (*arrows*) despite the complete loss of neural rim tissue, indicating that this pigment is in the lamina cribrosa.

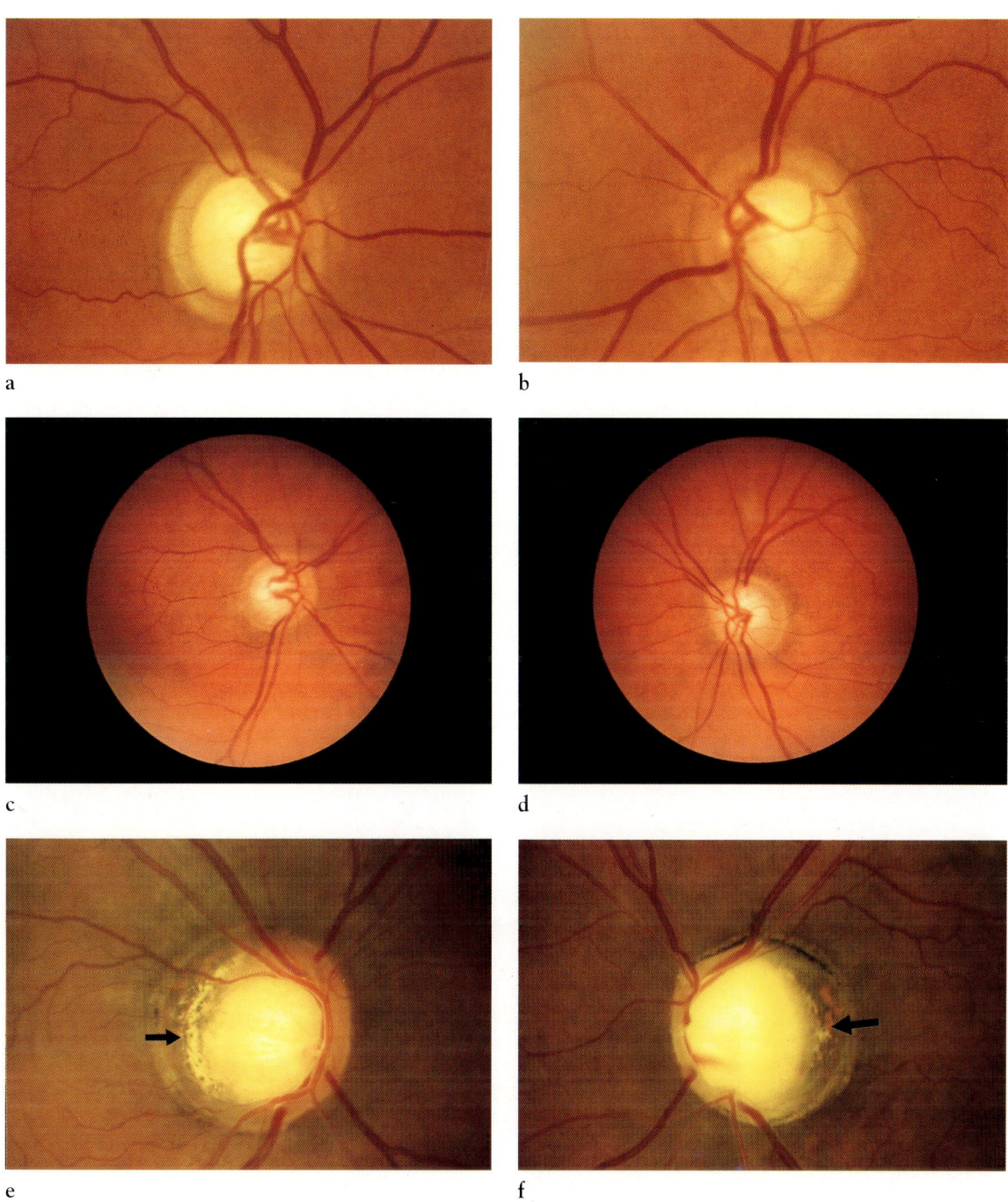

a

b

c

d

e

f

OPTIC NERVE HEAD

The Optic Nerve Head in Myopia

I19a–b.   The patient with high myopia typically has changes in the appearance of the optic nerve head that may interfere with the early recognition of glaucomatous optic atrophy. The most striking of these changes is the oblique insertion of the optic disc, which creates an increase in the vertical-oval shape of the disc, with thinning of the temporal neural rim and a prominent temporal peripapillary halo. These photographs of the right and left eye of a patient with high myopia demonstrate all three features. It can also be seen, however, that this patient has superimposed features of glaucomatous optic atrophy, which include cup-disc asymmetry and baring of the circumlinear vessel in the superior quadrant of the right eye.

I19c–d.   This patient has high myopia with markedly oblique insertion of the optic nerve heads, an extremely wide temporal peripapillary halo and no visibility of the temporal neural rim. The best way to tell whether such a patient has superimposed glaucomatous optic atrophy is to look carefully at the neural rim in the superior and inferior quadrants. In this patient, the infero-temporal neural rim of the right eye is narrower than that of the left eye, suggesting glaucomatous optic atrophy.

I19e–f.   In another patient with high myopia, we again see markedly oblique insertion with temporal peripapillary halos. The patient also has obvious large cupping, with symmetrical superior neural rims, but nearly complete loss of the inferior neural rim in both eyes, again suggesting glaucomatous optic atrophy.

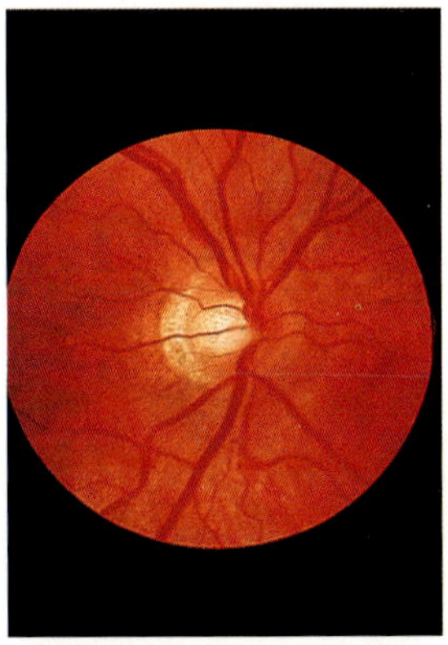

a

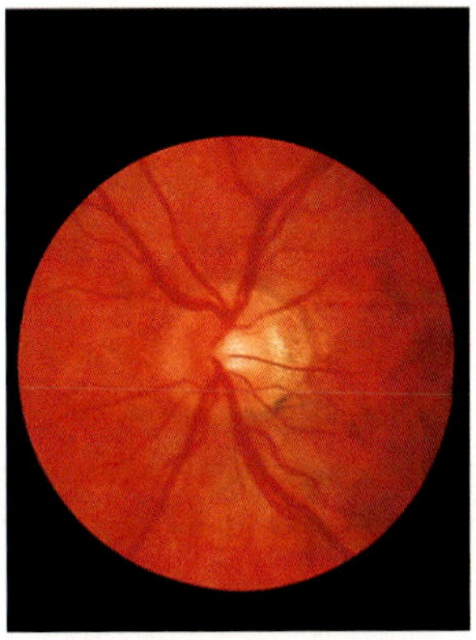

b

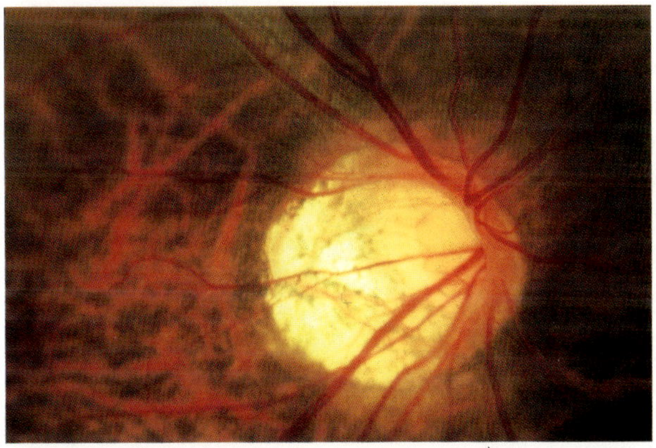

c

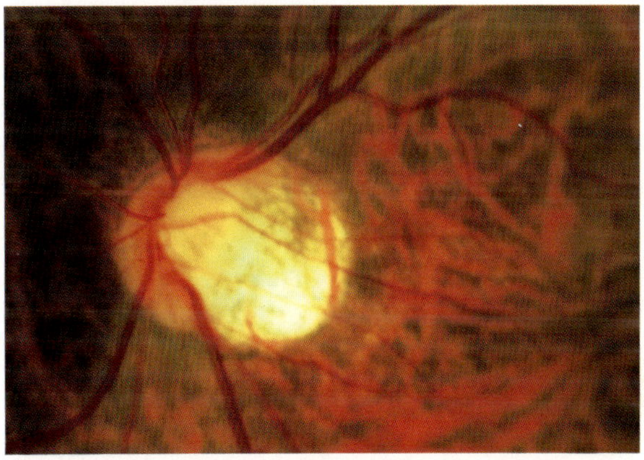

d

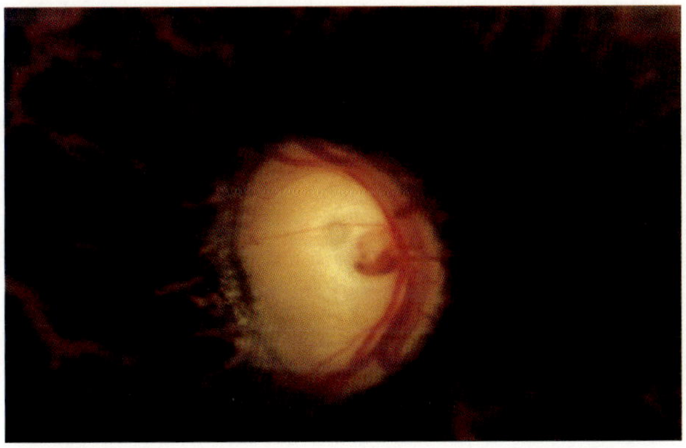

e

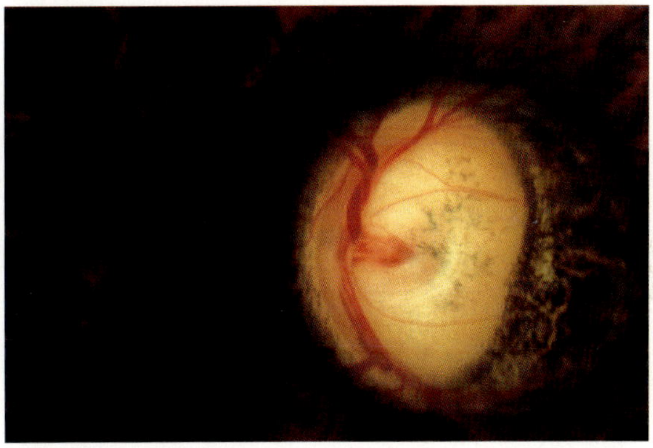

f

OPTIC NERVE HEAD

Tilted Disc Syndrome

120a–b. A variation of optic nerve head morphology, which is somewhat similar to the features of the myopic optic nerve head, has been referred to as the tilted disc syndrome. Unlike the myopic disc, which is tilted on a vertical axis, the discs in these cases are tilted on a horizontal axis, with a parapapillary crescent of atrophy in the inferior quadrant. A zone of chorioretinal atrophy may also extend inferiorly from the inferior crescent, as seen in both eyes of this patient. Another feature of the tilted disc syndrome is the tendency for sloping of the inferior neural rim, which may be difficult to distinguish from the inferior focal saucerization of early glaucomatous damage.

120c–d. Another example of the tilted disc syndrome is seen in a patient with large cups. The neural rim, however, is intact and relatively symmetrical between the two eyes, although the inferior sloping is again a concern for early glaucomatous damage.

120e. This patient appears to have a milder degree of the tilted disc syndrome, and it is difficult to distinguish from early glaucomatous optic atrophy with inferior cupping and a corresponding inferior zone of parapapillary atrophy. Even with low normal intraocular pressures, these patients must be followed closely as glaucoma suspects.

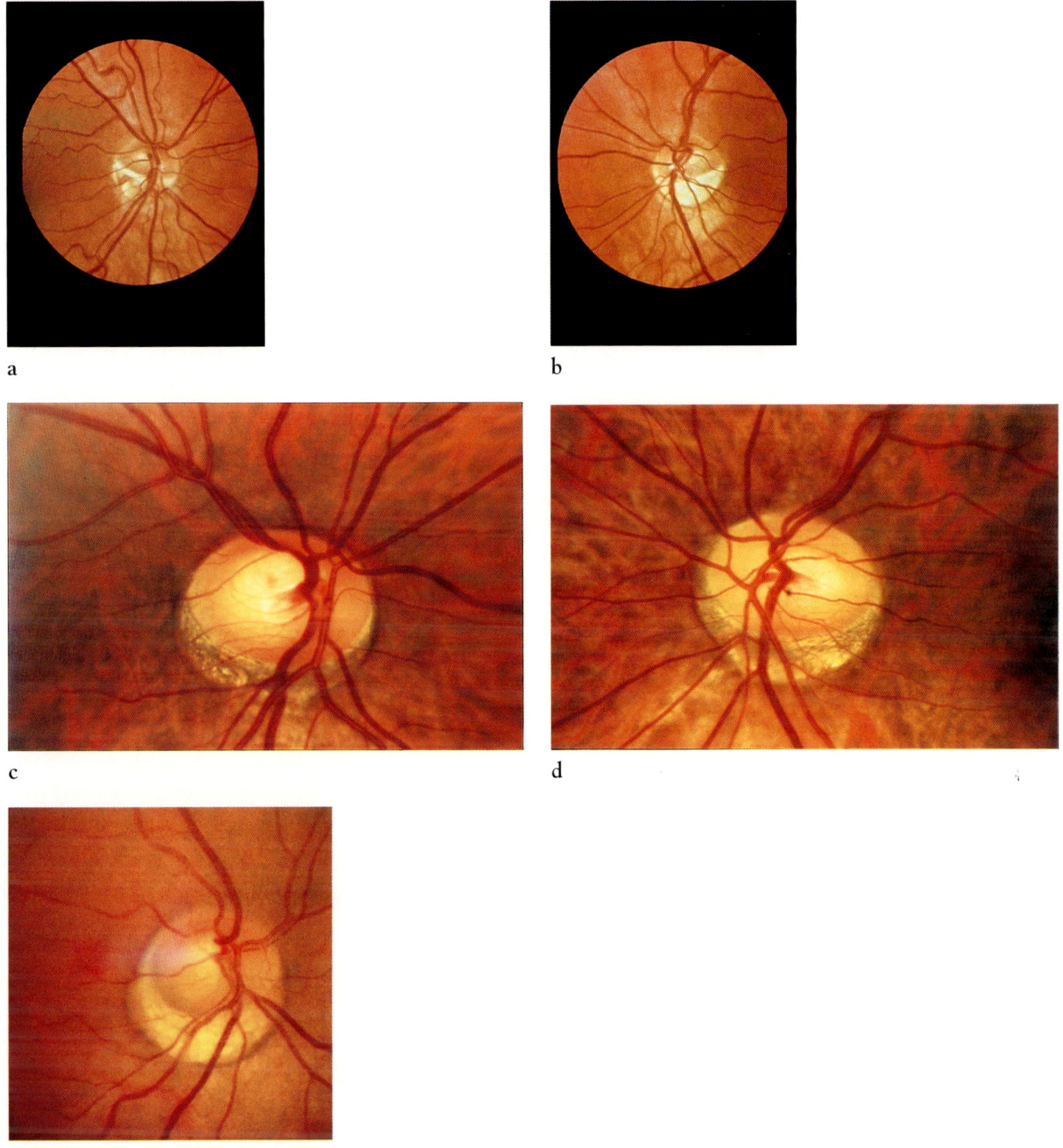

a

b

c

d

e

OPTIC NERVE HEAD

Giant Drusen of the Optic Nerve Head

121a.   This photo shows the typical features of giant drusen of the optic nerve head, in which the calcific bodies are clearly seen surrounding the disc.

121b–c.   When giant drusen of the optic nerve head are present in a patient with glaucoma, it may be more difficult to recognize and follow the progression of the glaucomatous optic atrophy. In this patient with chronic open-angle glaucoma and giant drusen of the optic nerve head, a suggestion of asymmetry of the cup/disc ratio exists, although the details are difficult to interpret. To further compound the problem, patients with giant drusen of the optic nerve head may have visual field changes that may be difficult to distinguish from those of glaucoma.

121d–e.   In this patient with chronic open-angle glaucoma, the giant drusen of the optic nerve head are buried deeper in the optic nerve head, creating an elevation of each disc and adding to the difficulty of interpreting glaucomatous optic atrophy. In cases such as this, the appearance of the optic nerve head has limited benefit in following the glaucoma, and more emphasis must be placed on the visual field and intraocular pressure.

(Figure 121a was provided courtesy of Ruth Schirmer.)

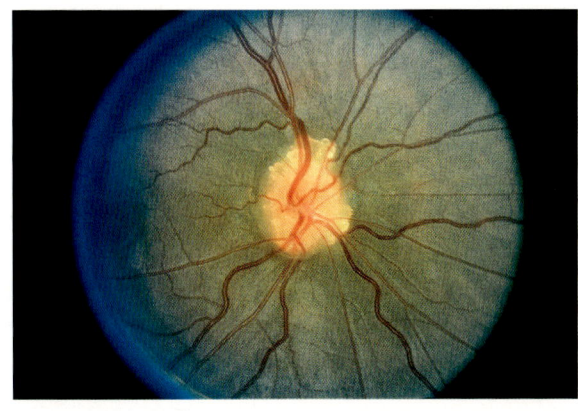

a

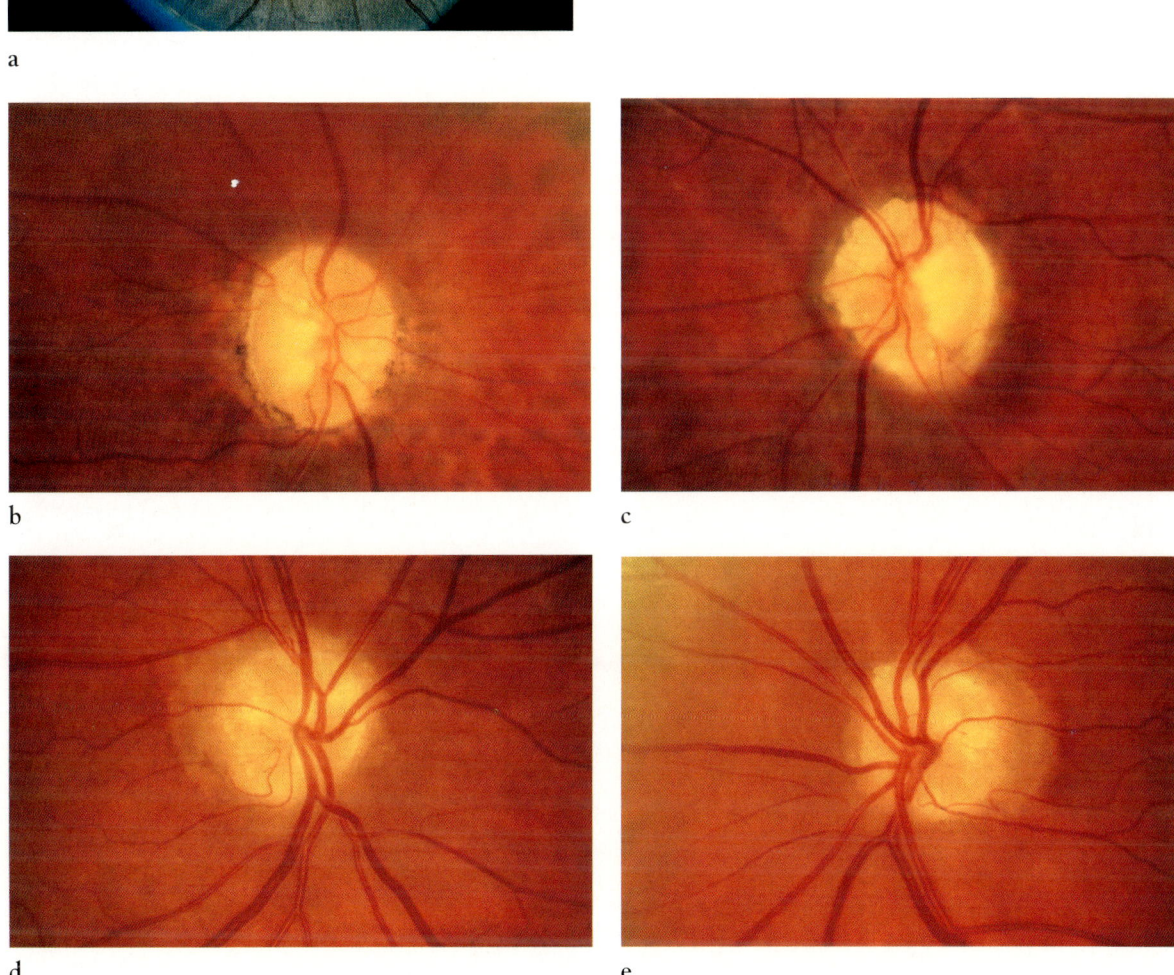

b

c

d

e

OPTIC NERVE HEAD

Developmental Anomalies

I22a–b.   Colobomas of the optic nerve head can simulate glaucomatous cupping. This patient would appear to have nearly total cupping and pallor, and yet the intraocular pressure was low normal and the visual fields were full with normal central vision.

I22c–d.   Another example is seen of a patient with colobomas involving the entire optic nerve head, which would be difficult to distinguish from total glaucomatous optic atrophy. Again, however, the patient had low normal pressures with normal central and peripheral vision. In cases such as this, the only way to distinguish a developmental anomaly from glaucomatous optic atrophy is the lack of progressive visual field loss in a developmental anomaly.

I22e.   Another example of a coloboma of the optic nerve head is seen, in which there appears to be a deeper, focal pit in the infero-nasal and possibly in the temporal quadrant.

(Figure I22e was provided courtesy of Ruth Schirmer.)

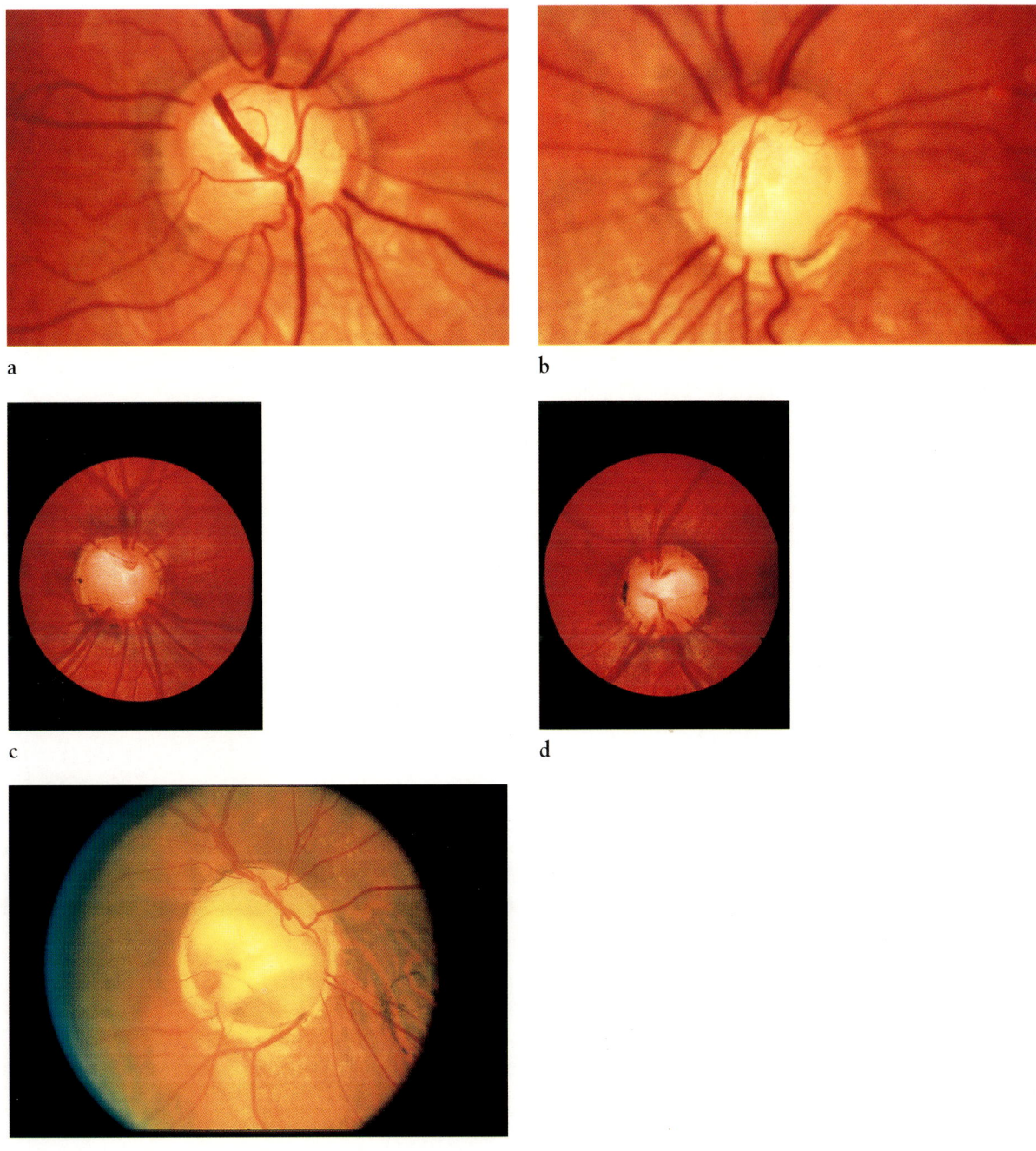

a

b

c

d

e

OPTIC NERVE HEAD

Developmental Anomalies

123a.   An anomaly of the optic nerve head, which may represent an atypical coloboma, is the congenital pit. It is seen in this patient as a focal area of depression and pallor adjacent to the temporal margin of the right optic nerve head. These may be difficult to distinguish from the focal cupping and pallor of glaucoma, although it is uncommon for glaucomatous optic atrophy to occur in the temporal quadrant with retention of healthy neural rim tissue in the superior and inferior quadrants, as seen in this photo.

123b.   In this case, the congenital optic pit involves the entire inferior quadrant, which is more difficult to distinguish from inferior glaucomatous cupping. In some cases, two optic pits may be present, as suggested in this photograph, which may help to distinguish it from glaucomatous optic atrophy.

123c.   Another variation of optic nerve head coloboma is called the morning glory syndrome. It is characterized by a large, funnel-shaped staphylomatous coloboma of the nerve head and peripapillary region with white central tissue, elevated peripapillary pigment disturbance and multiple radially orientated retinal vessels.

123d.   Patients with developmental anomalies of the optic nerve head, as in this patient with the morning glory syndrome (same eye as 123c), may have associated macular or extramacular serous detachment, which may lead to visual disturbances.

123e–f.   Another example of the morning glory syndrome is seen in this patient, with the large coloboma, radially oriented vessels, and peripapillary pigment disturbance. Figure 123f also shows some degree of retinal abnormality extending temporally toward the macula.

(Figure 123b was provided courtesy of Paul R. Singer, M.D.)

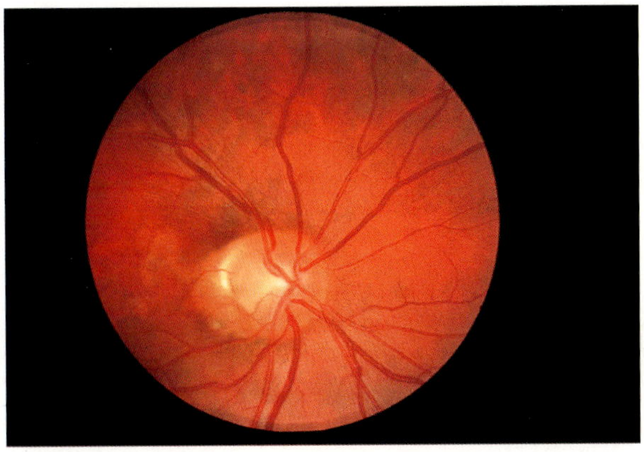

a

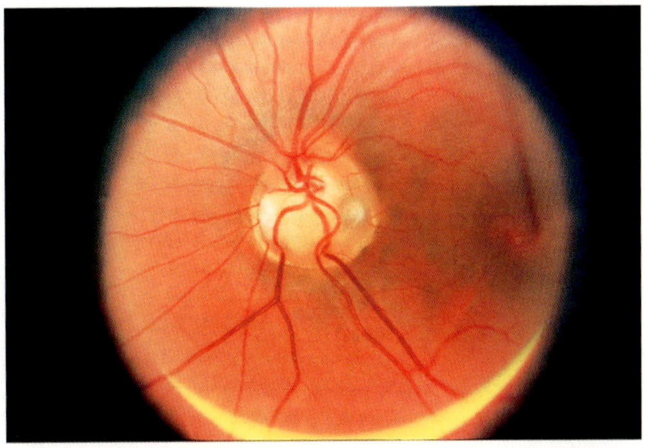

b

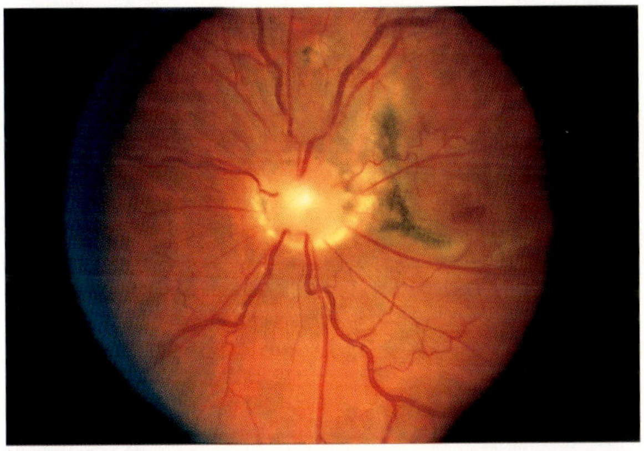

c

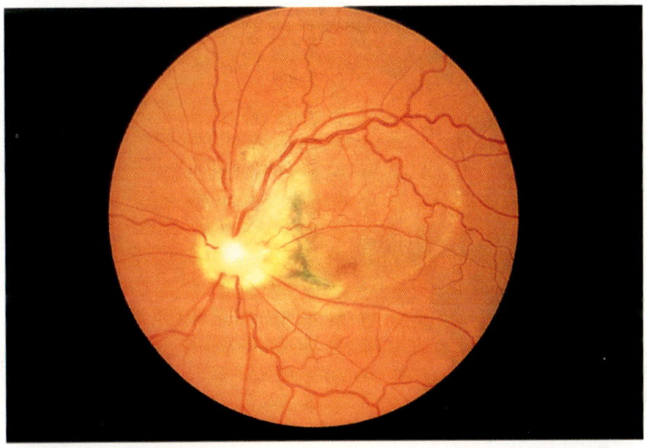

d

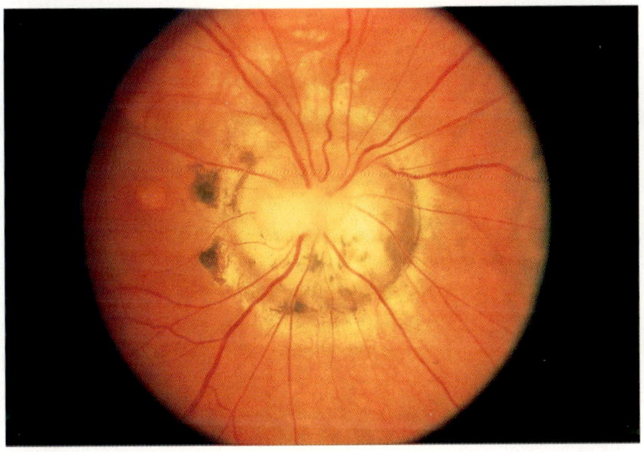

e

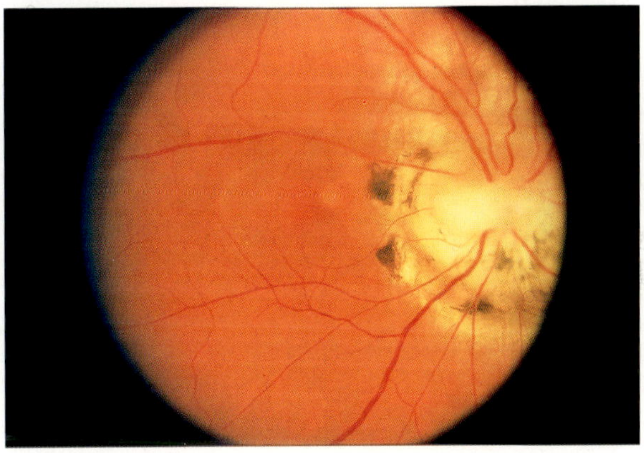

f

OPTIC NERVE HEAD

Evaluating and Recording Disc Findings

124a.   The preferred technique for evaluating the optic nerve head in the office is to use stereoscopic techniques, such as the Hruby lens slit-lamp attachment, as demonstrated in this photograph.

124b.   A more popular technique for evaluating the optic nerve head is to use a 90 diopter lens, or similar lens, at the slit lamp. This lens provides an inverted image, but excellent magnification and stereopsis.

124c.   Although the appearance of the optic nerve head, as evaluated in the office, should be recorded by description and drawings, these do not take the place of optic nerve head photographs, which are critical in following subtle changes in the disc over time. One fundus camera that is useful for this purpose is the Nidek, which provides simultaneous stereo images.

124d.   This photograph shows a typical simultaneous stereo image of the optic nerve head obtained with the Nidek fundus camera. The images are viewed with a stereo viewer.

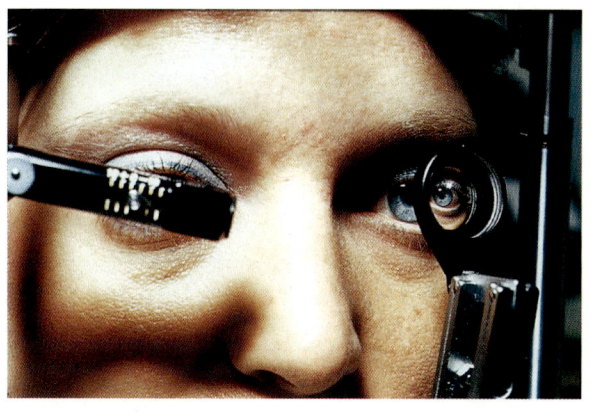

a

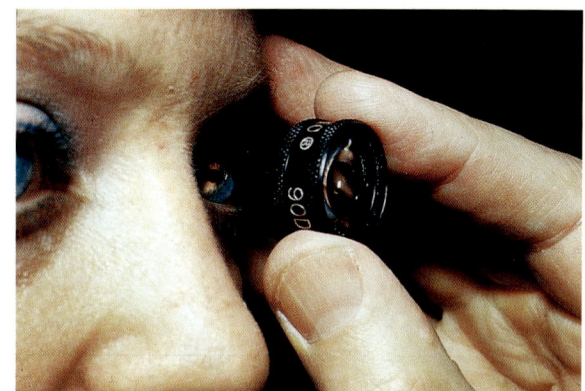

b

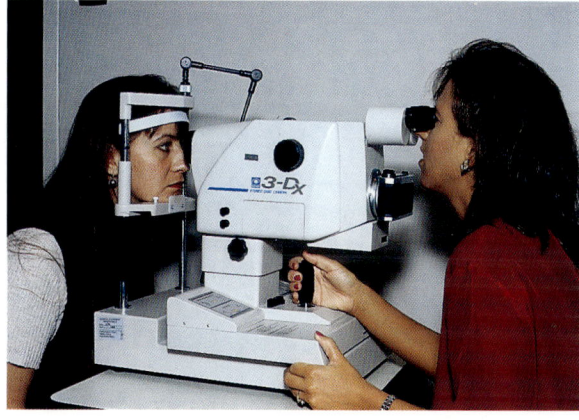

c

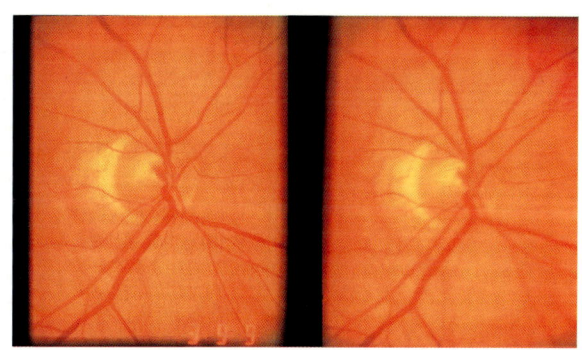

d

OPTIC NERVE HEAD

Computerized Image Analysis

Efforts to refine the assessment of the subtle findings of the optic nerve head and retinal nerve fiber layer have included computerized image analysis of the topography of these structures. Several instruments have been developed for this purpose; they are based on the principles of stereophotogrammetry, rasterstereography, or confocal laser scanning. Instruments based on the first two principles are shown on this page.

125a–b. The first generation of computerized image analyzers uses the basic principles of stereopsis, in which disparity between corresponding points of stereo pair images are used to generate contour lines and three-dimensional contour maps. One of the earliest instruments in this group is the Topcon Imagenet (formally the PAR IS 2000), shown in 125a. 125b shows an image from the television monitor of the Imagenet, giving the method of determining cup/disc ratio in the upper two images and a three-dimensional grid pattern of the optic nerve head topography in the lower portion of the screen. At the present time, this is the only commercially available instrument that uses the principle of stereophotogrammetry.

125c–d. Two other instruments that also use the principle of stereophotogrammetry, but are no longer commercially available, are the Rodenstock Optic Nerve Head Analyzer (125c) and the Humphrey Retinal Analyzer (125d). The Optic Nerve Head Analyzer differed from the other two instruments in that it projected vertical light stripes on the disc and peripapillary retina and used disparity between corresponding points along the light stripes of stereo pairs to generate vertical contour lines and three-dimensional contour maps. The other two instruments use disparity between existing structures in stereo images, rather than projected light stripes.

125e–f. The Glaucoma-Scope, as shown in these two figures, uses the principle of rasterstereography, in which a series of horizontal dark/light line pairs are projected on the disc and peripapillary retina at a fixed angle, and the computer scans a video image of the lines in a raster pattern (from side to side and from top to bottom). A computer algorithm translates deflections in the lines into depth numbers and creates a topographic map. 125f shows one of the printouts from the Glaucoma-Scope, which includes a three-dimensional grid contour (upper left), an estimation of disc and cup outlines (upper right), and horizontal and vertical cross-sections (lower right).

(Figures 125a and 125b were provided courtesy of George L. Spaeth, M.D., and Rohit Varma, M.D. Figure 125d was provided courtesy of Dr. Varma.)

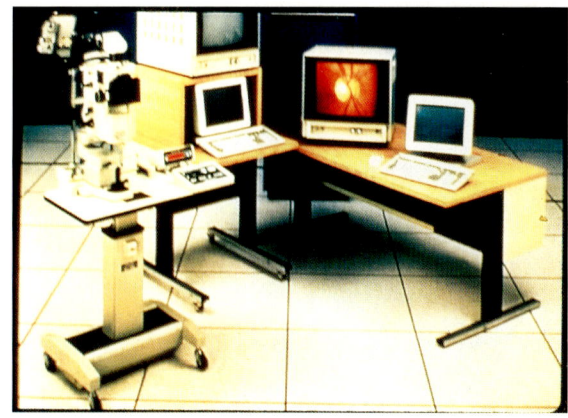

a

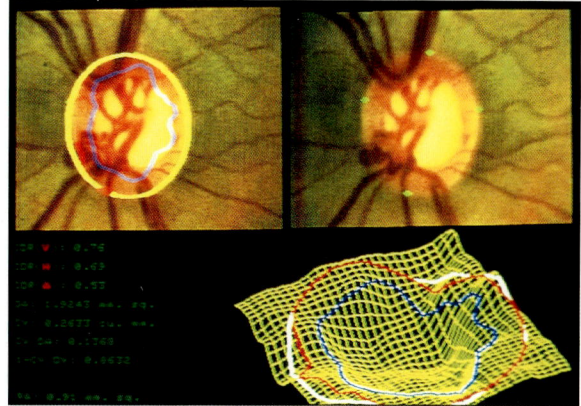

b

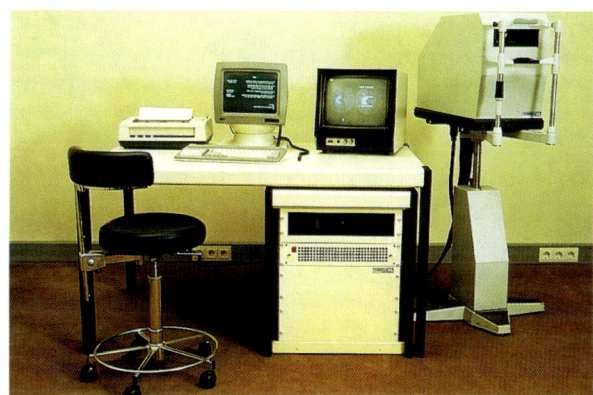

c

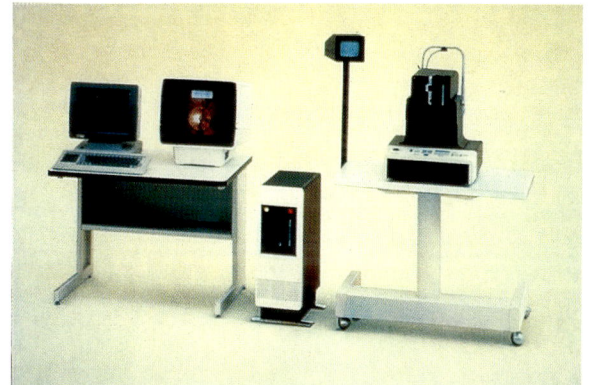

d

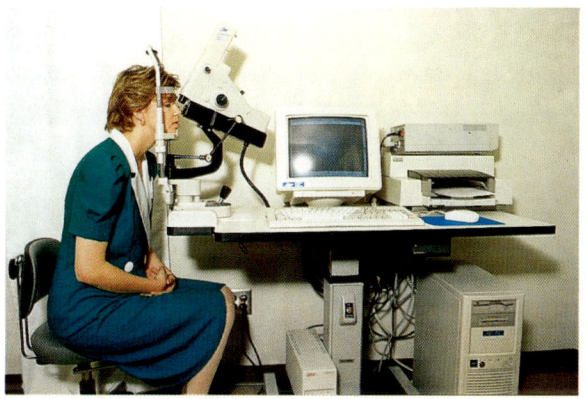

e

f

OPTIC NERVE HEAD

Computerized Image Analysis

The instruments shown on this page all use the principle of confocal laser scanning, which provides high resolution images by scanning the area of the fundus to be imaged with a focused laser beam. A confocal aperture, which is conjugate to the laser focus, eliminates scattered light and allows the photodetector to receive light from only a small spot on the fundus that is illuminated at any instant. By scanning the fundus with the laser, a two-dimensional image can be built up as an array of pixels.

126a–b. The principle of confocal scanning laser tomography uses a series of two-dimensional images, as described above, at successive planes of depth in the tissue, to construct a three-dimensional image. One example is the Heidelberg Retina Tomograph (HRT), shown in these two photographs. 126b shows an image from the HRT television monitor. The oval line surrounding the two disc images is 2.5 mm from the margin of the optic nerve head, and the green line in the lower portion of the screen shows the relative height of the nerve fiber layer along that 360° oval line (the profile starts in the temporal quadrant and moves superiorly).

126c–d. Another instrument that uses the principle of confocal scanning laser tomography is Laser Diagnostic Technologies' TopSS, as shown in these two photographs. 126d shows an image from the television monitor, with a vertical profile to the left and horizontal and circular profiles in the two upper frames. The three-dimensional image in the lower right frame can be changed to view the structure at different angles.

126e–f. The two instruments described above provide the relative height of the nerve fiber layer in relation to a reference point. Another confocal laser scanner, the Nerve Fiber Analyzer (NFA), measures the actual nerve fiber layer thickness by combining confocal laser scanning with the concept of scanning laser polarimetry. The latter is based on the principle that polarized laser light changes as it penetrates the birefringent nerve fiber layer, and the amount of change in the state of polarization, referred to as retardation, is linearly related to the thickness of the retinal nerve fiber layer. 126f shows an image from the television monitor of the NFA, in which the brighter colors represent a thicker nerve fiber layer. The profiles above and to the left of the left image provide horizontal and vertical contours, respectively. The profile in the upper right frame shows the circumferential profile with the typical "double hump" profile, because of the relatively thicker nerve fiber layer in the superior and inferior quadrants.

(Figures 126a and 126b were provided courtesy of Heidelberg Engineering; Figures 126c–f were provided courtesy of Laser Diagnostic Technologies, Inc.)

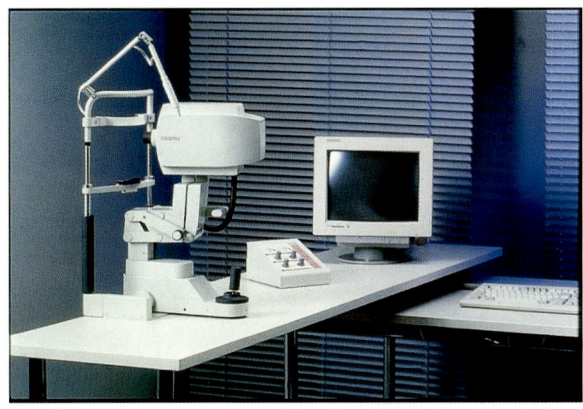

a

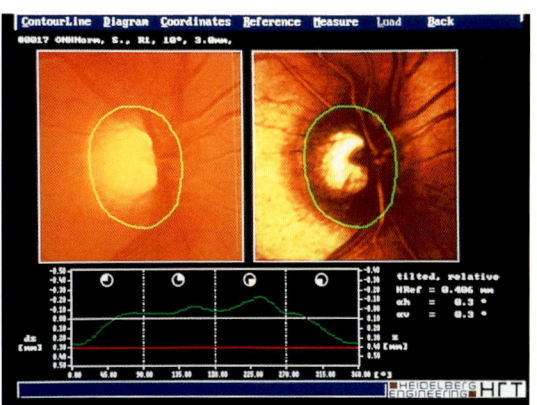

b

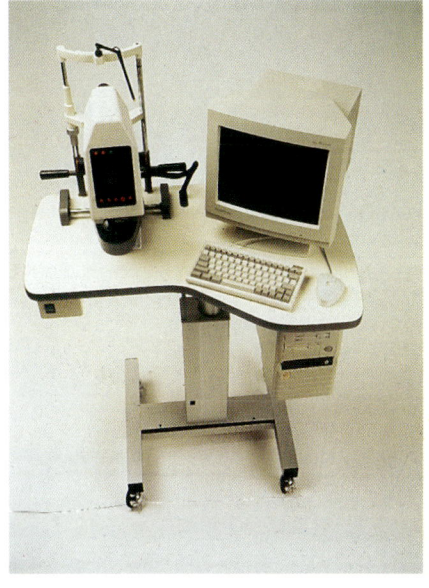

c

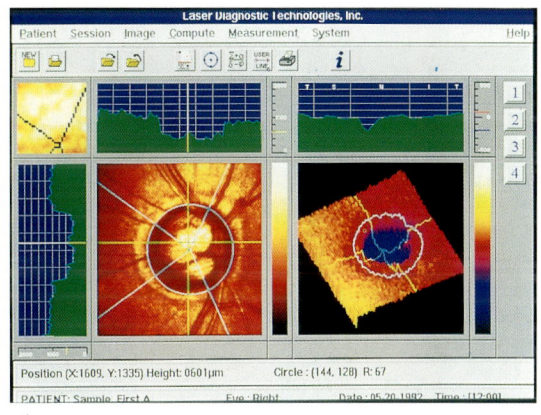

d

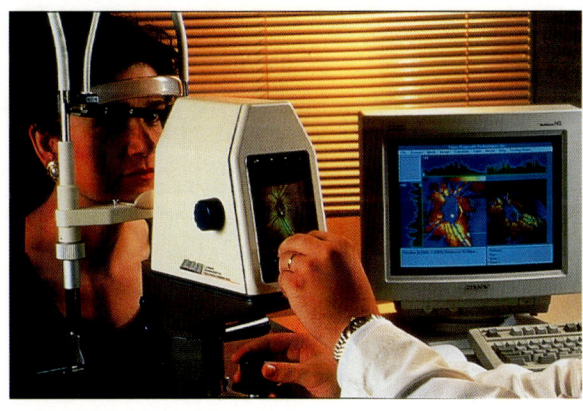

e

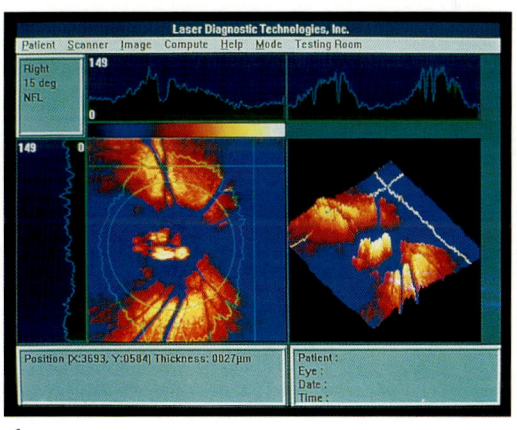

f

LIBRARY
POST GRADUATE CENTRE
KETTERING GENERAL HOSPITAL

OPTIC NERVE HEAD

Correlation with Visual Field

I27a–b. In glaucoma, a correlation typically exists between the glaucomatous optic atrophy and visual field loss. Failure to observe such a correlation should prompt the consideration of other possible disease processes. In these two photos, we see a good correlation between disc and field, which is consistent with glaucoma. The cup and pallor have extended to the inferior margin of the disc, and we see a corresponding complete superior arcuate scotoma. The superior neural rim remains reasonably healthy, and, as would be expected, the inferior visual field is full.

I27c–d. In these corresponding disc and visual field photos, more extensive glaucomatous damage is present. We see a broad area of cupping and pallor to the supero-temporal disc margin with a corresponding complete inferior arcuate scotoma. In addition, a small notch of cupping and pallor to the infero-temporal margin is seen with a corresponding superior paracentral scotoma.

I27e–f. In this visual field, we see an inferior nasal scotoma suggestive of a glaucomatous nasal step. The optic nerve head, however, has an intact neural rim, which does not correlate with the visual field. Further evaluation of the fundus reveals supero-temporal chorioretinal scarring as the explanation for the visual field loss. When neither disc nor retinal findings explain a visual field defect, a lesion posterior to the globe must be considered.

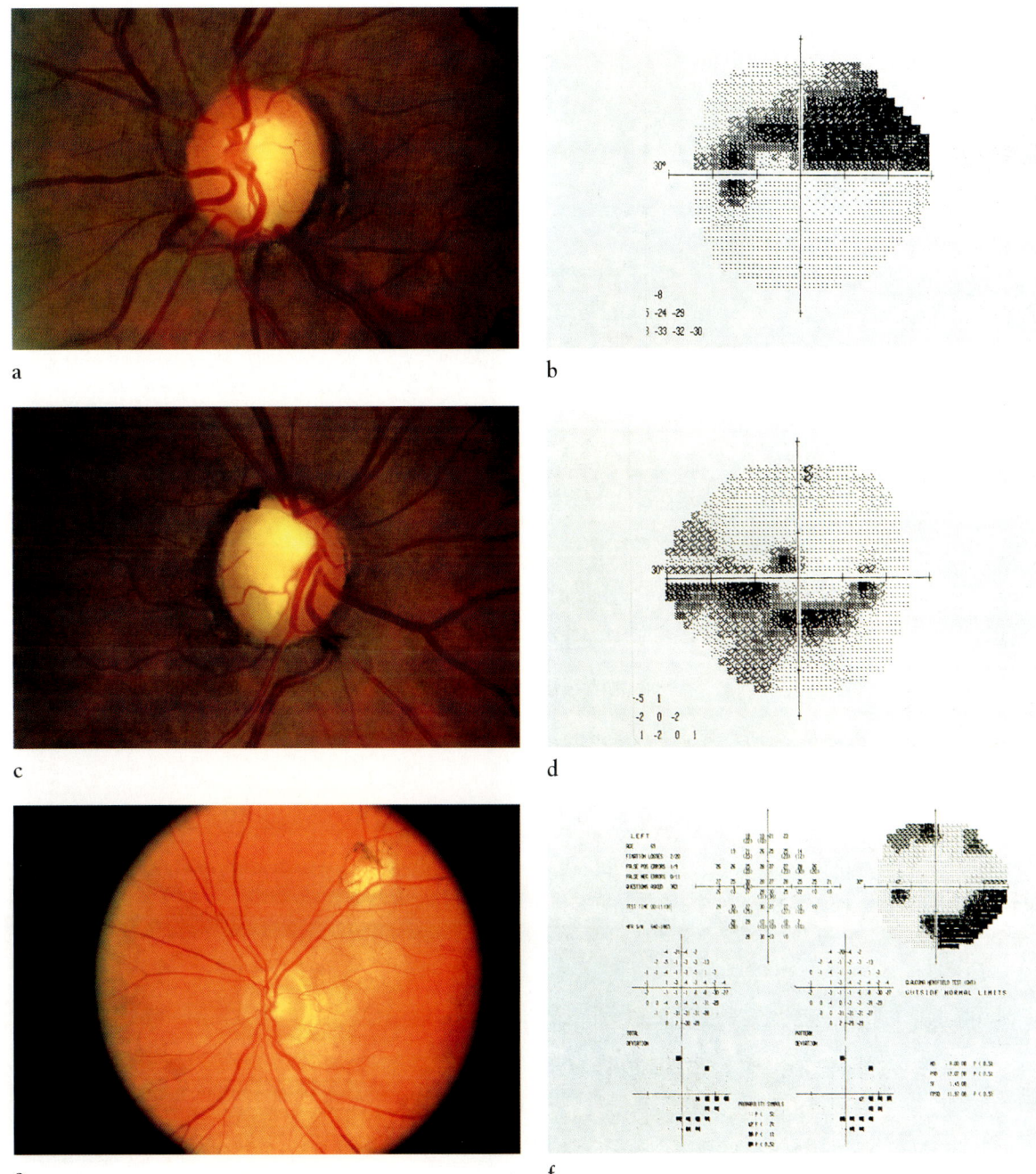

Section II

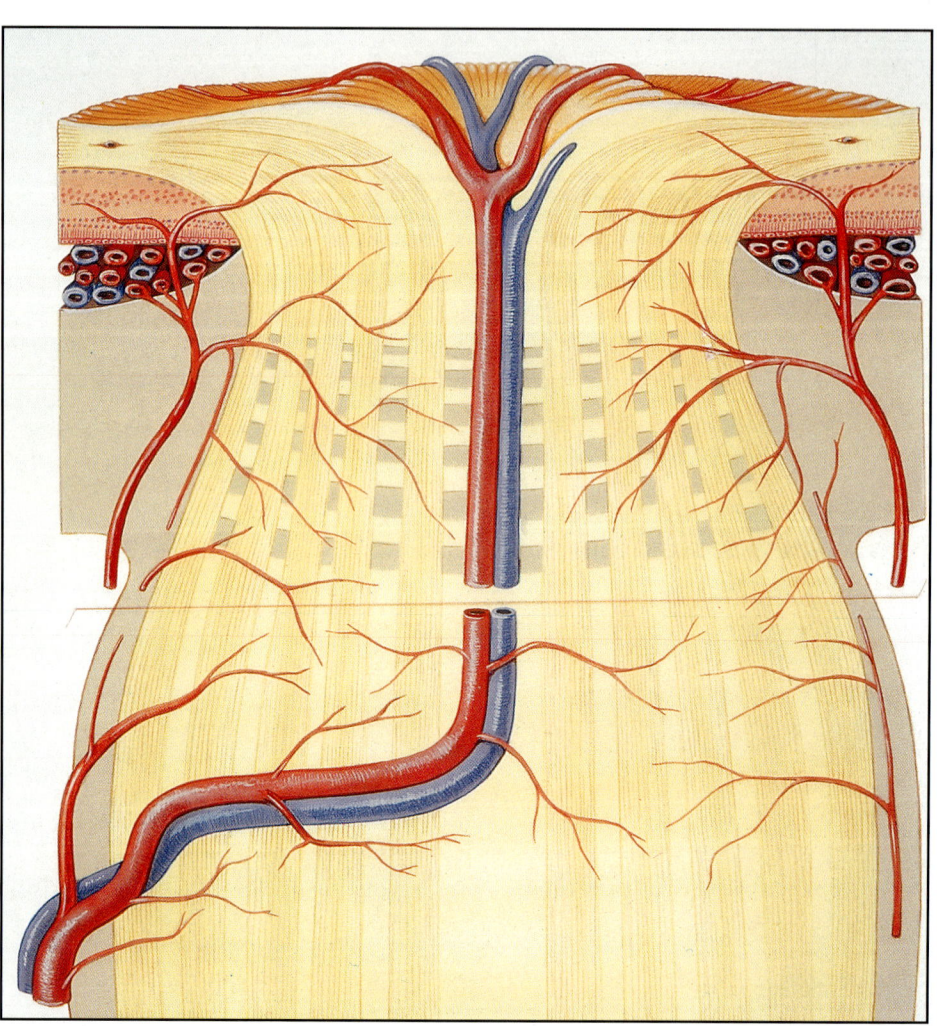

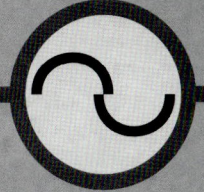

THE CLINICAL FORMS
OF
GLAUCOMA

PUPILLARY-BLOCK GLAUCOMAS

II2a.   This photo demonstrates three features of acute angle-closure glaucoma: 1) diffuse conjunctival hyperemia; 2) corneal clouding; and 3) a mid-dilated, fixed pupil, which is often vertically oval, as in this photo.

II2b.   After an acute attack, several clinical findings indicate the previous attack of acute angle-closure glaucoma. One of those, as seen in this photo, is glaukomflecken, which is the irregular white opacities in the anterior portion of the lens (*arrow*).

II2c.   Another finding in an eye that has had an acute attack of angle-closure glaucoma is sector atrophy of the iris, as seen in the superior quadrant in this photo.

II2d.   When a patient is suspected of being in angle-closure, or having had a previous angle-closure attack, or when evaluating the potential for angle-closure, it is essential to examine the depth of the peripheral anterior chamber. A screening test for this, which should be a routine part of the slit-lamp examination, has been referred to as the van Herick technique. With this test, the peripheral anterior chamber depth is estimated by comparing it with the thickness of the adjacent cornea. This is usually best performed in the temporal periphery, as demonstrated in this photo. When the peripheral anterior chamber depth is l/4 corneal thickness or less, gonioscopy should be performed (as shown on the next page).

(Figure II2a was provided courtesy of Saul H. Sugar, M.D.)

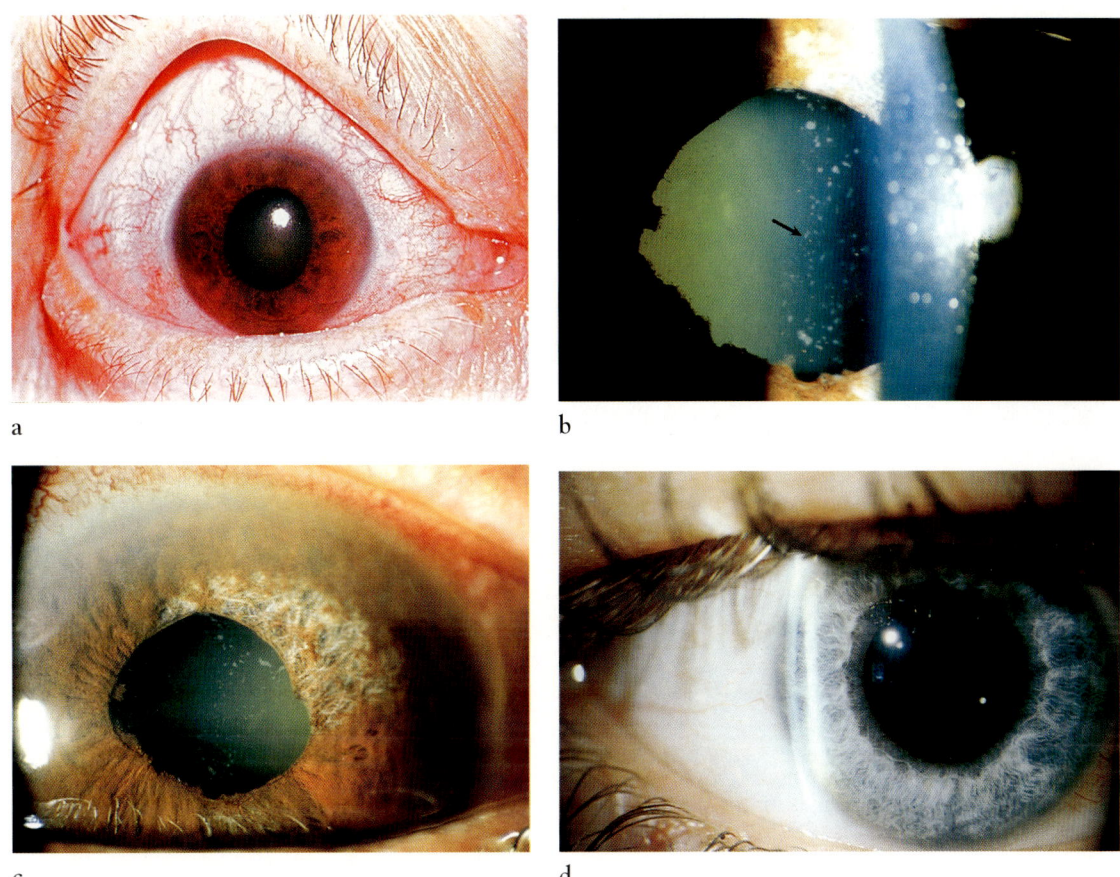

a

b

c

d

ANGLE-CLOSURE GLAUCOMAS

II3a. In this narrow angle, only the anterior portion of the trabecular meshwork (dark band) is visible. The iris is also bowed forward in the periphery, as is typical of pupillary-block glaucoma.

II3b. This patient with angle-closure glaucoma has an even narrower angle than in the previous case. In this gonioscopic view, only Schwalbe's line is visible, except for a possible thin rim of trabecular meshwork to the left of the view. The peripheral iris is again bowed forward.

II3c. This patient has chronic angle-closure glaucoma with broad peripheral anterior synechiae. We see less forward bowing of the peripheral iris, which appears to insert into the trabecular meshwork, leaving only a thin, irregular band of visible anterior meshwork.

II3d. This patient has the plateau iris syndrome. Notice that the pupil is dilated and the peripheral iris has several folds, which obscure visualization of all angle structures.

(All photographs on this page were provided courtesy of L. Frank Cashwell, Jr., M.D.)

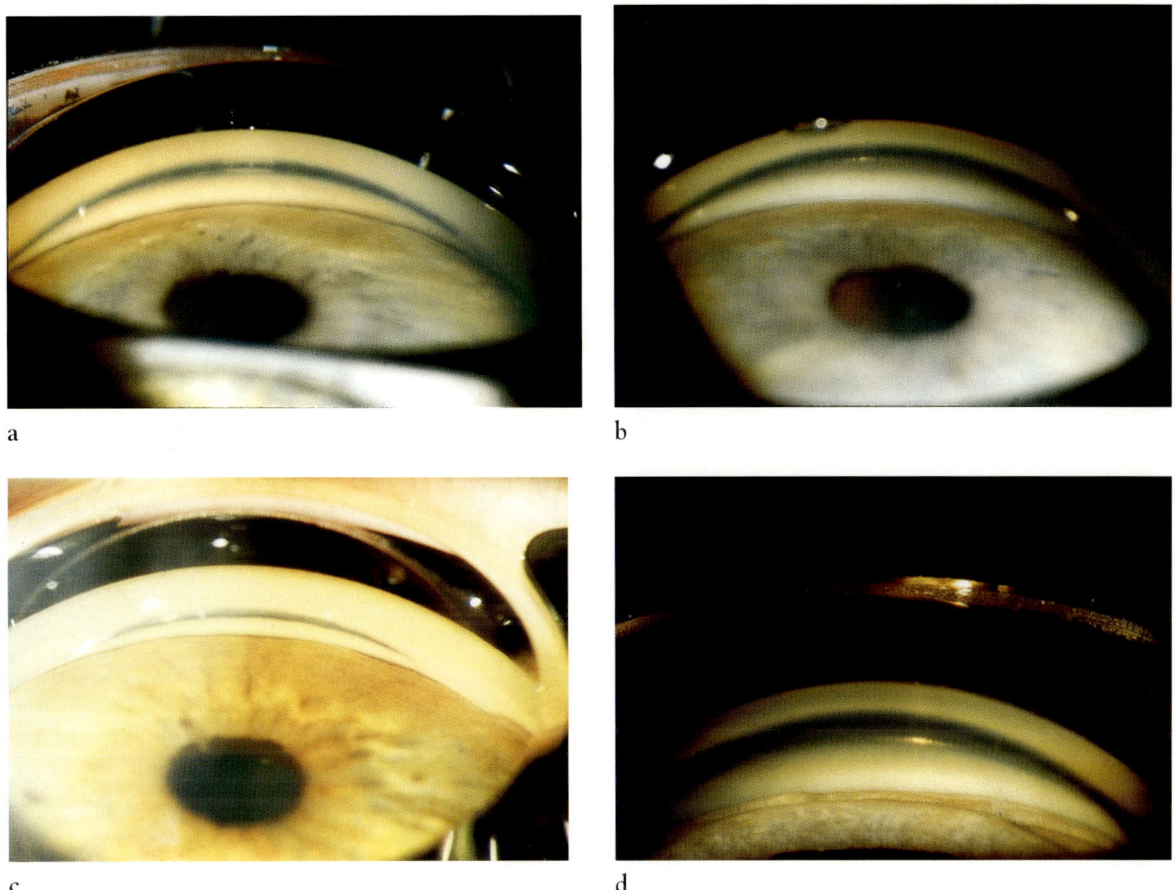

a

b

c

d

CONGENITAL GLAUCOMA

Embryology of the Anterior Chamber Angle

II4a.   A meridional section through the anterior segment of an 11-week fetus eye shows loosely arranged, spindle-shaped cells (mesenchymal cells of neural crest origin) occupying the ill-defined angular region. Schlemm's canal is unrecognizable, and the ciliary muscles and processes have not yet formed from the neuroectodermal fold of the optic cup. The corneal endothelium appears continuous with the cellular covering of the primitive iris.

II4b.   The angular region in the eye of a 6-month fetus now shows the easily recognizable trabecular meshwork and Schlemm's canal, which is functioning as an aqueous sinus. The ciliary processes are well formed. Meridional ciliary muscle fibers and scleral spur are defined, and radial circular fibers are also recognizable.

II4c.   The meridional section from the anterior chamber angle of an infant with congenital glaucoma shows an embryonic configuration. The characteristic features include: 1) anterior insertion of the iris; 2) rudimentary scleral spur; 3) direct insertion of ciliary muscle into trabecular meshwork; and 4) undifferentiated trabecular meshwork.

II4d.   This meridional section through the anterior chamber angle of an infant with congenital glaucoma shows a cellular layer ("Barkan's membrane"), which covers the inner aspect of the trabecular meshwork (*arrow*) and is contiguous with the corneal endothelium. Notice that the trabecular meshwork and Schlemm's canal otherwise look grossly normal.

(All photographs on this page were provided courtesy of Ramesh C. Tripathi, M.D., Ph.D.
    Figures II4a, II4b and II4d are reprinted with permission from Duane TD, Jaeger EA, eds. Congenital glaucoma: Embryology of the anterior chamber angle. Biomedical Foundations of Ophthalmology. Vol. 1. Philadelphia: Harper & Row, 1982.
    Figure II4c was reprinted with permission from Ritch R, Shields MB, Krupin T, eds. The Glaucomas. Vol. 1. 2nd edition, p. 34. St. Louis: CV Mosby, 1996.)

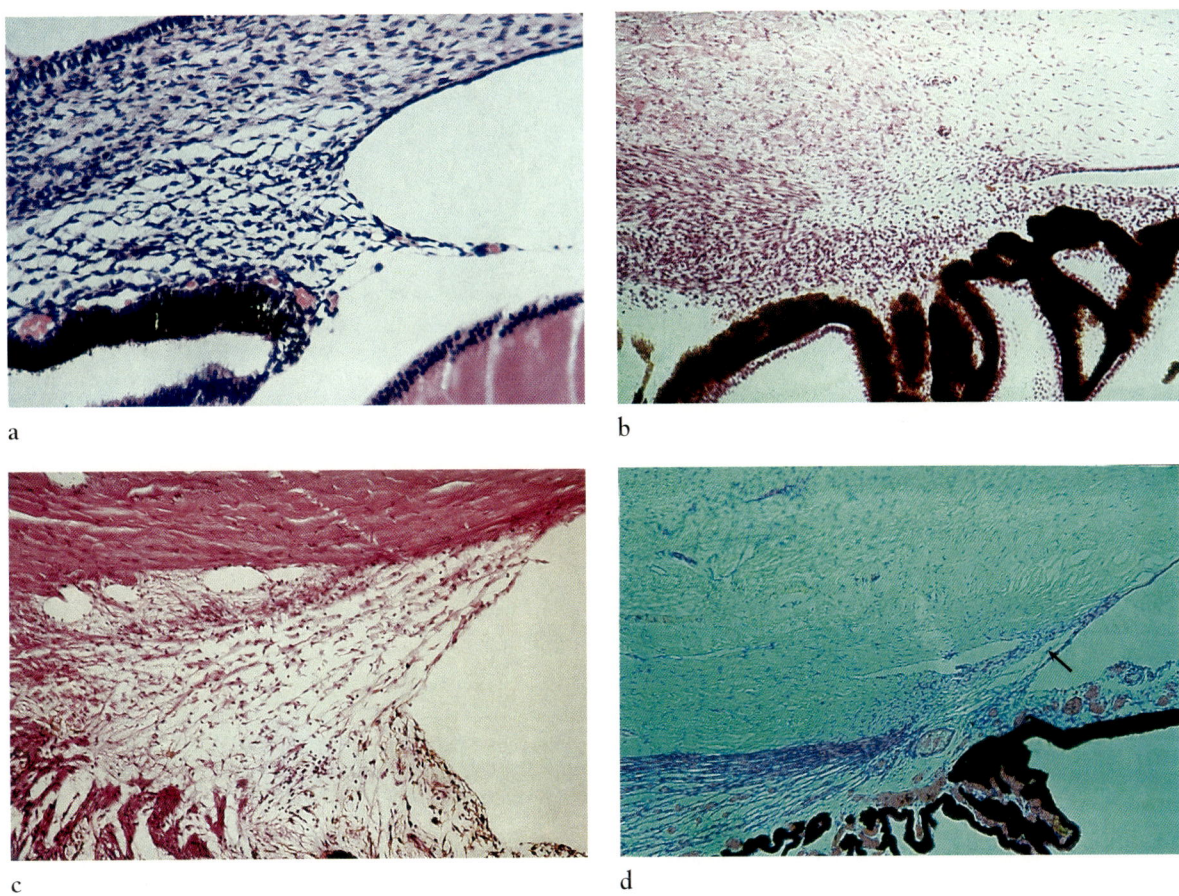

a

b

c

d

CONGENITAL GLAUCOMA

Infant Examination

II5a. The examination of an infant for congenital glaucoma is often done under anesthesia or sedation, although portions of the examination can sometimes be performed with the child awake. In this view we see the typical findings of congenital glaucoma in the left eye, in which the cornea is enlarged (buphthalmos) and mildly hazy.

II5b. The horizontal corneal diameter of each cornea is measured with calipers. The average horizontal corneal diameter at birth is approximately 10.5 mm, and a diameter over 12 mm in the first year of life is highly suspicious.

II5c. The intraocular pressure is being measured with a Perkins applanation tonometer. When performing the examination under anesthesia, it is advisable to perform the tonometry early, before the level of anesthesia is deep, which may influence the intraocular pressure.

II5d. The anterior segment of the eye is examined with a portable slit-lamp, looking primarily for characteristic changes in the cornea (discussed on the next page). The anterior chamber, iris, and lens are typically normal in congenital glaucoma, but may be abnormal in other types of developmental glaucoma.

II5e. The anterior chamber angle is examined next, using an infant Koeppe goniolens. The physician is holding the Barkan focal illuminator (foreground) and the biomicroscope, and the assistant is maintaining the position of the goniolens.

II5f. The final step of the examination is the funduscopy. This is usually done through an undilated pupil to avoid the influence of dilation on the intraocular pressure. Visualization of the disc may be helped by using a direct ophthalmoscope with the Koeppe lens on the cornea.

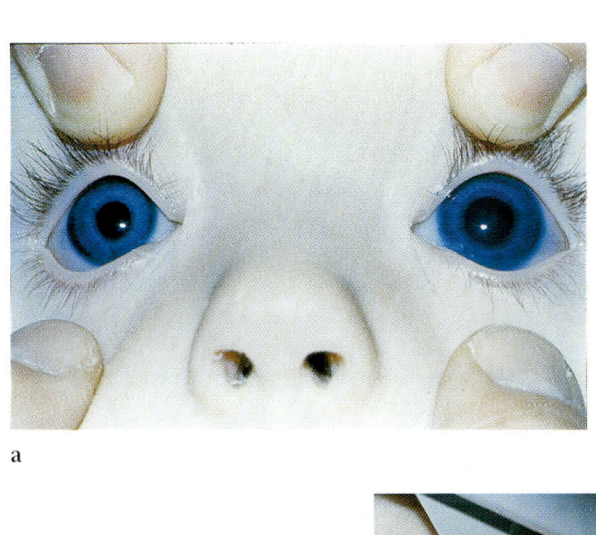

a

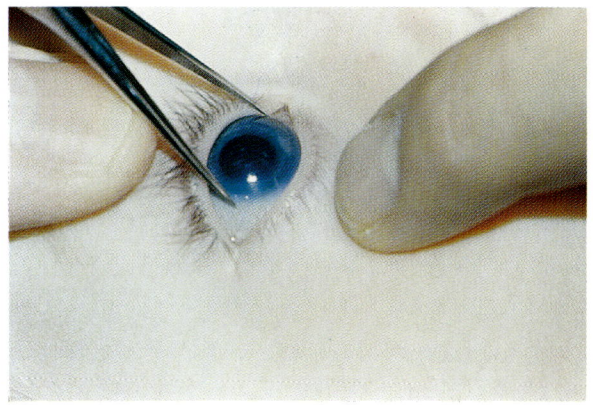

b

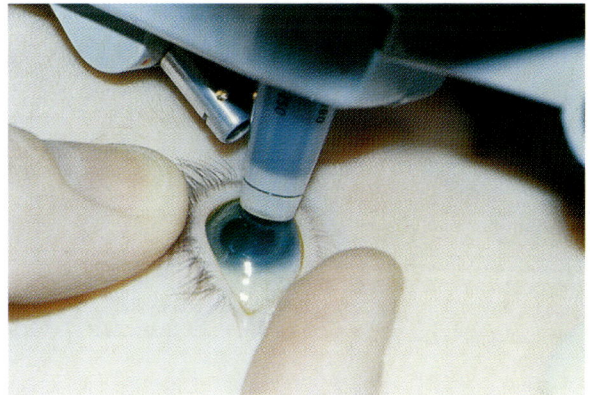

c

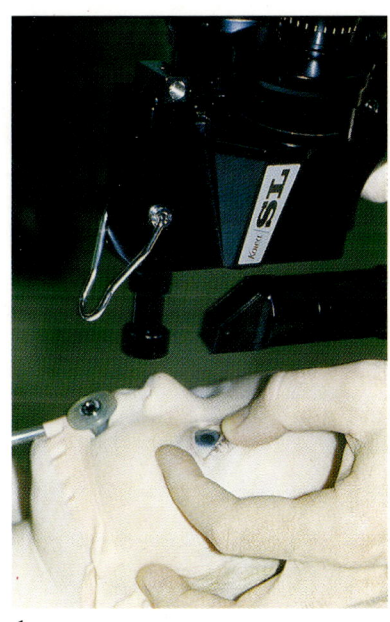

d

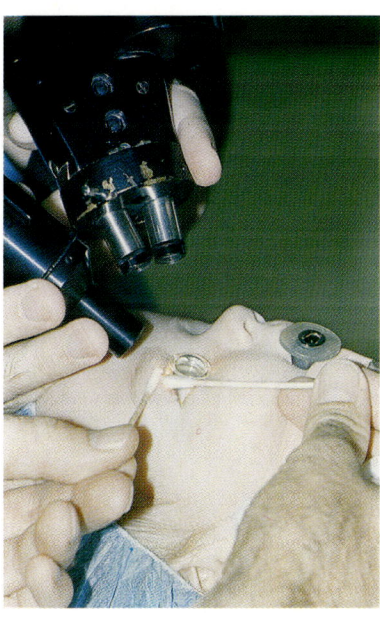

e

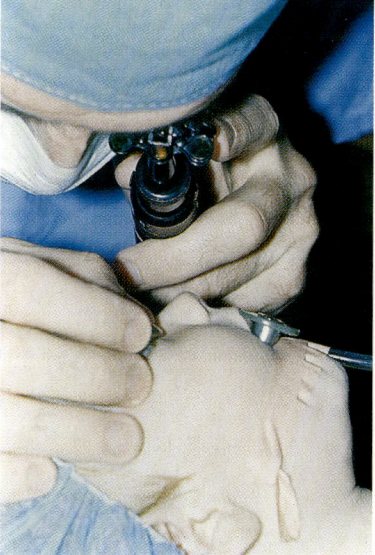

f

CONGENITAL GLAUCOMA

Corneal Abnormalities

II6a.   A common finding in the cornea of individuals with congenital glaucoma (or any glaucoma that develops during the first three years of life) is tears in Descemet's membrane (Haab's striae). These may be single or multiple and are characteristically oriented horizontally or concentric to the limbus.

II6b.   Another cause of tears in Descemet's membrane is birth trauma. This should be considered in the differential diagnosis of congenital glaucoma, although the tears can usually be distinguished from Haab's striae by the vertical or oblique orientation.

II6c.   Another common corneal abnormality in congenital glaucoma is corneal edema, which may produce a mild corneal haze that clears with normalization of the intraocular pressure or, as in this photo, may cause a dense opacification of the corneal stroma, which may persist despite reduction of the pressure.

II6d–f.   Several other causes of corneal clouding in infants are found that can be confused with that of congenital glaucoma and should be included in the differential diagnosis. The congenital corneal opacity in II6d is strikingly similar to that of the child with congenital glaucoma in II6c with the addition of the peripheral pannus. II6e shows the typical appearance of congenital hereditary corneal dystrophy, while II6f shows the cornea of a child with sclerocornea.

(Figures II6d and II6e were provided courtsey of John W. Reed, M.D.)

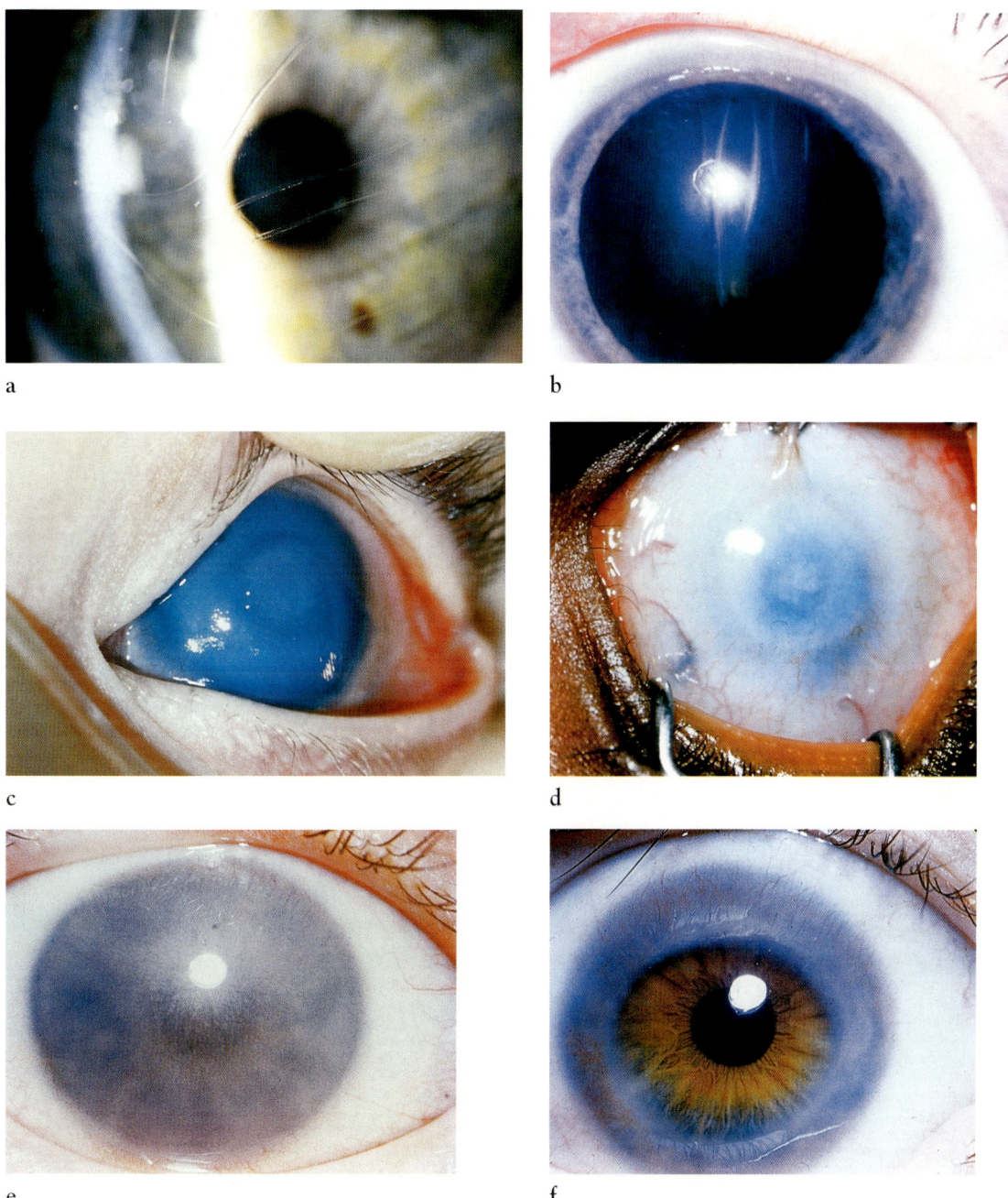

CONGENITAL GLAUCOMA

Gonioscopy

II7a.   The typical gonioscopic appearance of the child with congenital glaucoma is an open-angle, with a high insertion of the iris root, which obscures the view of the trabecular meshwork, as in this photo. Although the angle is usually avascular, loops of vessels from the major arterial circle may be seen above the iris root (*arrows*), which has been called the "Loch Ness monster phenomenon."

II7b.   In this gonioscopic photo of a child with congenital glaucoma, a portion of the faintly pigmented trabecular meshwork can be seen just above the high insertion of the iris. One vascular loop is also visible (*arrow*).

II7c.   In this older individual with congenital glaucoma, the high insertion of the iris obscures all angle structures.

II7d.   This individual has juvenile glaucoma. The angle is wide open, with visualization of the ciliary body band, scleral spur, and moderately pigmented trabecular meshwork, although numerous iris processes are present that obscure the structures in some areas and are confluent to the right of the gonioscopic view.

II7e–f.   Some children with congenital glaucoma or other forms of developmental glaucoma have more advanced developmental abnormalities, in which the anterior chamber angle is cicatrized, as shown in both of these photos, and occasionally vascularized, as shown in II7f. In addition, the peripheral iris may be covered by a fine, fluffy tissue that has been referred to as "Lister's morning mist."

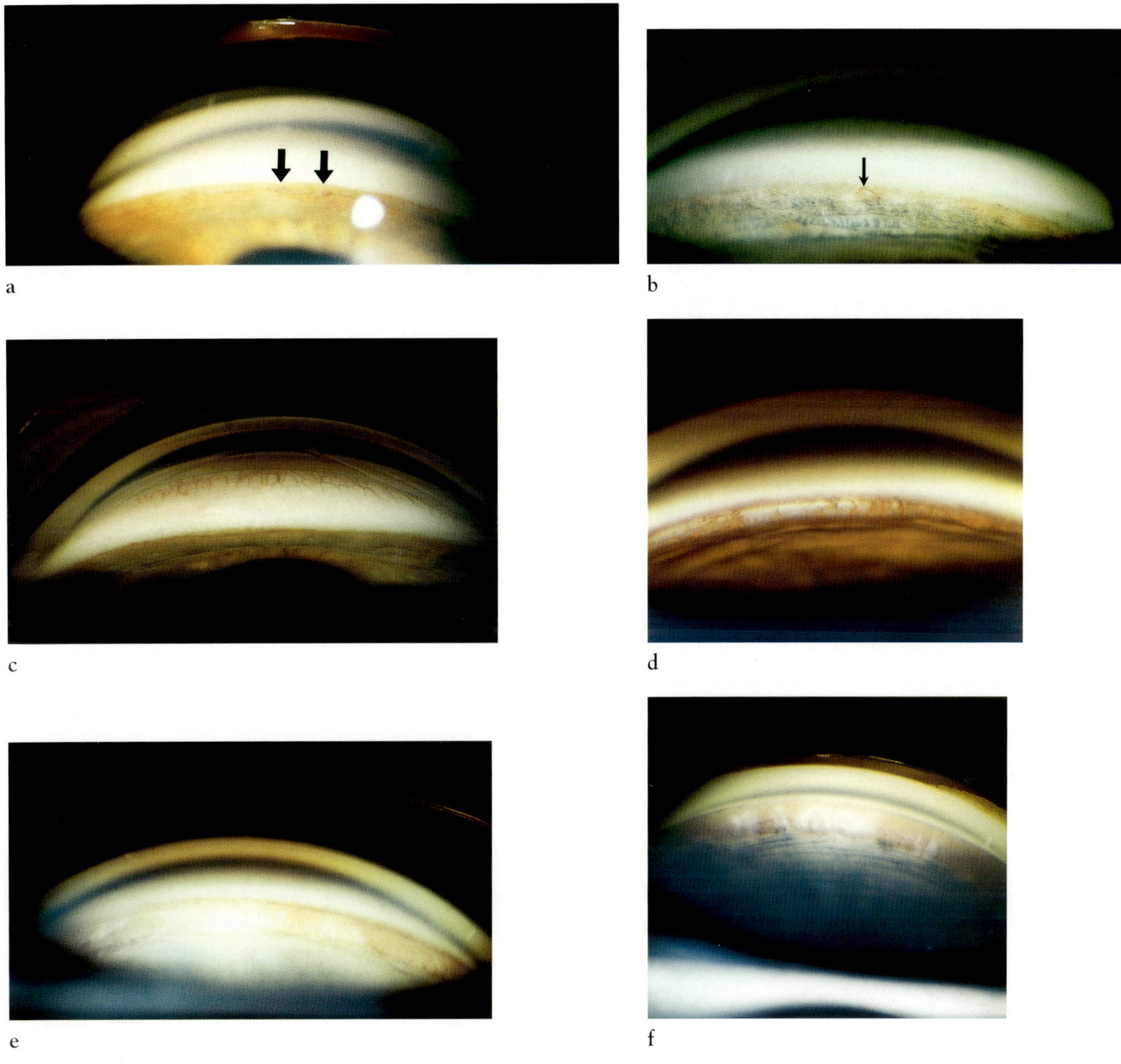

a

b

c

d

e

f

AXENFELD-RIEGER SYNDROME

Iris Features

II8a. The Axenfeld-Rieger (A-R) syndrome is a developmental disorder that includes anomalies of the peripheral cornea, anterior chamber angle and iris. In this photo, the typical iris features of corectopia and hole formation are seen best in the left eye.

II8b. A closer view of an eye with the A-R syndrome shows supero-nasal corectopia with marked thinning and large hole formation in the opposite quadrant.

II8c. Some individuals with the A-R syndrome may have ectropion uveae, which is present in all quadrants of this photo and extends to the peripheral iris in the left portion of the photo.

II8d. While lens abnormalities are not a typical feature of the A-R syndrome, a cataract, as seen in this photo behind the grossly abnormal iris, is one of many additional ocular abnormalities that may be seen in this spectrum of developmental disorders.

II8e. The red reflex from the retina further emphasizes the marked iris abnormality of the A-R syndrome, in which the pupil is distorted supero-nasally, with several iris holes temporally.

II8f. The abnormality that is believed to have caused the iris changes in the A-R syndrome, is the retention of a primordial endothelial layer on portions of the iris and anterior chamber angle. In this light microscopic photo, the endothelial layer is seen on the anterior surface of the iris. Contraction of the layer is believed to cause the changes in the iris, which includes the ectropion uveae as seen in this photo.

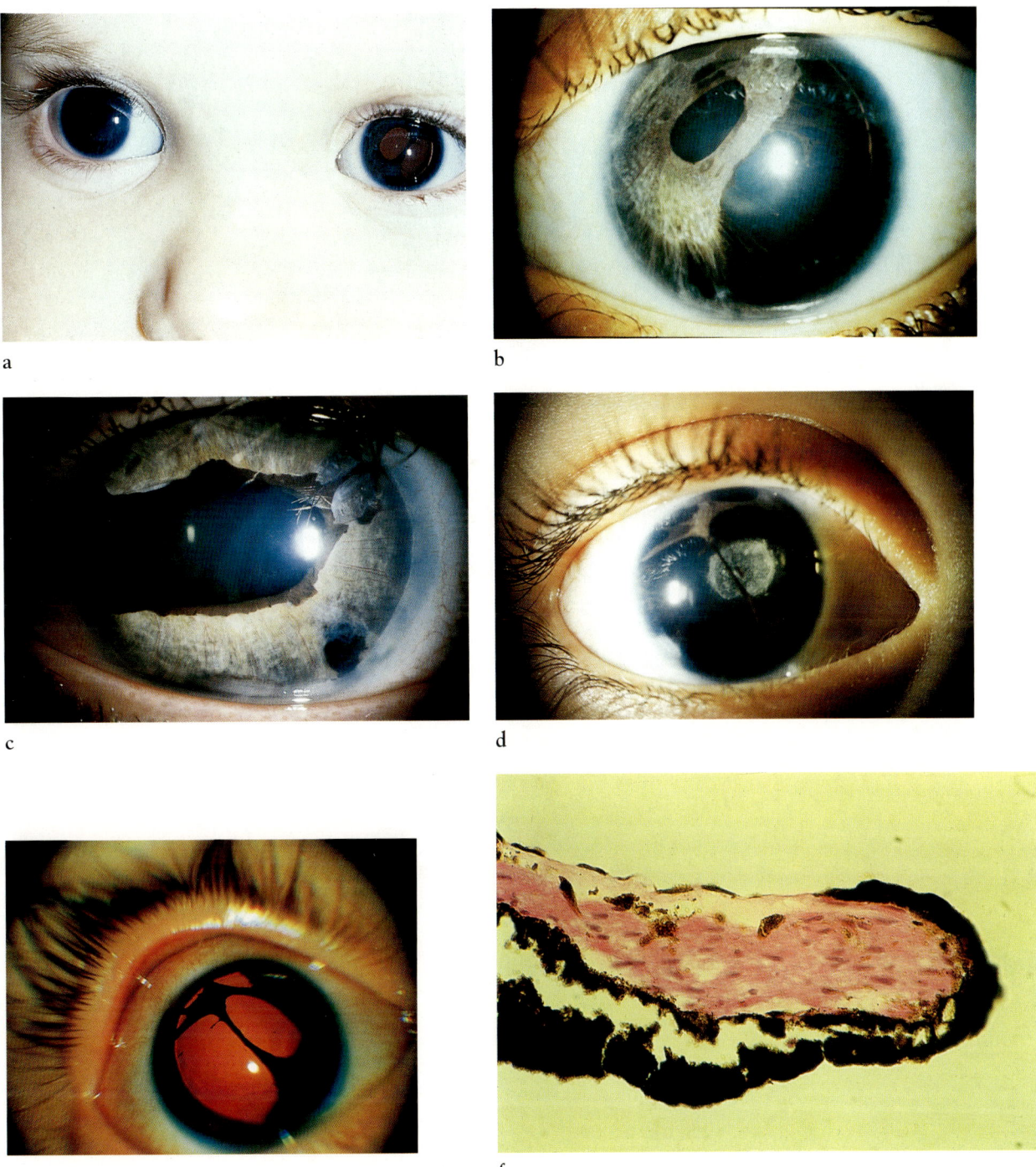

a

b

c

d

e

f

AXENFELD-RIEGER SYNDROME

Corneal Features

II9a. A characteristic abnormality of the cornea in the Axenfeld-Rieger (A-R) syndrome is a prominent, anteriorly displaced Schwalbe's line. This may be an isolated finding without the other features of the A-R syndrome in 8% to 15% of the general population. As in this photo, the isolated finding is seen as a white line usually in the temporal periphery (*arrow*), and is often referred to as posterior embryotoxon.

II9b–d. In a patient with the A-R syndrome, the prominent anteriorly displaced Schwalbe's line is typically seen in all quadrants, as in these three photos. In some cases, as in II9b, the iris features may be limited to minimal peripheral stromal atrophy, which was originally called Axenfeld's anomaly. In other cases, as in II9c, slight corectopia may be present as well as more advanced peripheral stromal iris atrophy, while other patients, as in II9d, may have marked corectopia.

II9e. A closer view of the prominent, anteriorly displaced Schwalbe's line in the A-R syndrome shows its typical location on the posterior cornea.

II9f. Another typical feature of the A-R syndrome is iridocorneal adhesions, which bridge the anterior chamber angle from the peripheral iris to the prominent Schwalbe's line (*arrow*). These iridocorneal adhesions are better appreciated by gonioscopy, which is shown on the next page.

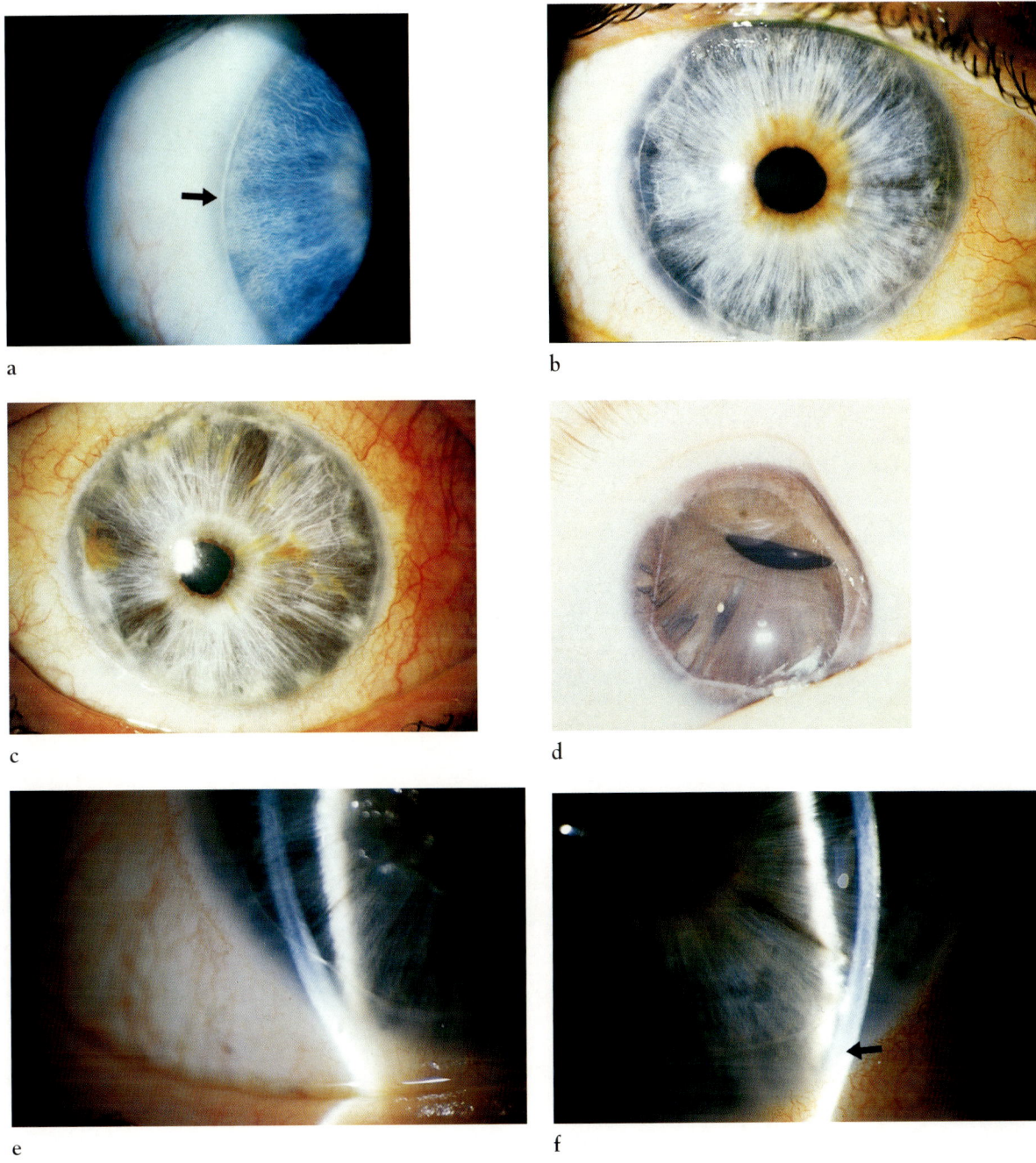

a

b

c

d

e

f

AXENFELD-RIEGER SYNDROME

Gonioscopic Features

II10a.   The gonioscopic appearance of an eye with the Axenfeld-Rieger (A-R) syndrome shows several iridocorneal adhesions extending from the peripheral iris to the prominent, anteriorly displaced Schwalbe's line (*arrows*).

II10b.   In this gonioscopic view of an eye with the A-R syndrome, the iridocorneal adhesions are so extensive that they allow visualization of only small portions of the prominent anteriorly displaced Schwalbe's line (*arrows*).

II10c–d.   These gonioscopic photos show further examples of the iridocorneal adhesions in the A-R syndrome. In II10c, the adhesions are extremely broad, allowing visualization of the prominent Schwalbe's line only in the far left of the view. In Il10d, we see one relatively broad adhesion to the left of the view, with two small, tented adhesions to the right.

II10e–f.   These light microscopic photographs show the prominent Schwalbe's line, which is composed of dense collagen and ground substance covered by a monolayer of spindle-shaped cells with a basement membrane. In II10e, an anterior insertion of the iris is present; this may be seen in several forms of developmental glaucoma. II10f shows an iridocorneal adhesion (*arrow*) extending from the peripheral iris to the prominent Schwalbe's line.

(Figure Il10e was provided courtesy of Ramesh C. Tripathi, M.D., Ph.D.)

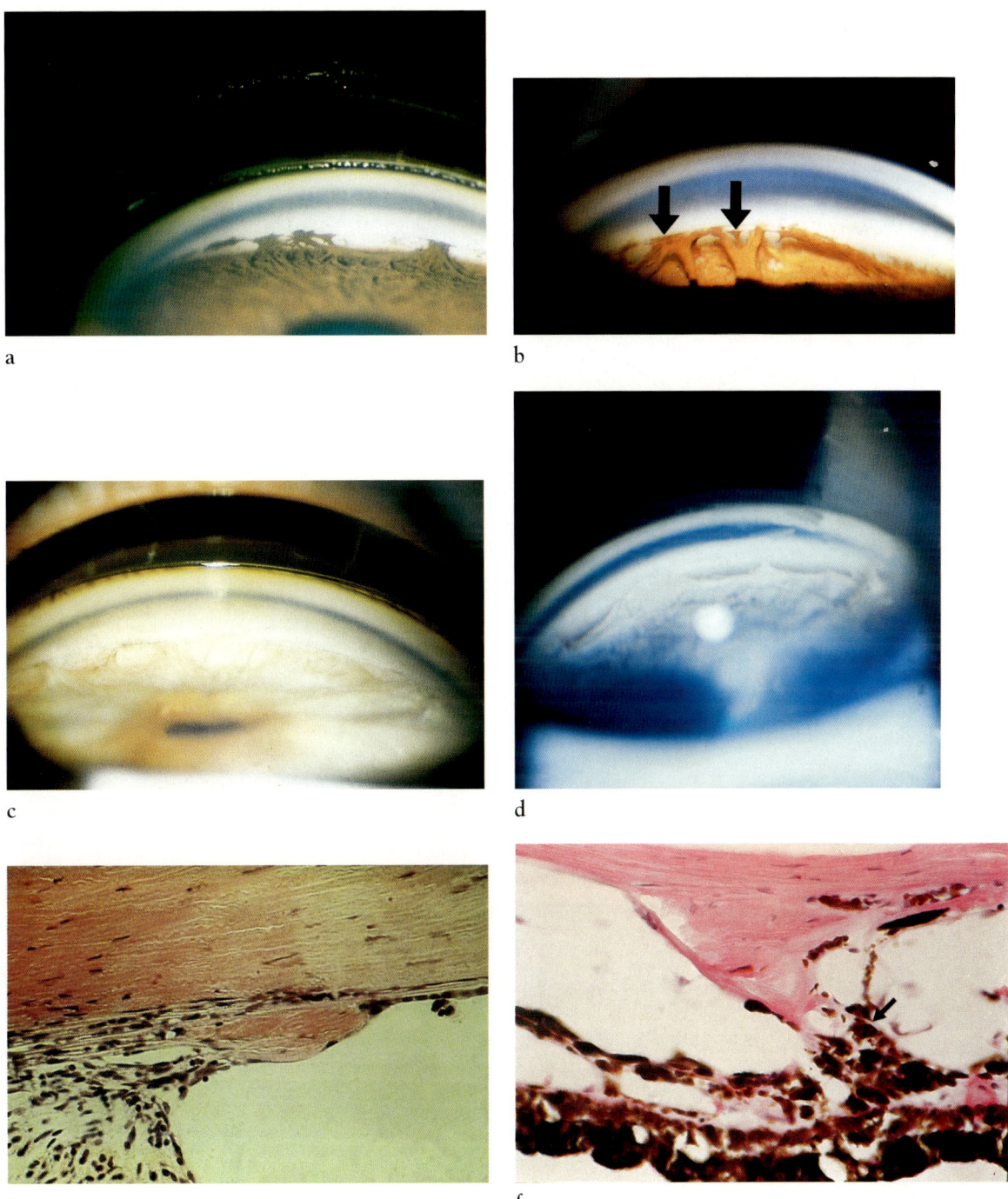

a

b

c

d

e

f

PETERS' ANOMALY

II11a.   Peters' anomaly is a bilateral, congenital disorder, characterized by central opacities of the cornea and lens, with adhesions from the central iris to the periphery of the corneal opacity.

II11b.   In this photo (same eye as II11a) the slit beam shows the adhesion of the central iris to the central cornea, which has a relatively faint posterior opacity. The central cataract can be seen to the right of the iris adhesion.

II11c.   In other patients with Peters' anomaly, the corneal opacity may be more prominent, sometimes obscuring most of the pupillary opening, as in this photo.

II11d.   In this photo (same patient as II11c) a sector iridectomy was performed during a trabeculectomy procedure to provide a better optical opening. Note the cataract just above the corneal opacity.

II11e.   This photo shows another patient with the central corneal opacity of Peters' anomaly. This condition was once classified with the Axenfeld-Rieger syndrome as a single category of developmental disorders. It is now known, however, that the two conditions are distinctly different, and Peters' anomaly appears to be a morphologic finding with more than one pathogenic mechanism.

II11f.   The histologic hallmark of Peters' anomaly is a central defect in Descemet's membrane and corneal endothelium, with thinning and opacification of the corresponding area of the corneal stroma, as seen in this light microscopic photo. In some cases, the cataractous lens is in contact with the abnormal cornea.

(Figures II11e and II11f were provided courtesy of George O. Waring, III, M.D.)

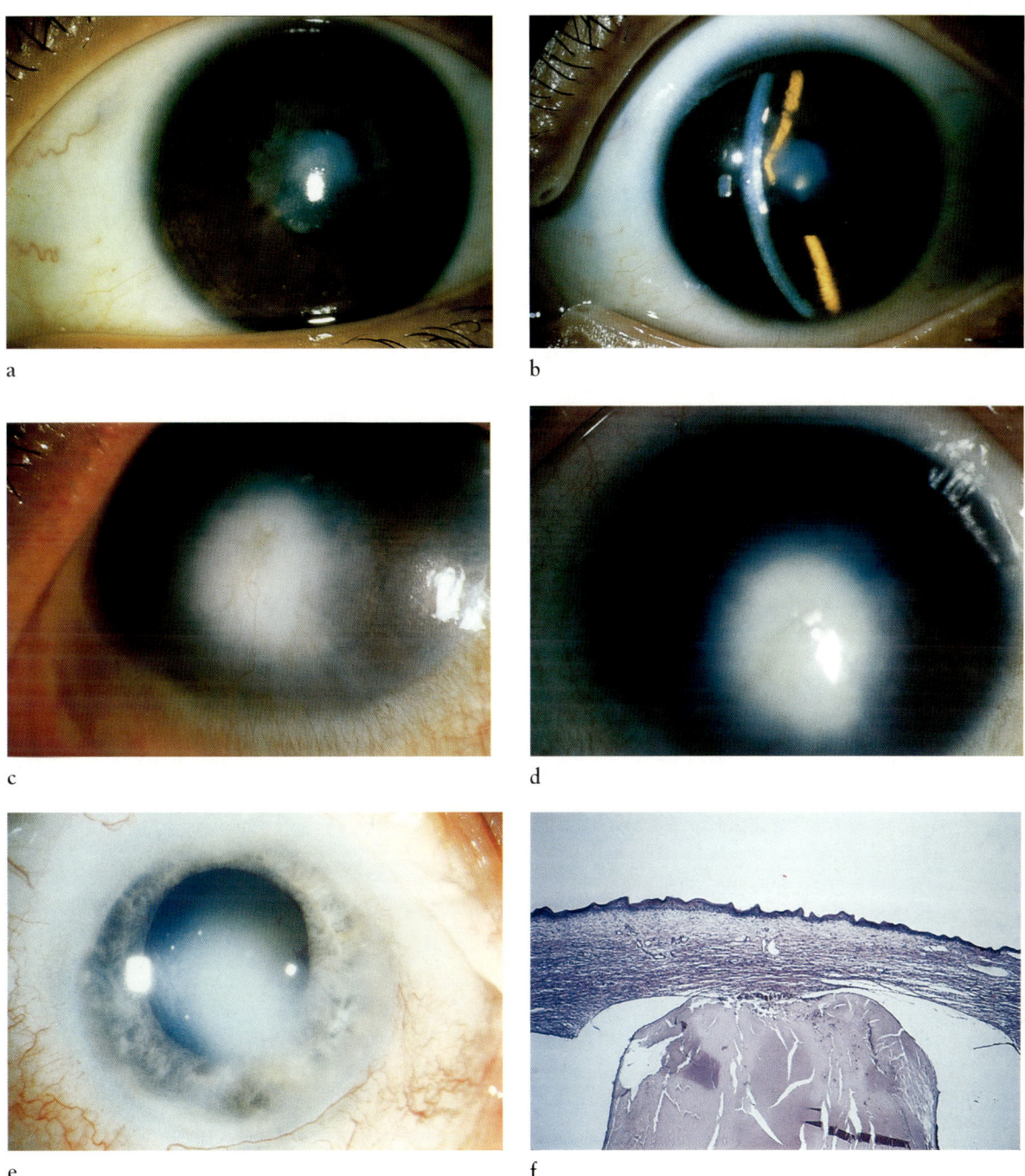

a

b

c

d

e

f

LIBRARY
POST GRADUATE CENTRE
KETTERING GENERAL HOSPITAL

ANIRIDIA

II12a.   Aniridia is a bilateral, developmental disorder, characterized by the partial absence of the iris, with a rudimentary stump of variable width. In some cases, as in this photo, the stump of iris is so short that none can be seen by external or slit-lamp examination.

II12b.   In other patients, as seen in this photo, a wider stump of rudimentary iris is easily seen.

II12c.   In addition to the characteristic iris abnormality, patients with aniridia may also have corneal pannus and opacity, foveal hypoplasia, and several abnormalities of the lens. Progressive cataract formation may lead to significant visual impairment. In addition, the lens may be subluxed, as seen in this photo.

II12d.   This higher magnification of the eye in II12c shows the stretched lens zonules against the red reflex. The stretching of the zonules may explain the subluxation of the lens in some patients with aniridia.

II12e.   This gonioscopy view of a patient with aniridia shows the rudimentary stump of iris. Ciliary processes are faintly visible beneath the iris. The appearance of the anterior chamber angle suggests a high insertion of the peripheral iris, which may be a mechanism of glaucoma in some patients, especially when it occurs early in life.

II12f.   A more common mechanism of glaucoma, which occurs in 50% to 75% of patients with aniridia, is a progressive angle-closure during the first 5 to 15 years of life, as the rudimentary stump of iris is pulled forward against the trabecular meshwork, possibly by the contraction of tissue strands between the iris and meshwork. In this photo, the peripheral iris has been pulled completely forward against the meshwork, exposing the pigment epithelial layer and the ciliary processes.

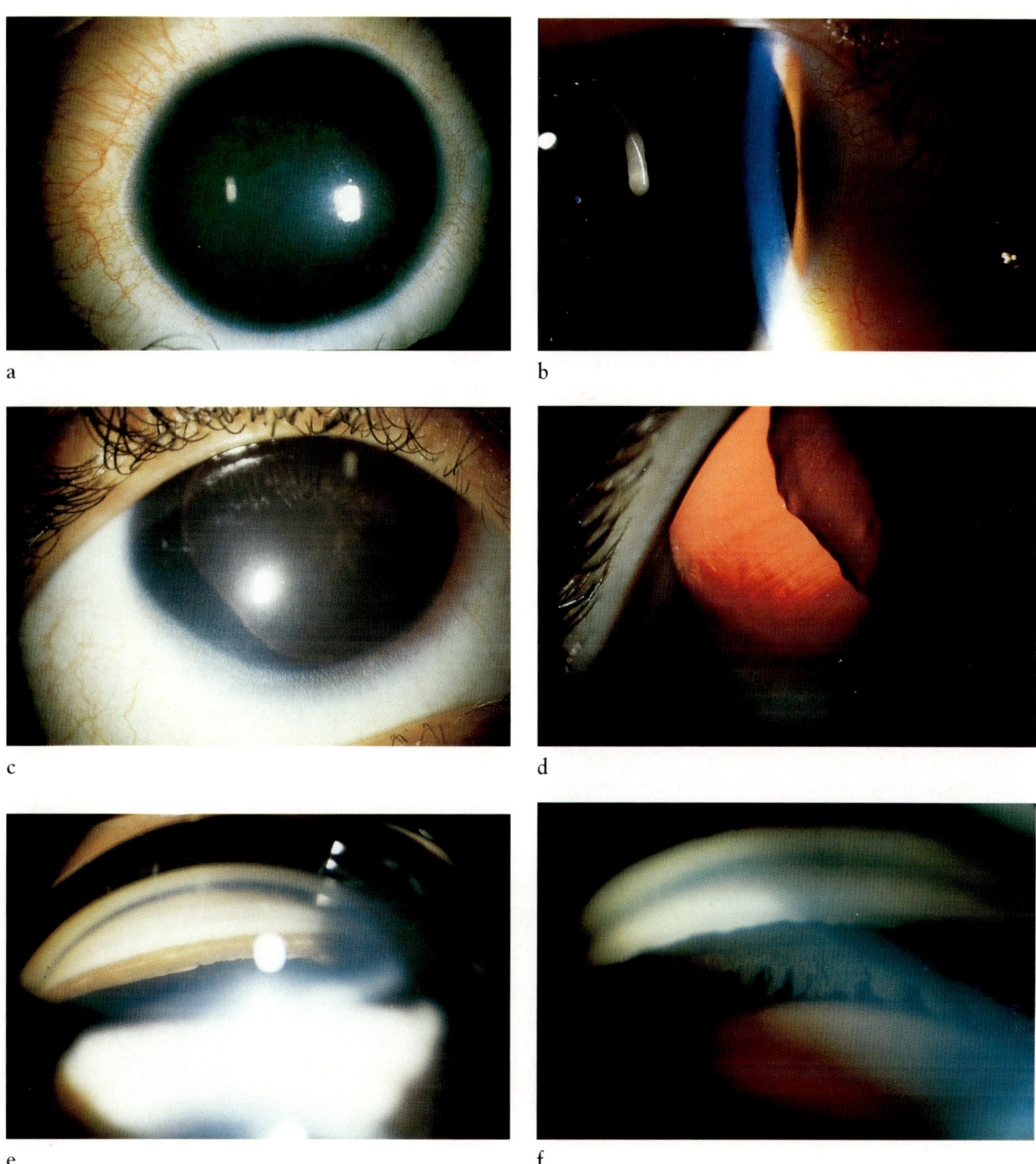

CONGENITAL ECTROPION UVEAE

II13a. Ectropion uveae, in which a variable portion of the iris pigment epithelium is pulled around the pupillary margin onto the stromal surface of the iris, may be associated with a wide range of developmental disorders, including the Axenfeld-Rieger syndrome, as previously discussed. In other cases, it may be found as an isolated developmental abnormality. Some of these cases may have associated glaucoma. In some patients, the ectropion uveae may be seen most prominently in one quadrant, as in this photo.

II13b. In other patients with congenital ectropion uveae, the developmental abnormality may appear for nearly 360° around the pupil, as in this photo.

II13c–d. In some patients, the ectropion uveae may be bilateral, as seen in a patient's right and left eye in these two photos

II13e–f. In other cases, the ectropion uveae may be unilateral, as seen in this patient, in which II13e shows 360° ectropion uveae, while the fellow eye in Il3f is normal.

(Figure II13b was provided courtesy of Charles M. Lederer, Jr., M.D.)

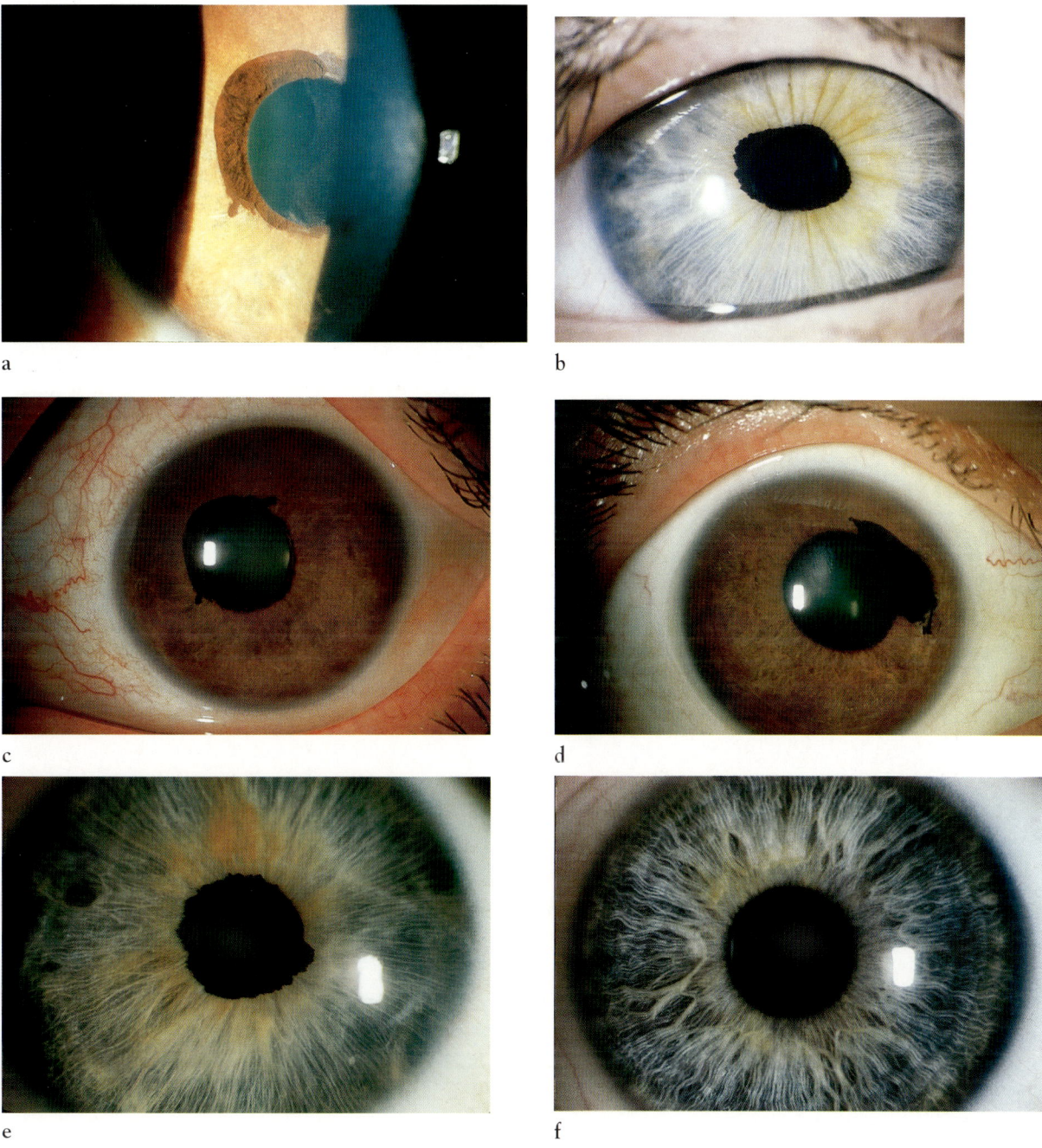

a

b

c

d

e

f

IRIDOCORNEAL ENDOTHELIAL SYNDROME

Corneal Features and Clinical Variations

II14a.   The iridocorneal endothelial (ICE) syndrome is a clinically unilateral ocular condition that is usually recognized in early to middle adulthood, with a predilection for women. A common feature in all patients with the ICE syndrome is a corneal endothelial abnormality, which may be seen by slit-lamp examination as a fine hammered silver appearance of the posterior cornea (*arrow*). It is similar in appearance to the endothelial changes of Fuchs' dystrophy, but less coarse.

II14b.   In some cases, the endothelial abnormality is the only corneal finding. In other patients, the endothelial abnormality may lead to corneal edema, as seen in this photo, with variable degrees of pain and reduced vision.

II14c.   Three clinical variations of the ICE syndrome have been described, with the distinguishing features based primarily on the appearance of the iris. In Chandler's syndrome, the iris may appear grossly normal, or may have minimal corectopia and mild peripheral iris stromal atrophy, as in this photo.

II14d.   Other patients with Chandler's syndrome have more obvious iris changes, with a distorted, displaced pupil and variable degrees of iris stromal atrophy, but no hole formation in the iris.

II14e.   A second variation of the ICE syndrome is referred to as progressive iris atrophy (previously called essential iris atrophy). These patients typically have more marked corectopia (the pupil is in the inferior quadrant in this eye), but the most distinguishing characteristic is the hole formation in the iris, which in this photo is quite extensive.

II14f.   The third variation of the ICE syndrome is called the Cogan-Reese syndrome. These patients may have any degree of corectopia and iris atrophy, but the distinguishing feature is the presence of pigmented, pedunculated nodules on the surface of the iris, as seen in this case.

(Figure II14d is reprinted with permission from Am J Ophthalmol 1978;85:749.)

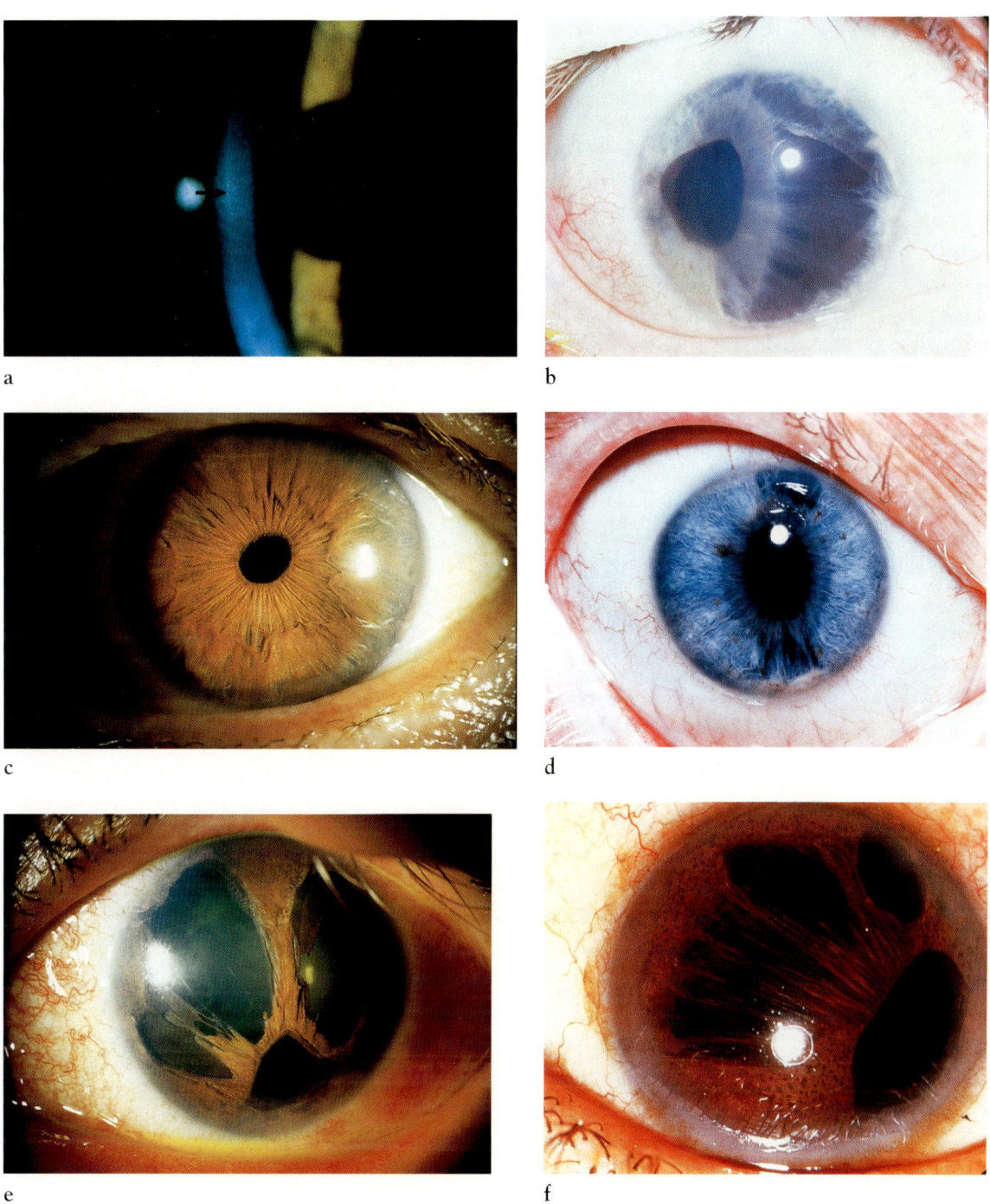

a

b

c

d

e

f

IRIDOCORNEAL ENDOTHELIAL SYNDROME

Iris Holes And Gonioscopic Features

II15a. Two types of iris holes may be seen in patients with progressive iris atrophy or the Cogan-Reese syndrome. The most common type is referred to as a "stretch hole," in which the iris is markedly thin in the quadrant away from the direction of the pupillary distortion and the hole develops within the area that is being stretched.

II15b. A less common type of hole formation has been referred to as a "melting hole," which develops without associated corectopia or thinning of the iris, as seen in this photo (*arrow*). Fluorescein angiographic studies suggest that these holes are associated with ischemia of the iris. Another feature of the ICE syndrome is ectropion uveae, which is seen in the superior quadrants of this photo.

II15c. Glaucoma occurs in a high percentage of patients with the ICE syndrome. In the vast majority of cases, the glaucoma is associated with peripheral anterior synechiae, which usually extend to or beyond Schwalbe's line.

II15d. This gonioscopic photo again shows the high peripheral anterior synechiae, especially in the center of the view, which also reveals a broad area of ectropion uveae.

II15e. The glaucoma in the ICE syndrome does not correlate precisely with the degree of synechial closure, and cases have been reported in which the angle was entirely open. In such cases, it is presumed that the trabecular meshwork is covered by a cellular membrane, consisting of a single layer of endothelial cells and Descemet's-like membrane (*arrow*).

II15f. The source of the cellular membrane, which grows over the anterior chamber angle and iris and subsequently contracts to produce the changes in these structures, is believed to be the corneal endothelium. This electronmicroscopic photo shows the posterior cornea in an advanced case of the ICE syndrome, in which markedly abnormal endothelial cells line a multi-layered collagenous tissue behind Descemet's membrane.

(Figure II15d was provided courtesy of William A. MacIlwaine, IV, M.D. Figure II15b is reprinted with permission from: Iris nodules in essential iris. Arch Ophthalmol 1976;94:406—410, and Figure II15f from Ophthalmology 1979;86:153.)

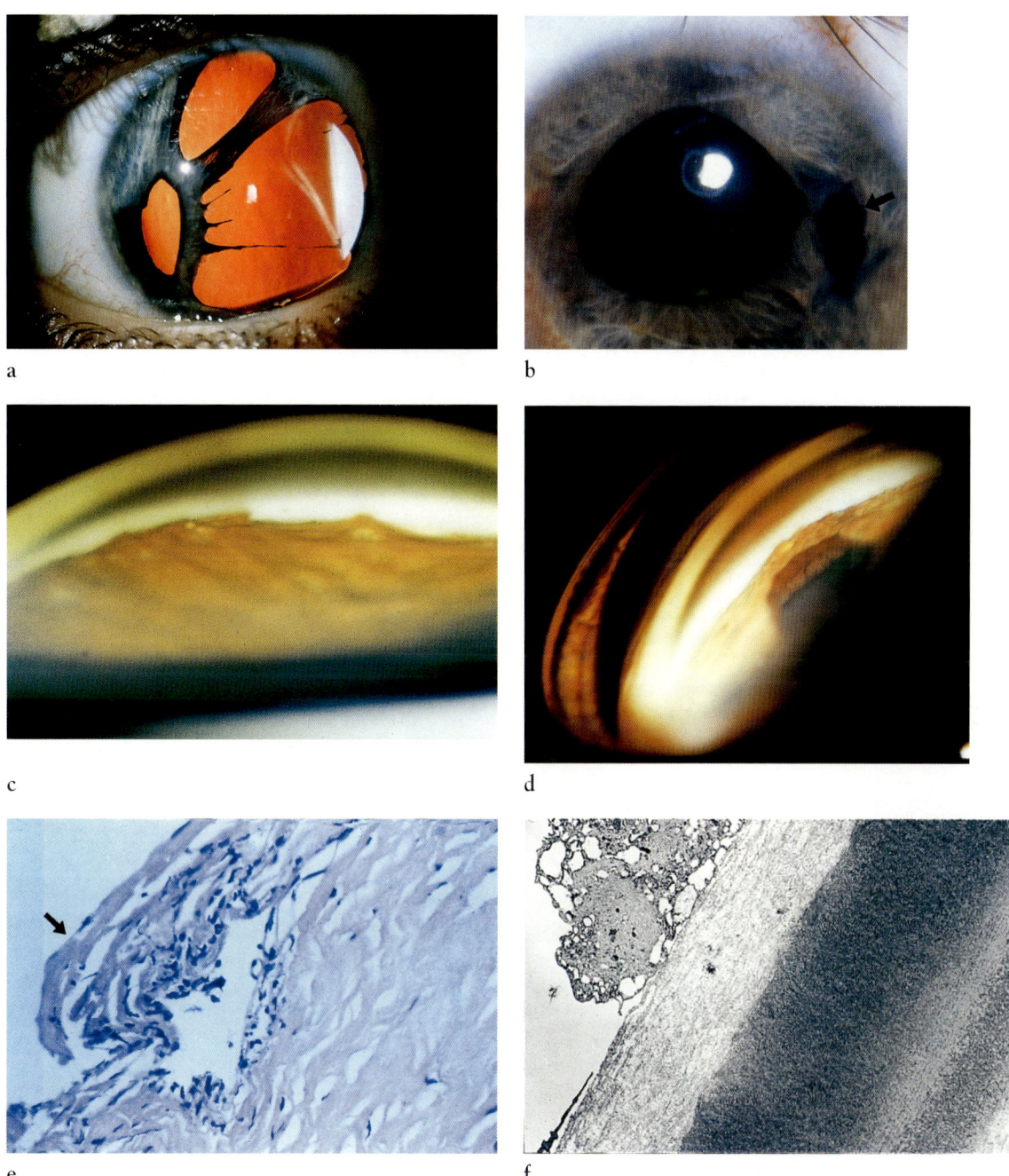

a

b

c

d

e

f

IRIDOCORNEAL ENDOTHELIAL SYNDROME

Cogan-Reese Syndrome

II16a. As previously noted, the hallmark of the Cogan-Reese variation of the iridocorneal endothelial syndrome (ICE) is the pigmented, pedunculated nodules on the iris. The surrounding iris has a characteristic flat appearance, as can be appreciated in this photo. Note also the ectropion uveae in the quadrant adjacent to the nodules and flattened iris.

II16b. Another patient with the Cogan-Reese syndrome reveals extensive pigmented nodules with slight corectopia and ectropion uveae and mild stromal iris atrophy in the quadrants opposite those containing the iris nodules.

II16c. This patient with the Cogan-Reese syndrome has more extensive corectopia and ectropion uveae, as well as more extensive iris atrophy with hole formation.

II16d. This gonioscopic view of an eye with the Cogan-Reese syndrome reveals the typical high peripheral anterior synechiae, the iris nodules, and extensive iris atrophy and hole formation.

II16e–f. The iris nodules in the Cogan-Reese syndrome (*large arrow*) have a histologic appearance similar to that of the underlying stroma of the iris and are always surrounded by the previously described cellular membrane (*small arrows*). Contraction of the cellular membrane is believed to cause the formation of the iris nodules, as well as the other iris and anterior chamber angle alterations in all clinical variations of the ICE syndrome. Note the ectropion uveae adjacent to the nodule in II16e.

(Figures II16a, II16b, II16d, and II16f are reprinted with permission from Arch Ophthalmol 1976;94:406.)

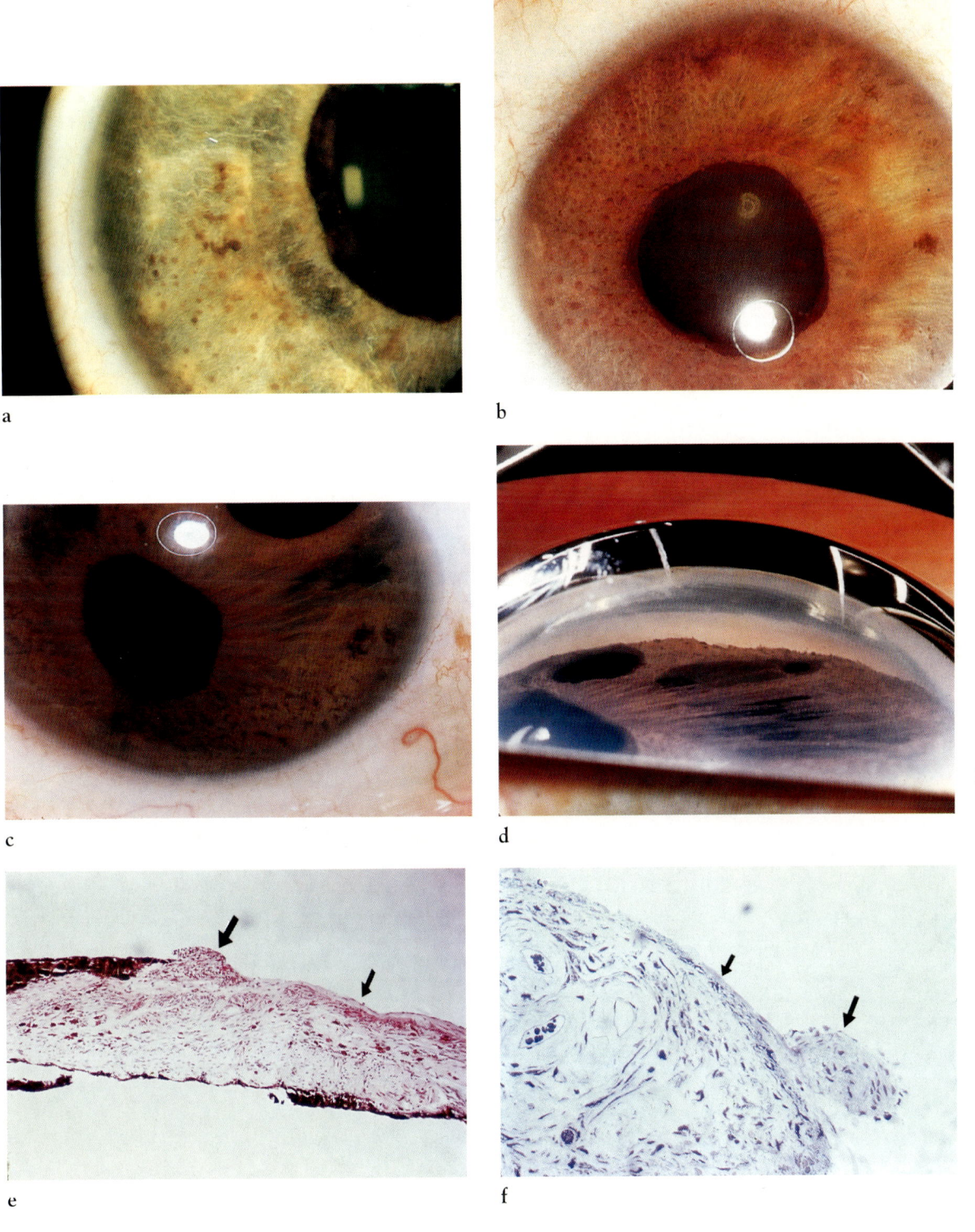

a

b

c

d

e

f

POSTERIOR POLYMORPHOUS DYSTROPHY

II17a. Posterior polymorphous dystrophy is a bilateral, familial disorder of the corneal endothelium. By slit-lamp examination, the posterior cornea has the appearance of blisters or vesicles at the level of Descemet's membrane.

II17b. In some patients with posterior polymorphous dystrophy, the vesicles on the posterior cornea may be linear or in groups and surrounded by an aureole of gray haze. In the vast majority of patients, as in this case, the iris and anterior chamber angle are normal, and glaucoma is not a typical feature.

II17c. A small number of patients with posterior polymorphous dystrophy may have glaucoma, associated with broad peripheral anterior synechiae extending to or beyond Schwalbe's line, with variable degrees of corectopia, ectropion uveae, and atrophy of the iris.

II17d. This patient with posterior polymorphous dystrophy has corectopia and atrophy of the iris stroma, which might be confused with the iridocorneal endothelial syndrome and should be considered in the differential diagnosis of the latter condition, especially when the findings are bilateral.

(Figure II17b was provided courtesy of Gary N. Foulks, M.D.)

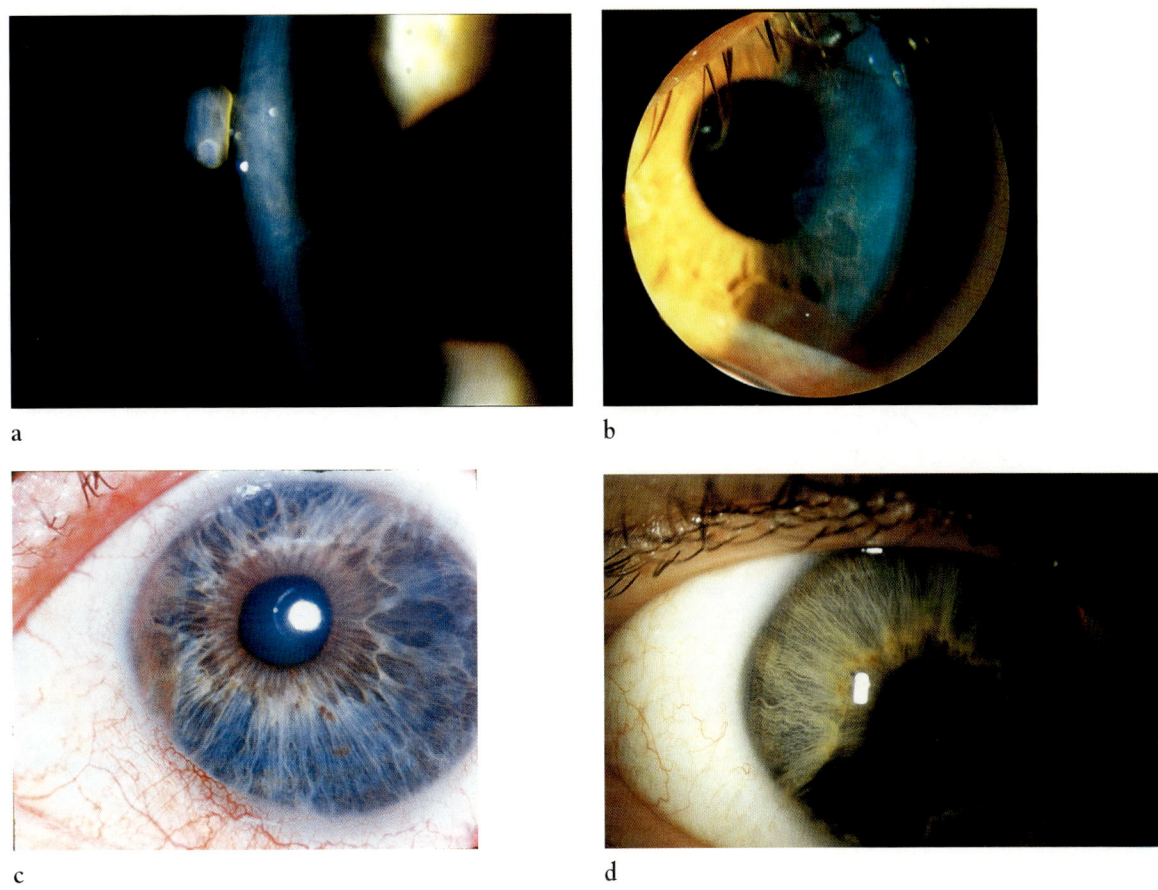

a

b

c

d

PIGMENTARY GLAUCOMA

Pigment Deposition on Iris and Cornea

II18a. Pigmentary glaucoma is a condition that typically effects young, myopic men. The hallmark of the disorder is a radial, spokelike pattern of transillumination defects in the mid-periphery of the iris. This feature can be seen in the photo, in which the light beam of the slit-lamp is directed through the pupil, perpendicular to the plane of the iris. These transillumination defects represent the sites of pigment loss from the iris pigment epithelium.

II18b. The pigment granules dislodged from the iris pigment epithelium are dispersed with the aqueous flow and deposited in many areas of the anterior ocular segment. In this photo, we see numerous pigment granules that have been deposited on the anterior surface of the iris stroma and are especially prominent in the circumferential folds of the peripheral iris.

II18c–d. The eyes of these two patients with pigmentary glaucoma also have extensive pigment deposition on the iris stroma. In addition, a faint band of pigment can be seen crossing the pupil in a vertically oblique orientation. The latter pigment is actually deposited on the posterior cornea and is called Krukenberg's spindles.

II18e–f. These two photos show further details of Krukenberg's spindle. In II18e, the characteristic, vertical orientation of the spindlelike pigment deposition can be seen (*arrow*). The higher magnification in II18f shows more detail of the vertical pigment deposition against the background of the illuminated iris.

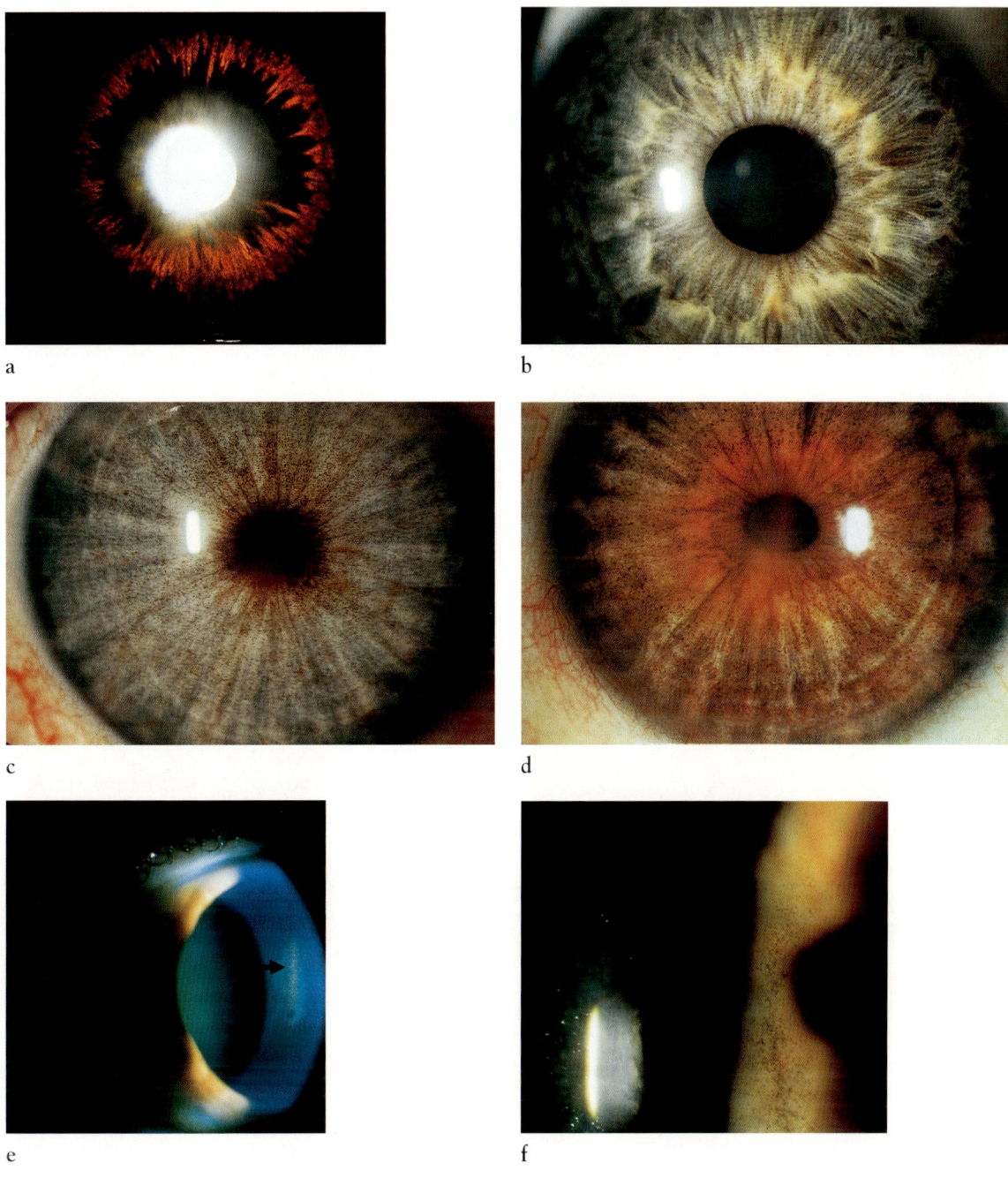

a

b

c

d

e

f

PIGMENTARY GLAUCOMA

Pigment Deposition in Angle and Elsewhere

II19a. In addition to the iris and cornea, several other anterior ocular structures exist on which the dispersed pigment may be deposited in pigmentary glaucoma. In this photo, we see pigment that has been deposited behind the lens as a result of aqueous flow in that direction.

II19b. In this photo, we see deposition of pigment on the equator of the lens (*large arrow*) and the lens zonules (*small arrows*). It is believed to be the rubbing of these lens zonules against the iris pigment epithelium that leads to the dispersion of pigment granules.

II19c–f. The most significant site of pigment deposition in pigmentary glaucoma is the trabecular meshwork, since it is here that the pigment granules obstruct aqueous outflow and lead to intraocular pressure elevation. These four gonioscopic photos show the typical appearance of the anterior chamber angle in pigmentary glaucoma, in which a dense, homogenous deposition is found in the trabecular meshwork (darkest band in each photo), and is typically found in all quadrants. Note also the increased amount of pigment deposition on Schwalbe's line just above the trabecular meshwork in each photo. In II19d, the peripheral iris has bowed posteriorly. This is the typical configuration of the iris in pigmentary glaucoma, and it is this configuration of the iris that is believed to cause the rubbing between the iris pigment epithelium and lens zonules, leading to the pigment dispersion and subsequent deposition in pigmentary glaucoma.

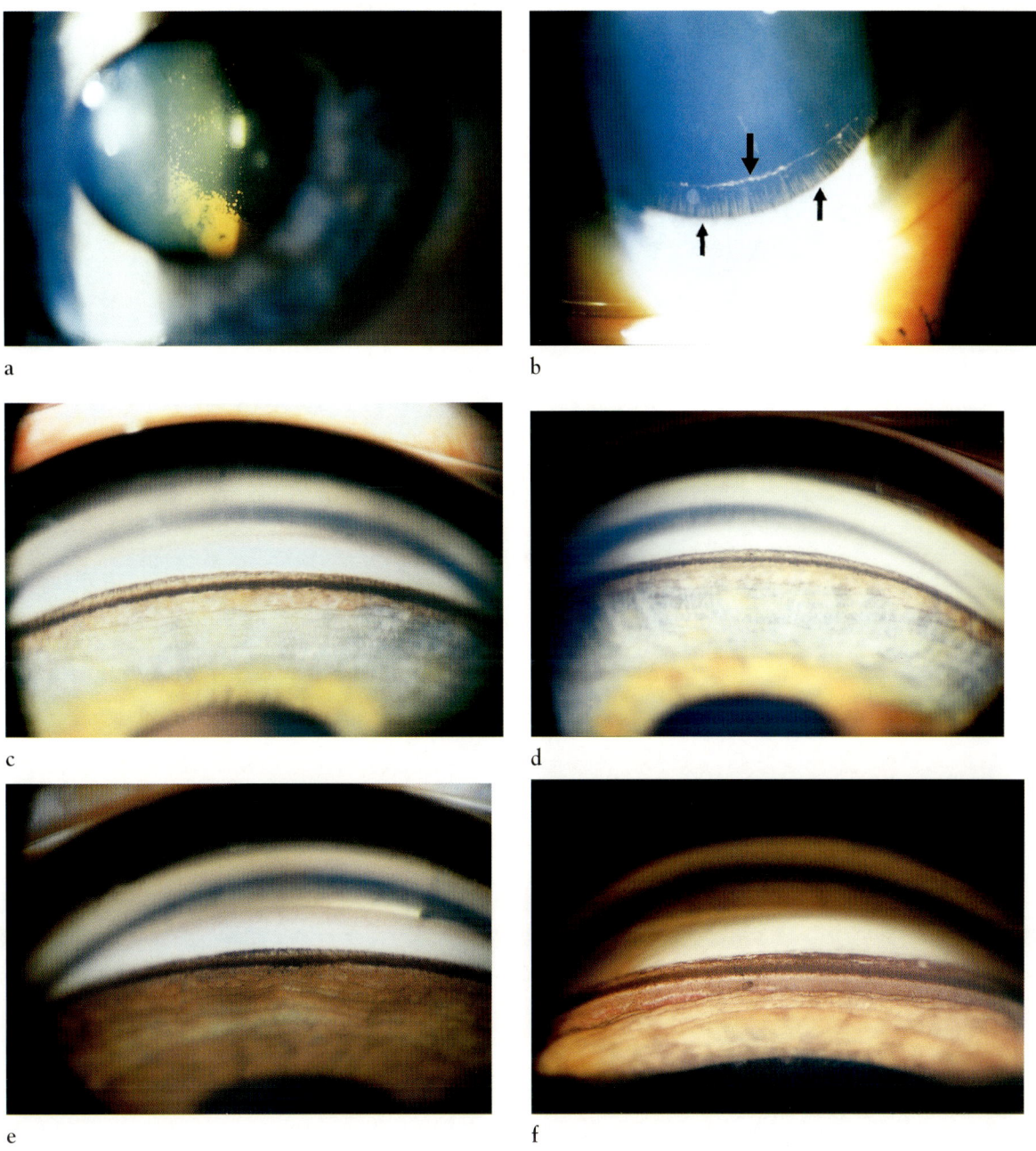

a

b

c

d

e

f

IRIDOSCHISIS

II20a–b. Iridoschisis is an uncommon condition that usually appears in the sixth or seventh decade of life, although it may be seen in younger individuals. As seen in these two photos of the same eye, the typical appearance is that of sheets or strands of iris stroma that have partially separated from the rest of the iris, especially in the inferior quadrants.

II20c. In some cases of iridoschisis, the loose tissue may touch the corneal endothelium, as in this photo, which can lead to edema of the adjacent cornea.

II20d. By gonioscopy, the strands of iris tissue may obscure the view of the anterior chamber angle, as in this photo. Approximately half of the patients with iridoschisis will have glaucoma, which may be because of obstruction of the trabecular meshwork by either the shredded iris stroma or pigment that has been released from the iris. In other cases of iridoschisis and glaucoma, an angle-closure mechanism may be present.

II20e. This photo shows another patient with more extensive iridoschisis in the inferior and temporal quadrants.

II20f. This atypical case of iridoschisis in the superior quadrant occurred in a young adult woman with chronic iritis.

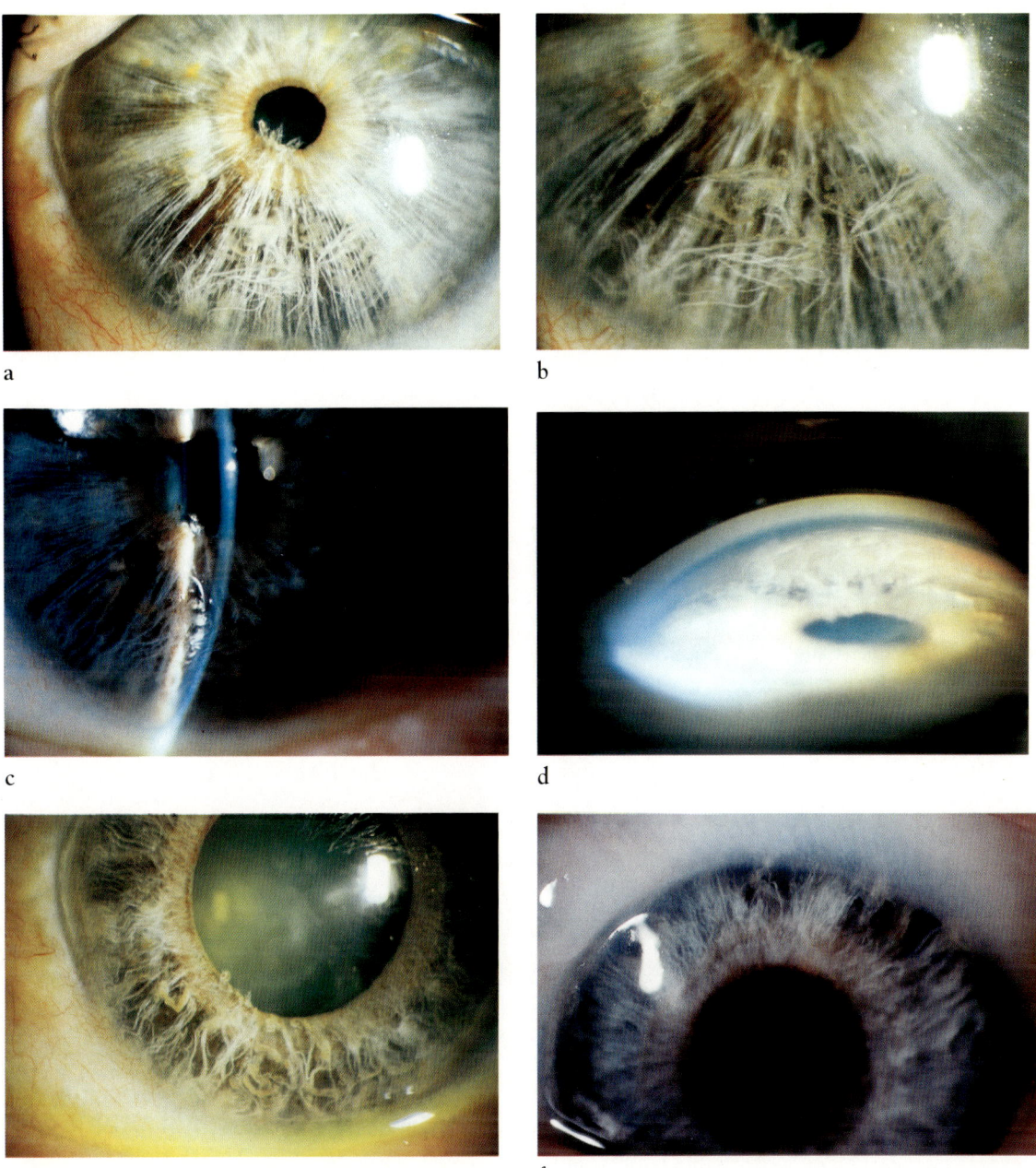

a

b

c

d

e

f

EXFOLIATION SYNDROME

Iris and Lens Features

II21a.   The exfoliation syndrome typically afflicts older individuals in their late 60s or beyond, and may be unilateral or bilateral. The clinical hallmark is a white material on the anterior lens capsule. This is usually not apparent with the undilated pupil. Even in these cases, however, the white material can usually be seen on the pupillary margin, as in this case.

II21b.   Higher magnification shows more clearly the deposition of the exfoliation material on the pupillary margin, especially to the left in the photo. Other iris features in the exfoliation syndrome include loss of pigment at the pupillary ruff and a "moth-eaten" pattern of iris transillumination near the pupillary sphincter.

II21c.   With dilation of the pupil, the exfoliation material on the anterior lens capsule can be seen. In this photo, it is a thin, irregular line of white tissue just central to the pupillary margin for 360°.

II21d.   The characteristic appearance of the exfoliation material on the anterior lens capsule has three distinct zones: 1) a translucent, central disc with occasional curled edges; 2) a clear middle zone, which probably corresponds to contact with the moving iris; and 3) a peripheral granular zone, which may have radial striations. In this photo, all three zones are visible, with a connection between the central and peripheral zones in the upper righthand quadrant of the view.

II21e–f.   In these two photos of the same eye, the three zones of exfoliation material on the anterior lens capsule are clearly seen. In II21e, the central disc is sharply outlined by the curled edges of the exfoliation material. This zone is completely surrounded by the middle clear zone. The peripheral zone can be seen for nearly 360°, with curled edges in several areas. The higher magnification in II21f shows better detail of the curled edges of both the central and peripheral zones of exfoliation material. It is believed that the hippus movement of the iris (rhythmical pupillary dilation and constriction) causes the sphincter portion of the iris to rub the exfoliation material off the lens capsule in the middle zone (which appears to be consistent with the curling of material away from both sides of the middle zone, as seen in this photo).

(Figure II21c was provided courtesy of Ruth Schirmer. Figure II21d was provided courtesy of William E. Layden, M.D., and is reprinted with permission from Ritch R, Shields MB, eds. The Secondary Glaucomas, p. 105. St. Louis: CV Mosby, 1982.)

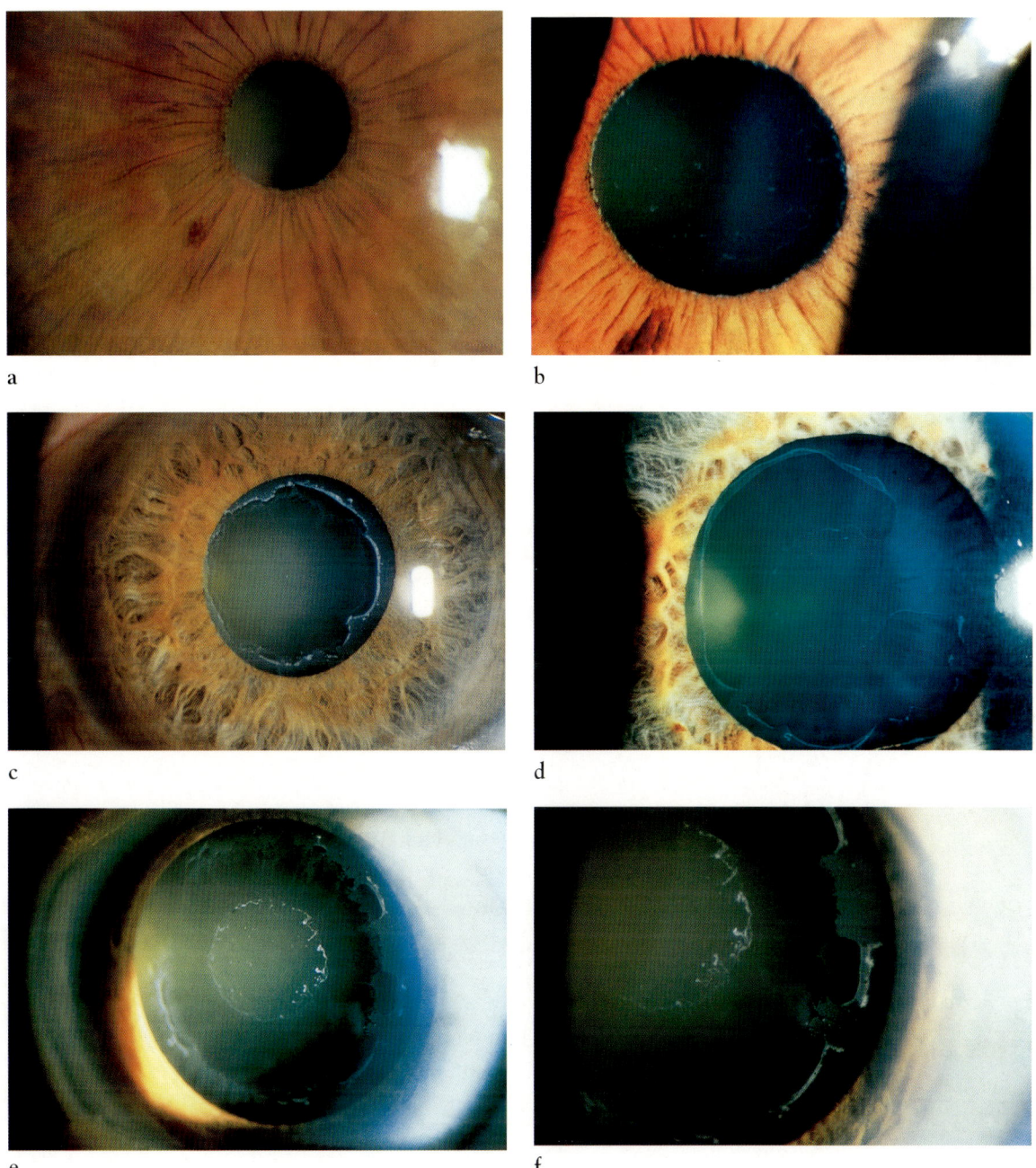

a

b

c

d

e

f

EXFOLIATION SYNDROME

Gonioscopic and Other Features

II22a. This photo shows the peripheral zone of exfoliation material on the anterior lens capsule, which is believed to be the primary source of exfoliation material on many structures in the anterior ocular segment.

II22b. In the anterior chamber angle, it is the deposition of exfoliation material and pigment granules (both presumably from rubbing between the iris and lens) that leads to obstruction of aqueous outflow with elevation of intraocular pressure and associated glaucoma in the exfoliation syndrome. The typical gonioscopic appearance is one of increased pigmentation of the trabecular meshwork, although the pigmentation has a more uneven distribution than is seen in pigmentary glaucoma and may be associated with flecks of exfoliation material, as seen in this photo. In addition, pigment may accumulate along Schwalbe's line, as is also seen in this photo, which has been referred to as Sampaolesi's line.

II22c. The exfoliation material may be deposited on many other anterior ocular structures. In this photo, the white dots within the pupil represent exfoliation material on the posterior lens capsule several years after cataract extraction. Such observations suggest other sources of the exfoliation material, the most likely of which is the iris.

II22d. The irregular flecks of exfoliation material within the slit-lamp beam in this photo are actually deposited on the posterior corneal endothelium. This finding is much less common than the deposition of pigment granules on the posterior cornea in pigmentary glaucoma.

II22e. In this gonioscopic photo, the exfoliation material is seen on the lens zonules. It is not clear whether this represents an additional primary source of exfoliation material or another site of secondary deposition.

II22f. This photo shows an unusual feature of the exfoliation syndrome, in which the exfoliation material has completely obstructed a laser iridotomy. The exfoliation material was easily dislodged from the iridotomy site with an application of Nd:YAG laser.

(Figure II22e was provided courtesy of William E. Layden, M.D.)

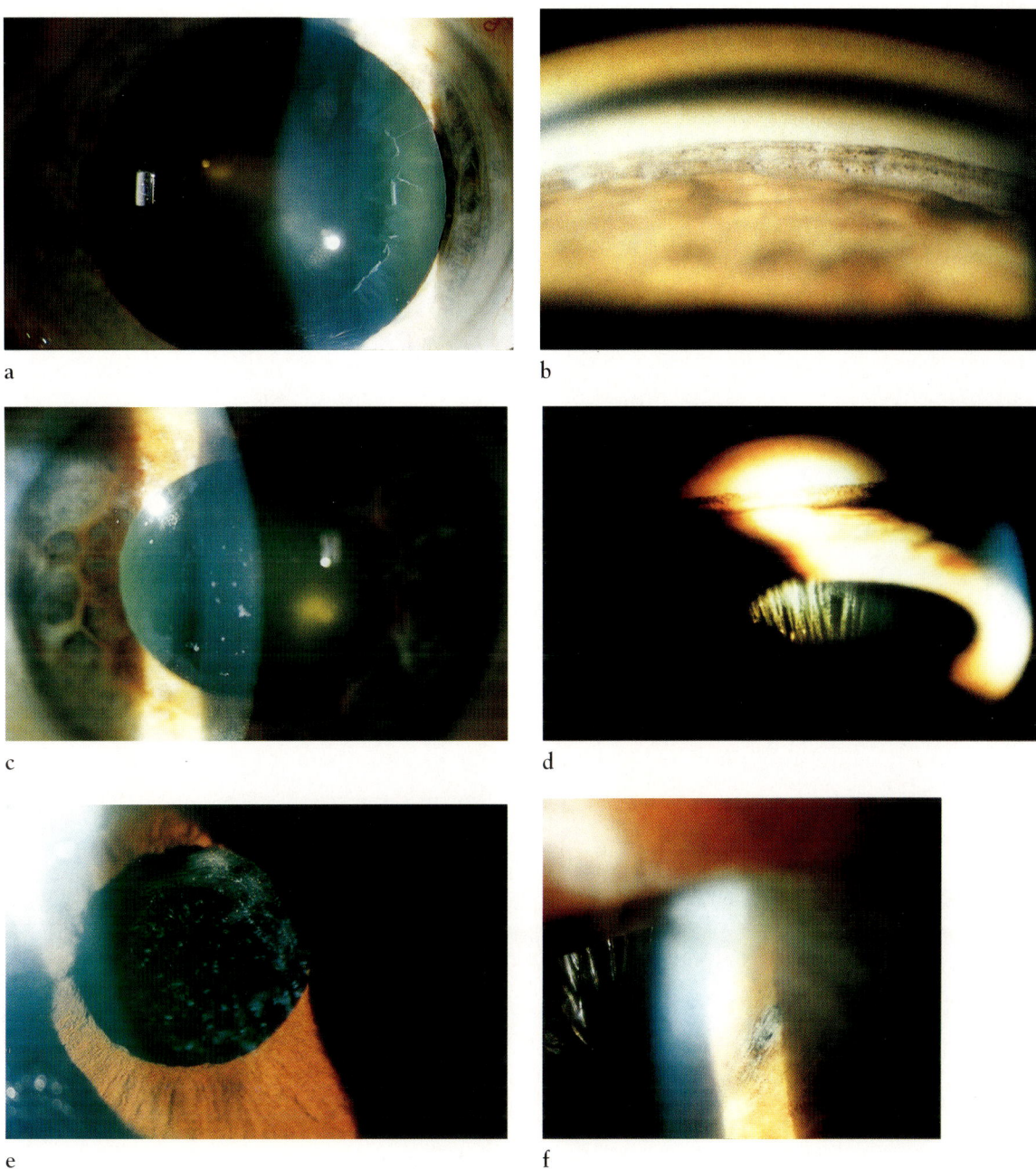

a

b

c

d

e

f

GLAUCOMAS ASSOCIATED WITH DISLOCATION OF THE LENS

II23a. Dislocation of the lens can result from a variety of disorders and can lead to glaucoma by several mechanisms. This photo shows a rare, autosomal recessive condition called ectopia lentis et pupillae, which is characterized by small, subluxed lenses and oval or slitlike pupils that are displaced usually in the opposite direction from that of the lenses.

II23b. The most common cause of a displaced lens is trauma, which is seen most commonly in young men. In this photo, the lens has dislocated laterally, revealing the equator of the lens.

II23c. Several inherited conditions are associated with dislocation of the lens. One of the more common is Marfan's syndrome, which is an autosomal dominant disorder characterized by a tall, slender individual with long, slender fingers and toes and frequent cardiovascular disease. The dislocation of the lens is rarely complete, and is usually seen as an upward subluxation, as in this photo. Another condition that must be distinguished from Marfan's syndrome is homocystinuria, in which the dislocation of the lens is more often in a downward direction.

II23d. In the Weill-Marchesani syndrome, the patient has a short, stocky habitus, in contrast to that of the individual with Marfan's syndrome. Partial lens dislocation is common in this condition, which results from loose lens zonules, as shown against the red reflex in this photo. The loose zonules also allow the lens to assume a typical small, round shape (microspherophakia).

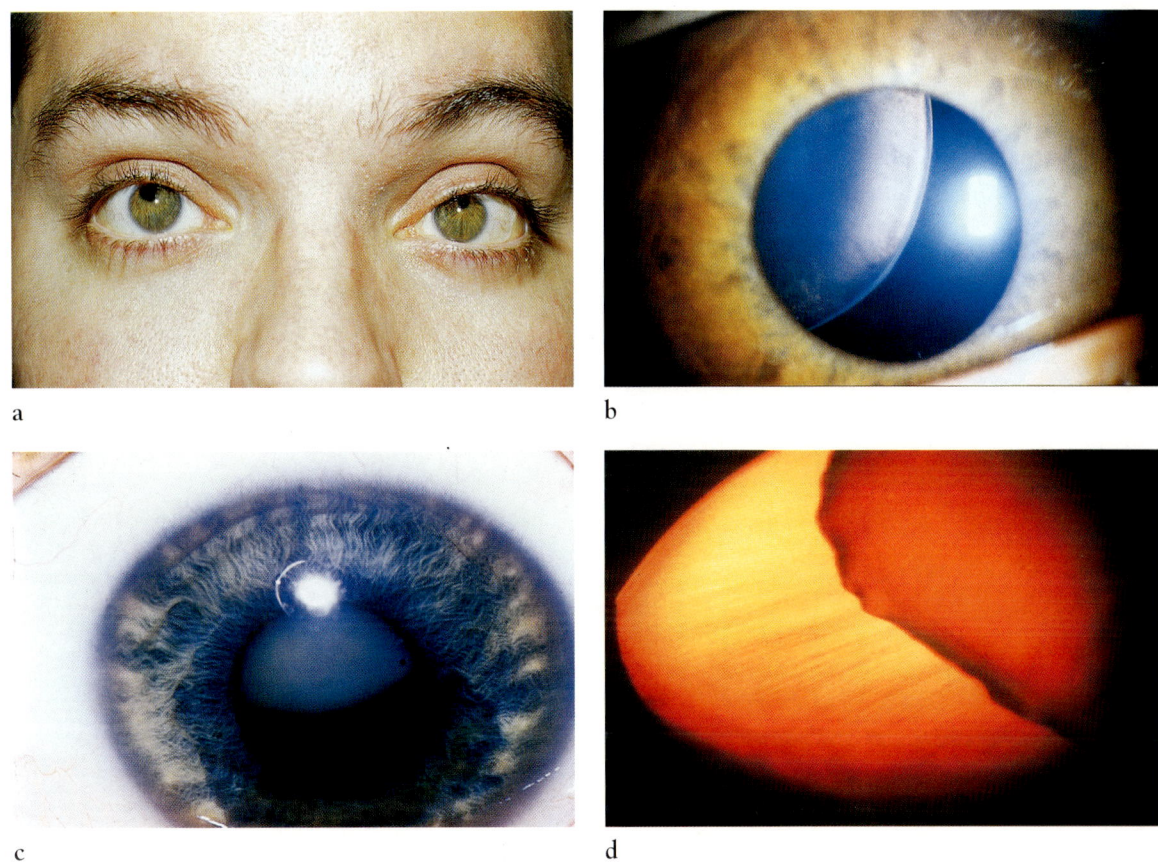

a

b

c

d

GLAUCOMA ASSOCIATED WITH CATARACT FORMATION

II24a.   When a lens becomes cataractous, it may lead to glaucoma by one of several mechanisms. The most common of these has been referred to as phacolytic glaucoma, in which the cataract is typically mature or hypermature. These patients usually present with the acute onset of monocular pain and redness, and the examination reveals a high intraocular pressure, conjunctival hyperemia and diffuse corneal edema. The anterior chamber is typically deep with a heavy flare, often associated with iridescent or hyperrefringent particles.

II24b.   This high magnification, slit-lamp view of a patient with phacolytic glaucoma shows the characteristic iridescent particles in the aqueous (the white, cloudy cornea is seen to the right and the brown iris to the left of the view). These particles represent either calcium oxalate or cholesterol crystals and are a helpful diagnostic sign in phacolytic glaucoma.

II24c.   Another slit-lamp photo of a patient with phacolytic glaucoma shows the heavy flare in the deep anterior chamber. This flare has been shown to include heavy molecular-weight soluble lens protein, which can obstruct aqueous outflow.

II24d.   The exact mechanism of intraocular pressure elevation in phacolytic glaucoma has been in dispute. The original theory held that macrophages, laden with phagocytosed lens material, blocked the trabecular meshwork to produce the acute glaucoma. In this light microscopic photo, numerous macrophages are seen in the anterior chamber angle (bottom of picture) adjacent to the trabecular meshwork. An alternative theory is that the heavy molecular-weight soluble lens protein is primarily responsible for the obstruction of aqueous outflow, and this has led to the alternative title of lens protein glaucoma.

II24e–f.   Another form of cataract-induced glaucoma is called lens particle glaucoma. This condition is typically associated with disruption of the lens capsule either by cataract extraction or a penetrating injury. The elevated intraocular pressure usually occurs soon after the primary event and the clinical appearance is that of "fluffed-up" lens cortical material in the anterior chamber, as seen in these two photos.

Other mechanisms of cataract-induced glaucoma include phacoanaphylaxis, which is a rare, delayed hypersensitivity reaction to lens protein, and phacomorphic glaucoma, in which an intumescent lens leads to angle-closure glaucoma.

(Figures II24b and II24c were provided courtesy of L. Frank Cashwell, Jr., M.D., and Figures II24e and II24f were provided courtesy of Brooks W. McCuen, II, M.D.)

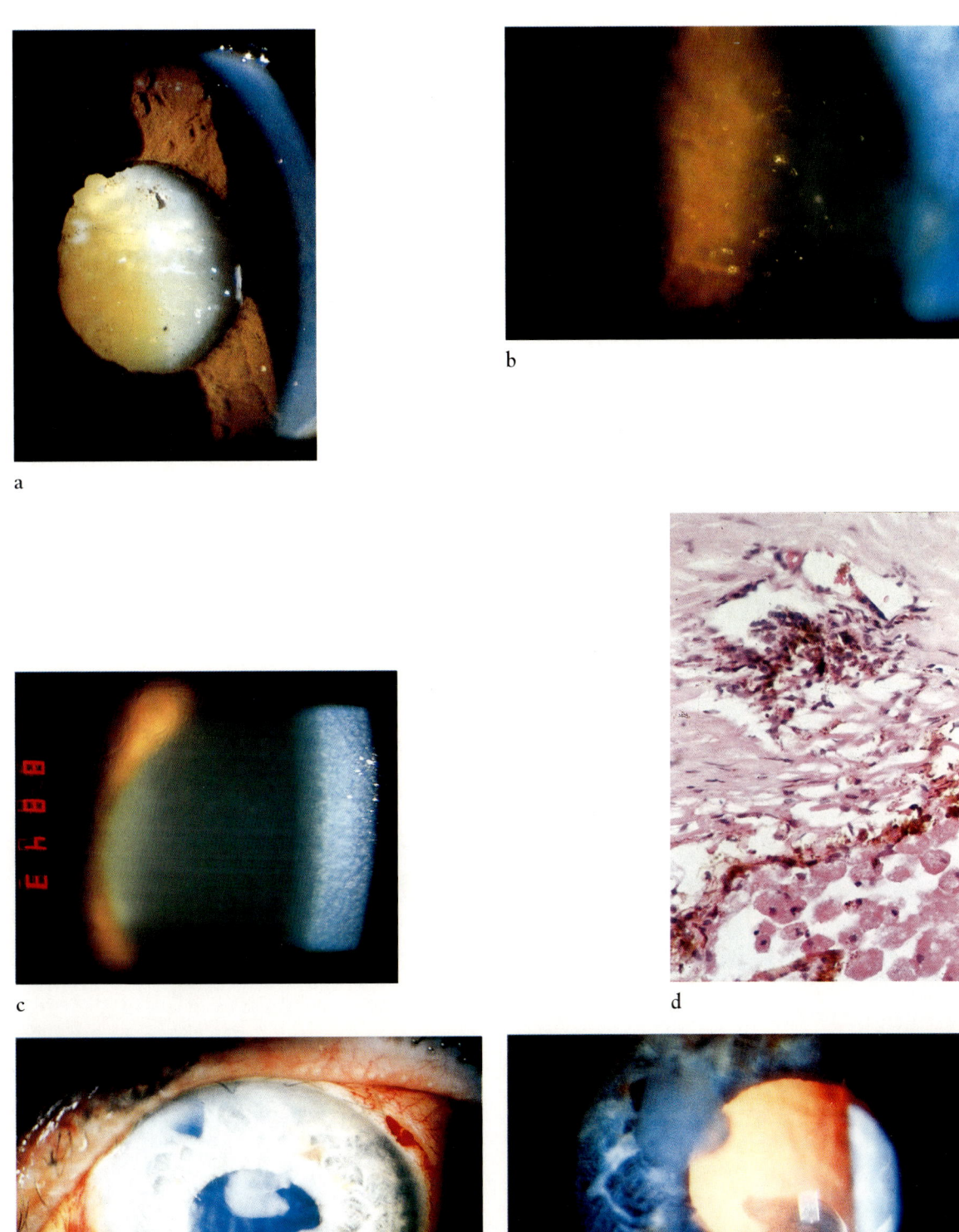

a

b

c

d

e

f

NEOVASCULAR GLAUCOMA

Iris Features

II25a. Neovascular glaucoma is characterized by neovascularization of the iris (rubeosis iridis) and anterior chamber angle, which leads to elevated intraocular pressure that is typically difficult to control. Several stages occur in the natural course of neovascular glaucoma. The first is a pre-rubeosis stage, in which a predisposing factor, such as diabetic retinopathy or central retinal vein occlusion, creates a high risk for developing rubeosis iridis. The second stage is the pre-glaucoma stage, in which the new vessels are seen on the iris and in the angle, but have not yet led to intraocular pressure elevation. This photo shows the pre-glaucoma stage, in which rubeosis iridis is seen in the peripupillary portion of the iris. In most cases, the new vessels are seen on the iris before they are found in the angle.

II25b. The third stage of neovascular glaucoma is the open-angle glaucoma stage. In this stage, a fibrovascular membrane has developed over the iris and the anterior chamber angle. It is the presence of this membrane, covering the open anterior chamber angle, that leads to obstruction of aqueous outflow and elevation of the intraocular pressure. At this stage, the new vessels may be seen throughout the iris, as in this photo.

II25c. As the course of neovascular glaucoma progresses, the new vessels may become larger and "angrier" in appearance, and the pupil may become distorted as the fibrovascular membrane begins to contract, all of which is seen in this photo. The contraction of the fibrovascular membrane also leads to progressive angle-closure, as the disorder progresses into the final or angle-closure glaucoma stage.

II25d. In some cases of advanced neovascular glaucoma, the fibrovascular membrane may grow across the pupillary margin onto the anterior surface of the lens, as demonstrated in the inferior quadrant of this eye.

II25e. Some patients with either the open-angle or angle-closure stage of neovascular glaucoma may present with a hyphema, as seen in this photo. It was for this reason that an earlier term for neovascular glaucoma was hemorrhagic glaucoma.

II25f. In this advanced case of angle-closure neovascular glaucoma, the contraction of the fibrovascular membrane has not only caused complete synechial closure of the anterior chamber angle with intractable glaucoma, but has also caused a flattening of the iris stroma with corectopia and ectropion uveae, as seen in this photo.

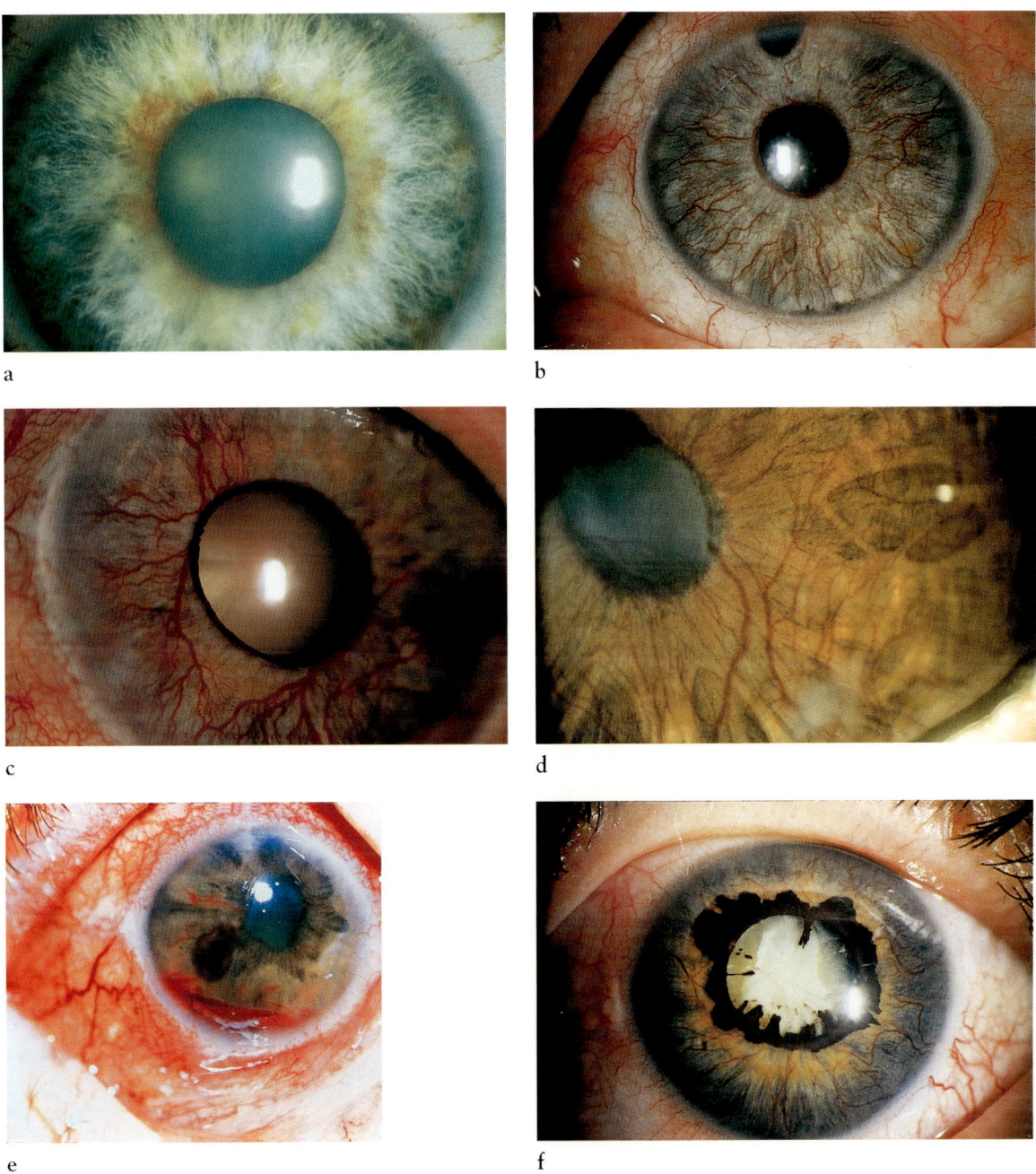

a

b

c

d

e

f

NEOVASCULAR GLAUCOMA

Gonioscopic Features

II26a–b.   The stages of neovascular glaucoma, as discussed on the previous page with regard to iris features, are also seen in the anterior chamber angle. These two photos represent patients in the pre-glaucoma stage, in which the anterior chamber angles are open and only a few new vessels cross the ciliary body band and scleral spur to the trabecular meshwork (*arrows*).

II26c–d.   In these two photos, the neovascular glaucoma is in the open-angle glaucoma stage. Although the angles are still open in both patients, we see a heavy accumulation of new vessels associated with the fibrous membrane, causing obstruction to aqueous outflow and elevated intraocular pressure.

II26e.   This patient also has open-angle neovascular glaucoma, with heavy neovascularization of the open angle. The angle, however, is beginning to close, as seen by the low synechia to the left of the view.

II26f.   This patient has advanced angle-closure neovascular glaucoma, in which total synechial closure of the anterior chamber angle has occurred. The contraction of the fibrovascular membrane has not only caused the angle closure, but has also caused a mechanical dilation and forward retraction of the iris, allowing the ciliary processes to be seen.

(Figure II26c was provided courtesy of Brooks W. McCuen, II, M.D.; Figure II26e was provided courtesy of L. Frank Cashwell, Jr., M.D.)

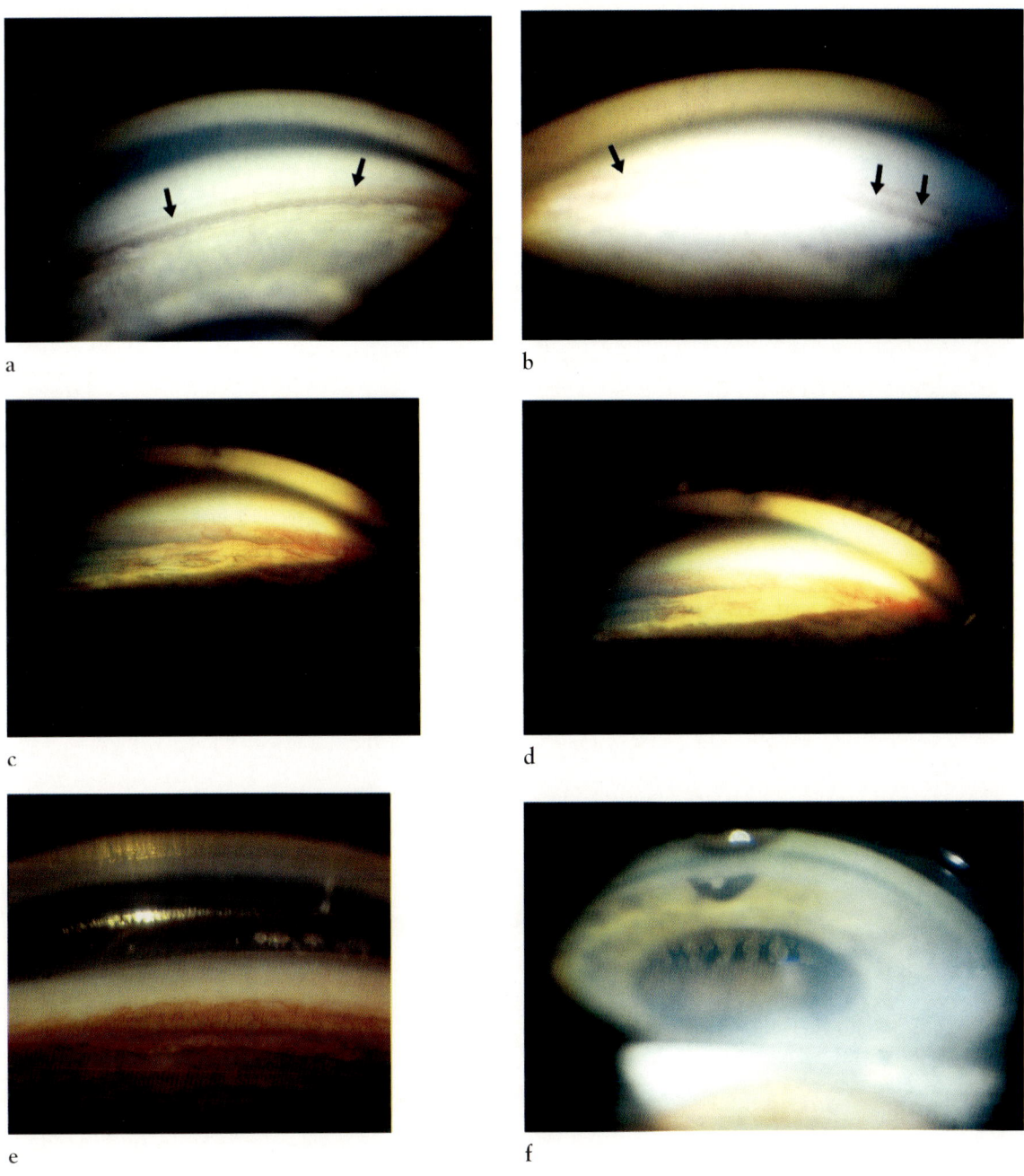

a

b

c

d

e

f

GLAUCOMAS ASSOCIATED WITH ELEVATED EPISCLERAL VENOUS PRESSURE

II27a.   Elevated episcleral venous pressure may result from obstruction to venous flow or arteriovenous fistulas, or it may be idiopathic. In any of these situations, the elevated episcleral venous pressure may lead to elevated intraocular pressure and associated glaucoma. One of the more common causes of the venous obstruction-type of elevated episcleral venous pressure is thyrotropic ophthalmopathy, with the characteristic exophthalmos, as seen in this photo.

II27b.   The anterior chamber angle in the patient with glaucoma associated with episcleral venous pressure is typically open and grossly normal in appearance. In some cases, however, blood reflux may be present in Schlemm's canal, as seen in this photo.

II27c–f.   In this series of photos of a patient with idiopathic elevated episcleral venous pressure and glaucoma, the characteristic features of the dilated, tortuous episcleral vessels are shown in the four quadrants of the same eye (superior, nasal, temporal, and inferior). Notice how the episcleral veins begin as small, tapered vessels just behind the limbus and become larger as they coalesce and move posteriorly. This is in contrast to the anterior ciliary arteries, which are more tortuous than the episcleral veins in the normal state and end abruptly just behind the limbus. One such artery is seen in the upper portion of II27d. Normally, these arteries are more prominent than the episcleral veins. With the elevation of the episcleral venous pressure, however, the veins become the most prominent vascular system.

Another relatively common cause of elevated episcleral venous pressure is the Sturge-Weber syndrome, which is discussed later under the heading of Phakomatoses.

(Figure II27a was provided courtesy of Jonathan J. Dutton, M.D., Ph.D.)

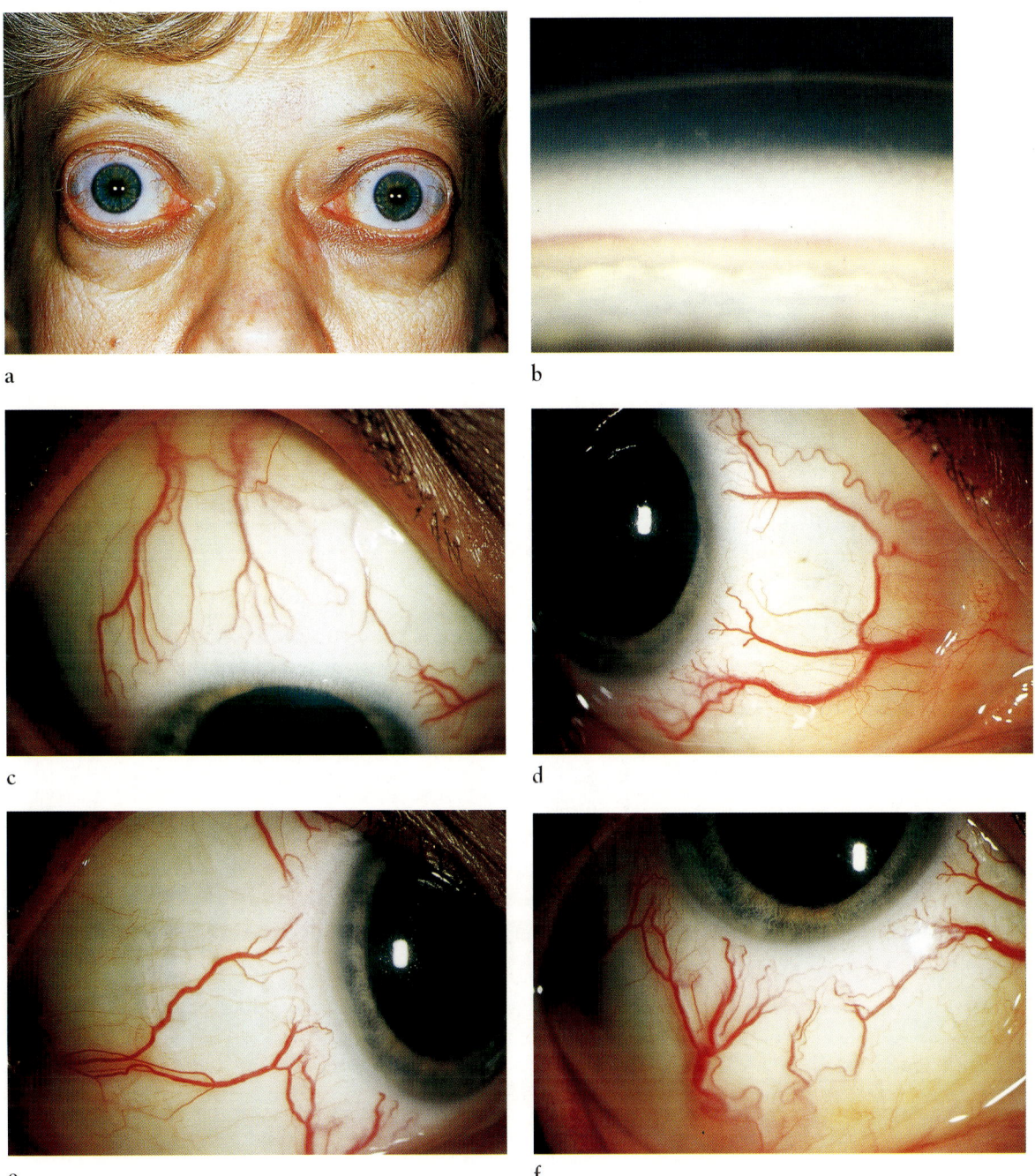

a

b

c

d

e

f

GLAUCOMAS ASSOCIATED WITH INTRAOCULAR TUMORS

Iris Melanomas

II28a–d. Glaucoma may be associated with melanomas of the iris, ciliary body, or choroid, although it is more commonly seen with the anterior uveal melanomas. Iris melanomas, as compared with ciliary body melanomas, tend to be less invasive and less likely to cause glaucoma, although they can do both. The diagnostic problem is compounded by the difficulty of distinguishing an iris melanoma from an iris nevus. This patient presented with a pigmented iris lesion in the inferior temporal quadrant with associated glaucoma (II28a). A trabeculectomy was performed in the superior temporal quadrant and a biopsy of the pigmented iris lesion was obtained at the same time (II28b). It was not possible to distinguish between iris nevus and iris melanoma in the initial biopsy specimen. Five years after the initial surgery, the patient returned with extensive new tumor formation in the anterior chamber angle (II28c and II28d). A repeat biopsy confirmed the diagnosis of malignant melanoma, and the eye was enucleated.

II28e–f. Some iris melanomas are amelanotic. This patient was referred with a preliminary diagnosis of neovascular glaucoma. The only explanation for the new vessel formation on the iris was a small, lightly pigmented iris lesion (II28e). The elevation of this lesion can be seen better by gonioscopy (II28f). The iris lesion was excised and was found to be an iris melanoma by histologic examination. The rubeosis resolved after removal of the melanoma, which was apparently the stimulus for the neovascularization.

(Figures II28e and II28f are reprinted with permission from: Neovascular glaucoma associated with an iris melanoma. Arch Ophthalmol 1987;105:672–674. Copyright 1987, American Medical Association.)

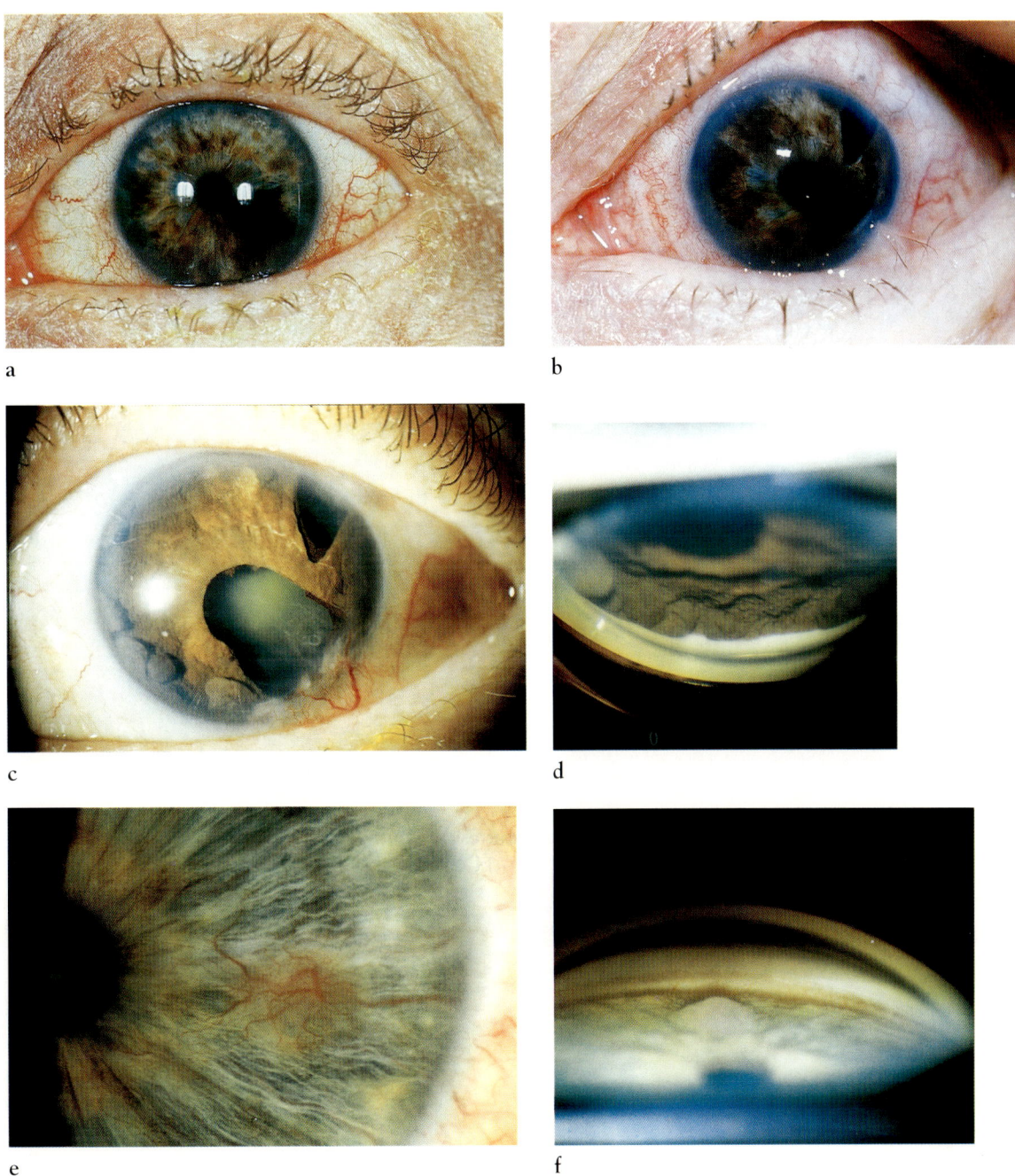

a

b

c

d

e

f

GLAUCOMAS ASSOCIATED WITH INTRAOCULAR TUMORS

Ciliary Body Melanomas

II30a. This gonioscopic view shows elevation of the peripheral iris in a patient with a ciliary body melanoma (note the similarity to II29e on the previous page).

II30b. After wide dilation of the eye in II30a, a solid mass with irregular pigmentation is seen between the iris and lens (*arrow*). This finding is highly suspicious of a ciliary body melanoma.

II30c. This patient had been known to have iris melanosis (note the darker half of the iris) for most of his life. He was subsequently found to have a mass lesion of the anterior chamber angle in the area of melanosis. Ciliary body melanoma was suspected, and the eye was enucleated.

II30d. Light microscopy of the eye in II30c shows a melanoma in the anterior chamber angle, which was felt to have extended from the ciliary body. This case emphasizes the potential for malignant growth from benign melanotic lesions.

II30e. Iris melanomas, as previously noted, may be amelanotic, although the same may be true of ciliary body melanomas that have extended through the angle to the iris. In this large, elevated, heavily vascularized tumor with associated ectropion uveae, the differential diagnosis between iris and ciliary body melanoma was difficult.

II30f. In this gonioscopic photograph, we see another patient with an amelanotic mass on the iris and in the anterior chamber angle. It is nodular and diffuse and could represent either a primary iris or ciliary body melanoma. Further examination, however, also revealed a primary malignant melanoma of the ciliary body.

(Figure II30e was provided courtesy of David G. Campbell, M.D.; Figure II30f is reprinted with permission from Ritch R, Shields MB, eds. The Secondary Glaucoma, p. 195. St. Louis: CV Mosby, 1982.)

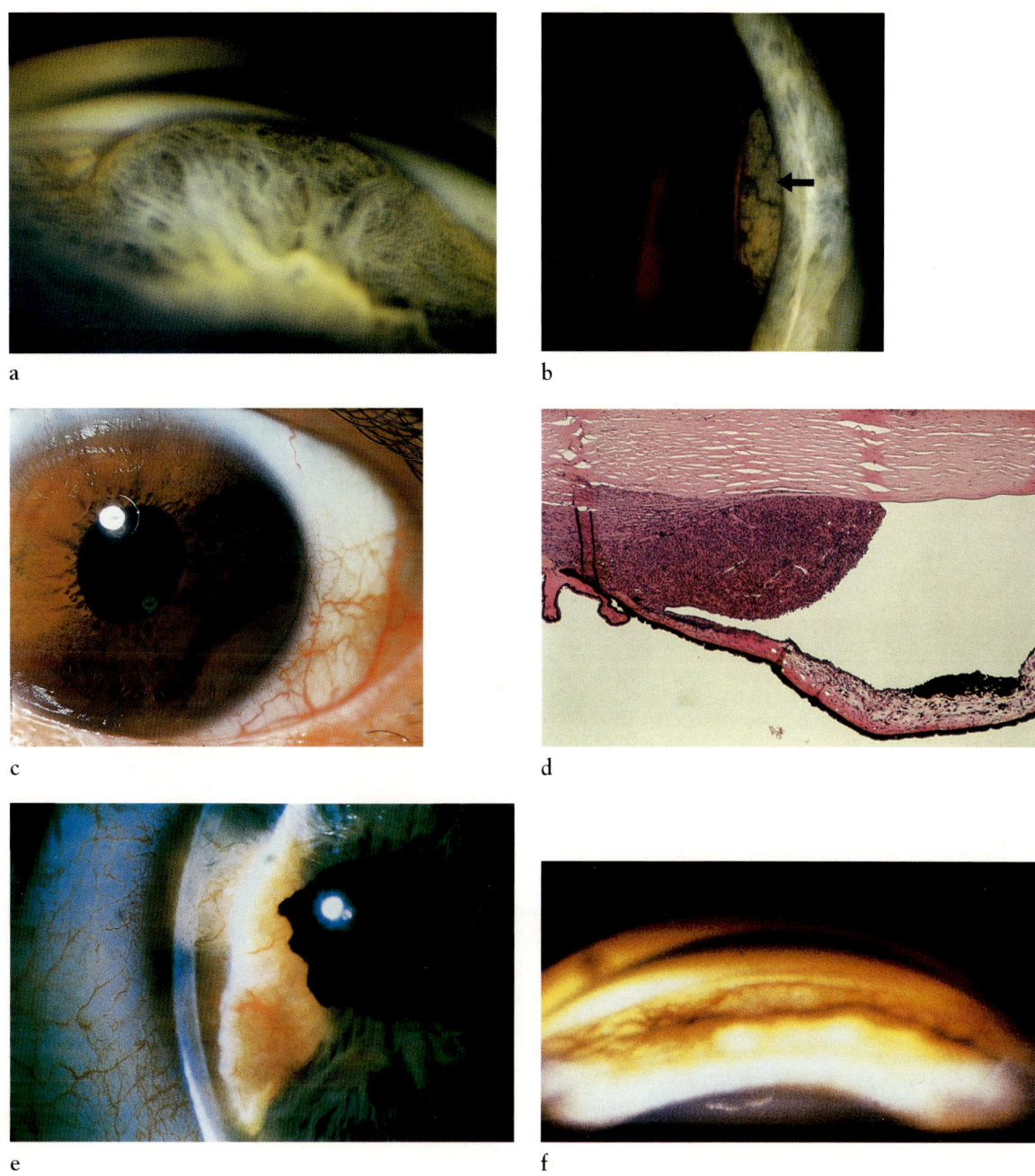

a

b

c

d

e

f

GLAUCOMAS ASSOCIATED WITH INTRAOCULAR TUMORS

Mechanisms of Associated Glaucoma

II31a–b.   As previously noted, anterior uveal melanomas may obstruct aqueous outflow, with subsequent intraocular pressure elevation and associated glaucoma, by direct extension of the tumor into the anterior chamber angle. Such mechanisms are seen in these two cases, in which ciliary body melanomas extended through the anterior chamber angle to obstruct the trabecular meshwork.

II31c.   In this light microscopic photo, an anterior uveal melanoma has extended into the anterior chamber angle, and tumor cells are seen invading the trabecular meshwork posteriorly.

II31d.   Other mechanisms of obstruction to aqueous outflow by anterior uveal melanomas include seeding of tumor cells or melanin granules. In this light microscopic view, we see numerous tumor cells in the anterior chamber angle, some of which have extended into the trabecular meshwork.

II31e.   When tumor cells are felt to be circulating freely in the anterior chamber, it may be possible to obtain a specimen by aqueous aspiration. The cells can then be preserved with a Millipore filter and prepared with Papanicolaou stain for histologic examination. This light microscopic view shows melanoma cells that were aspirated with the aqueous of an eye with an anterior uveal melanoma.

II31f.   In this eye of a patient with anterior uveal melanoma, the tumor cells have not only extended through the trabecular meshwork into Schlemm's canal, but can also be seen in an intrascleral outlet channel (*arrow*). This represents a potential route for extraocular metastasis.

(Figures II31a and II31f are reprinted with permission from Ophthalmology 1980;87:503; Figure II31e is reprinted with permission from Ritch R, Shields MB, eds. The Secondary Glaucomas, p. 196. St. Louis: CV Mosby, 1982.)

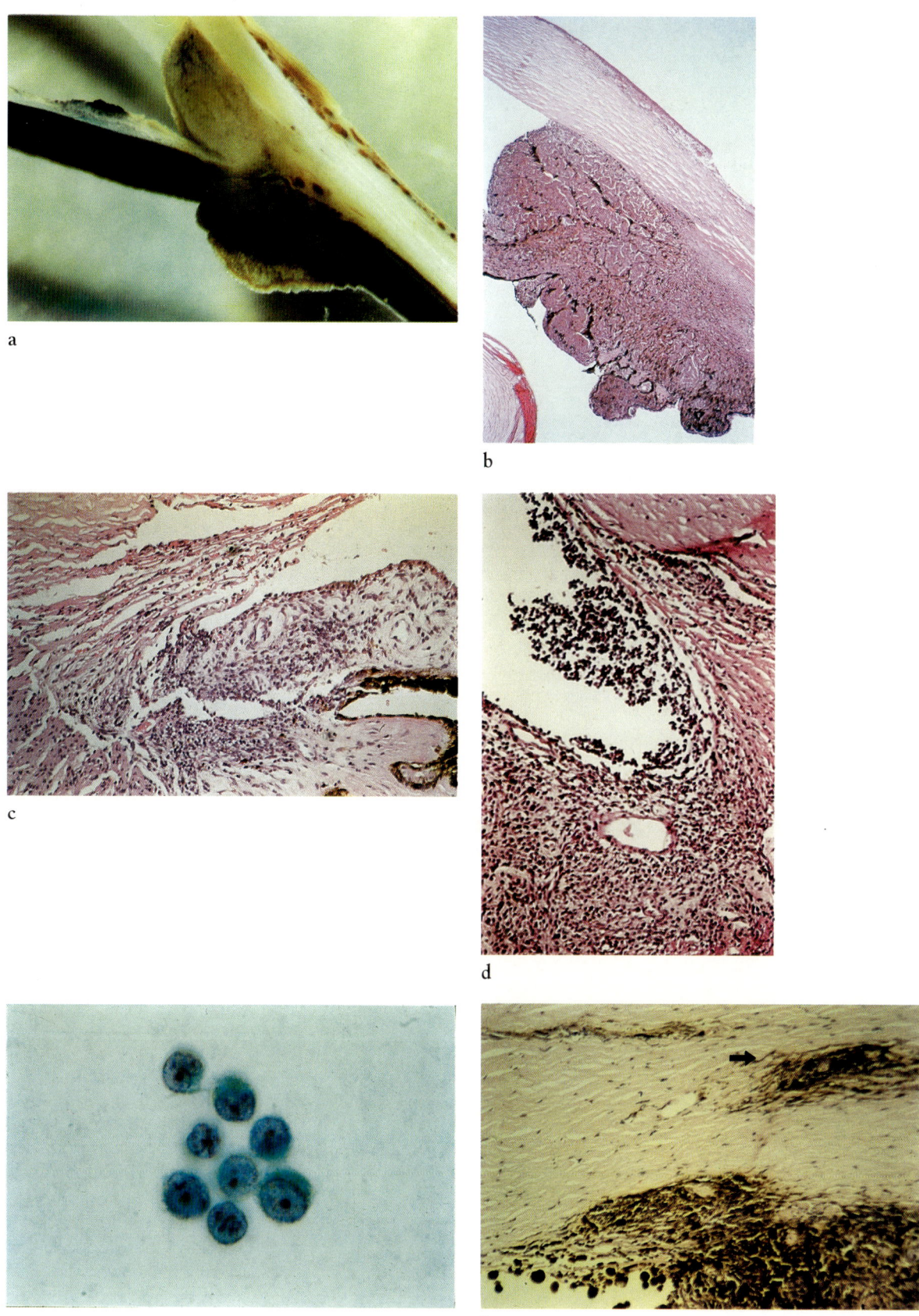

GLAUCOMAS ASSOCIATED WITH INTRAOCULAR TUMORS

Retinoblastoma

II32a. Although glaucoma is not commonly recognized clinically in children with retinoblastoma, histopathologic studies suggest that it is a frequent complication of this disease. In this 22-month-old child, we see the characteristic leukocoria of the right eye. This finding may be associated with several intraocular conditions of childhood, although the first that must be ruled out is retinoblastoma.

II32b. This 14-month-old child has heterochromia iridis, in which the darker right eye was found to have a retinoblastoma. The heterochromia in such cases is usually caused by iris neovascularization, the most common cause of glaucoma associated with retinoblastoma.

II32c–d. These two photos show the basic patterns of tumor growth with retinoblastoma: 1) endophytic, in which the tumor grows into the vitreous space and is seen ophthalmoscopically (II32c), and 2) exophytic, in which the growth is primarily subretinal giving rise to a retinal detachment (II32d).

II32e. In this eye with a diffuse endophytic retinoblastoma, the tumor has seeded into the anterior chamber producing a pseudohypopyon. This is another possible mechanism for glaucoma associated with retinoblastoma.

II32f. This light microscopic photo shows the anterior chamber angle of an eye with a retinoblastoma and associated neovascular glaucoma, with a fibrovascular membrane on the iris and extensive synechial closure of the anterior chamber angle.

(All figures on this page were provided courtesy of Jerry A. Shields, M.D.)

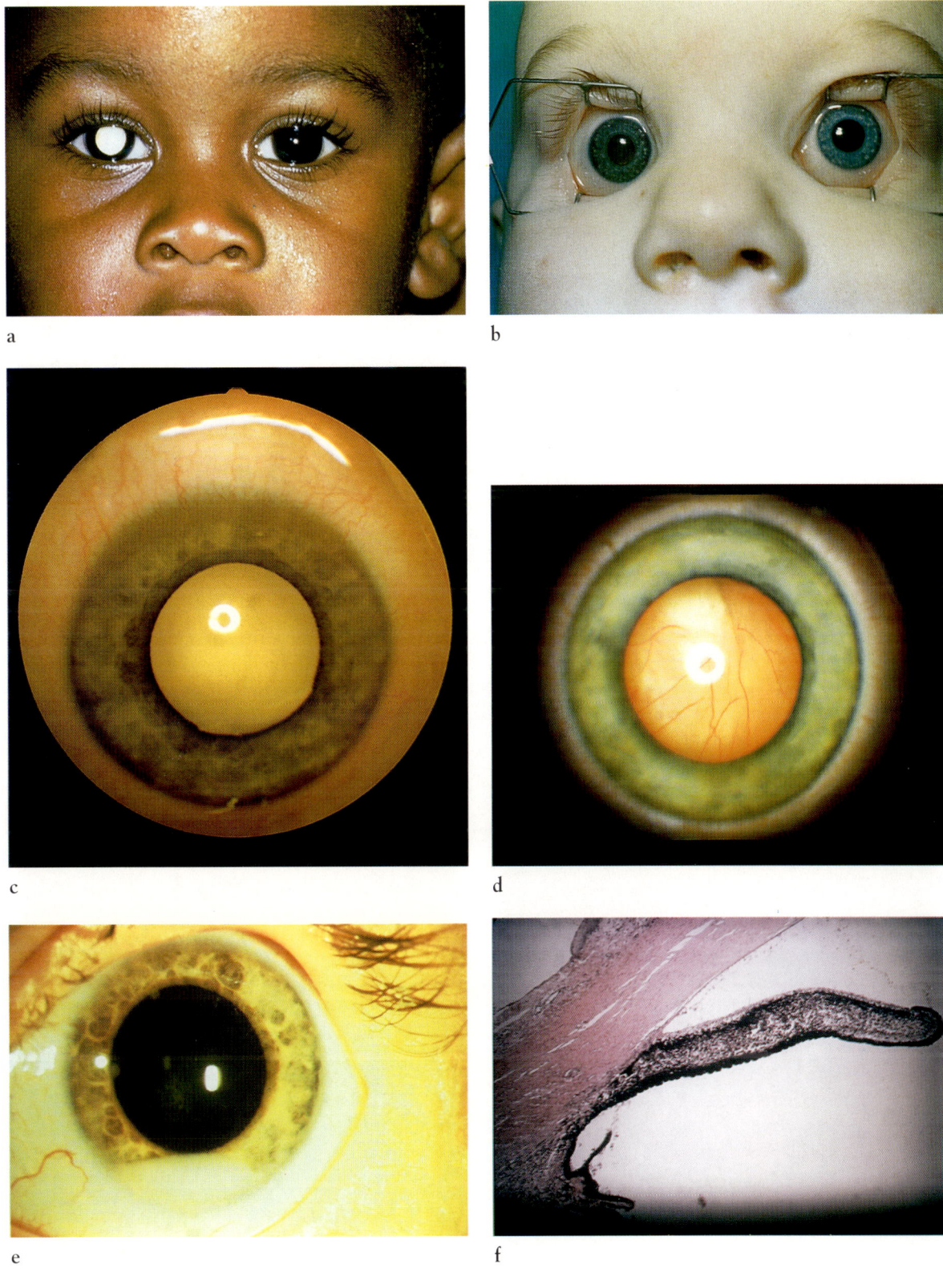

a

b

c

d

e

f

GLAUCOMAS ASSOCIATED WITH PHAKOMATOSES

Sturge-Weber Syndrome

II33a.   The phakomatoses are a group of disorders characterized by hamartomas, which primarily involve the eye, skin, and nervous system. Some of these conditions are frequently associated with glaucoma. One such example is the Sturge-Weber syndrome, characterized by the port wine hemangioma of the skin along the trigeminal distribution. This is usually unilateral, as seen in this child, and the associated glaucoma will always be on the side of the hemangioma.

II33b.   Much less often, the findings of the Sturge-Weber syndrome may be bilateral, as in this child. One side, however, is usually more involved than the other, as in the left side in this case, and it is typically that side that will have the associated glaucoma.

II33c–d.   Individuals with the Sturge-Weber syndrome typically have a dense episcleral vascular plexus. This is often associated with elevated episcleral venous pressure, which is one mechanism of the associated glaucoma. In other cases, the associated glaucoma may be related to developmental abnormalities of the anterior chamber angle.

II33e.   In addition to the episcleral vascular plexus, some patients with the Sturge-Weber syndrome may have ampulliform dilation of conjunctival vessels, as seen near the limbus in this case.

II33f.   This intraoperative photo during a trabeculectomy for glaucoma associated with the Sturge-Weber syndrome provides a direct view of the episcleral vascular plexus beneath the conjunctiva and Tenon's capsule, which have been reflected. This photo also demonstrates a common complication of filtering surgery in patients with the Sturge-Weber syndrome, in which intraoperative choroidal effusion causes herniation of uveal tissue through the fistula.

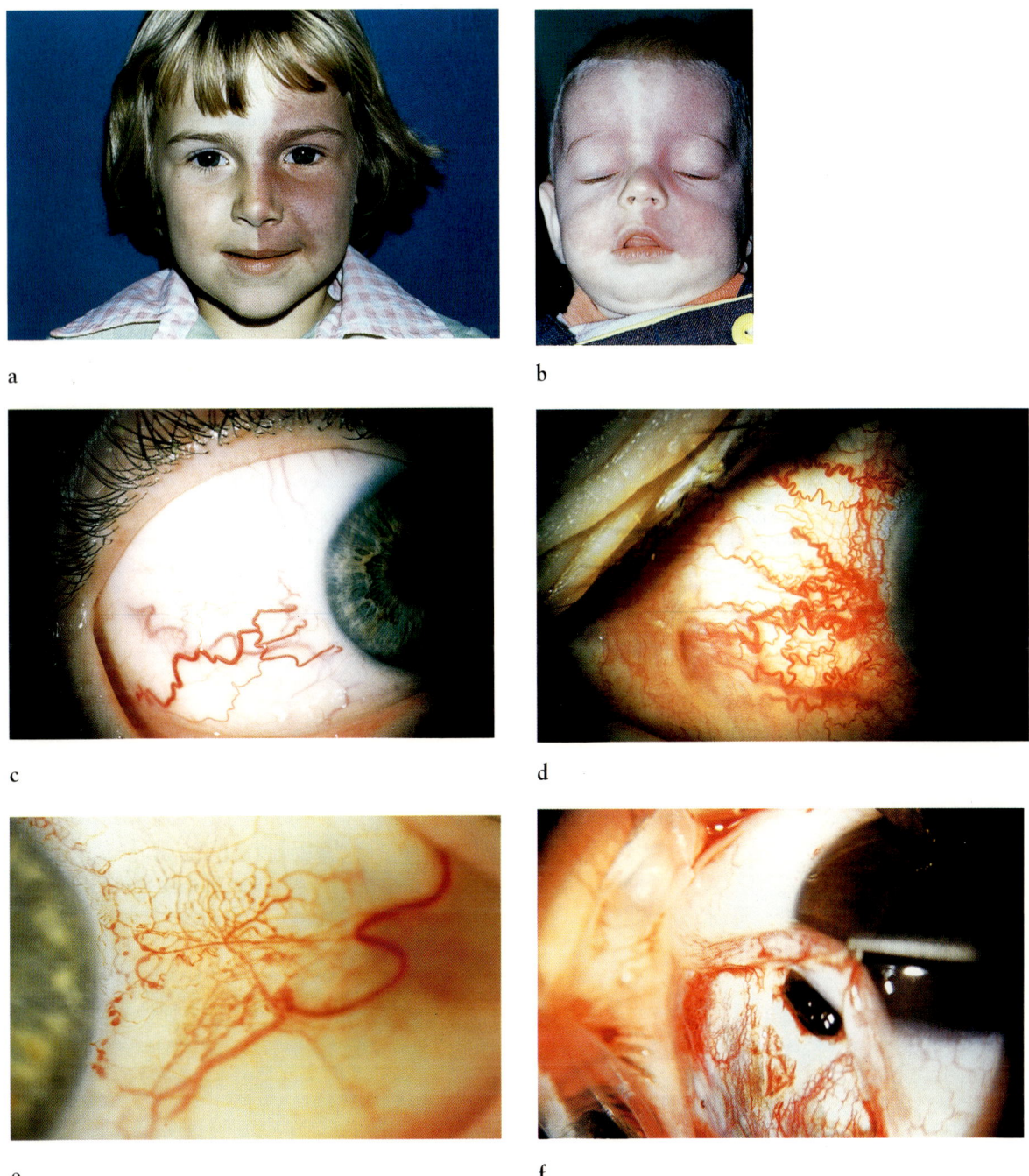

a

b

c

d

e

f

GLAUCOMAS ASSOCIATED WITH PHAKOMATOSES

Nevus of Ota

II35a.   The nevus of Ota (oculodermal melanocytosis) is not included in all reported classifications of the phakomatoses, but does fit the broader definition of this disease group. The hamartoma in this case is a unilateral accumulation of melanocytes in ocular tissues and the skin in the distribution of the trigeminal nerve, as noted on the left side of this individual.

II35b.   The most common site for the accumulation of melanocytes in the ocular tissues in the nevus of Ota is the episcleral, as shown in this photo.

II35c–d.   Another ocular site for accumulation of melanocytes in the nevus of Ota is the iris, which may produce heterochromia iridis, as in this patient in whom the right eye (II35c) is normal, while the involved left eye (II35d) is heavily pigmented.

II35e.   The mechanism of glaucoma in the nevus of Ota is believed to be the accumulation of melanocytes in the trabecular meshwork, as seen in this gonioscopic photo.

II35f.   The glaucoma associated with the nevus of Ota can lead to extensive optic atrophy, as seen in this case, in which increased pigmentation of the fundus and lamina cribrosa also have occurred.

(Figures II35a, II35b, and II35f are reprinted with permission from Ann Ophthal, American Society of Contemporary Ophthalmology, 1977;9:1299; Figures II35c, II35d, and II35e are reprinted with permission from: Glaucoma associated with the nevus of Ota. Arch Ophthalmol 1995;113:1208–1209. Copyright 1995, American Medical Association.)

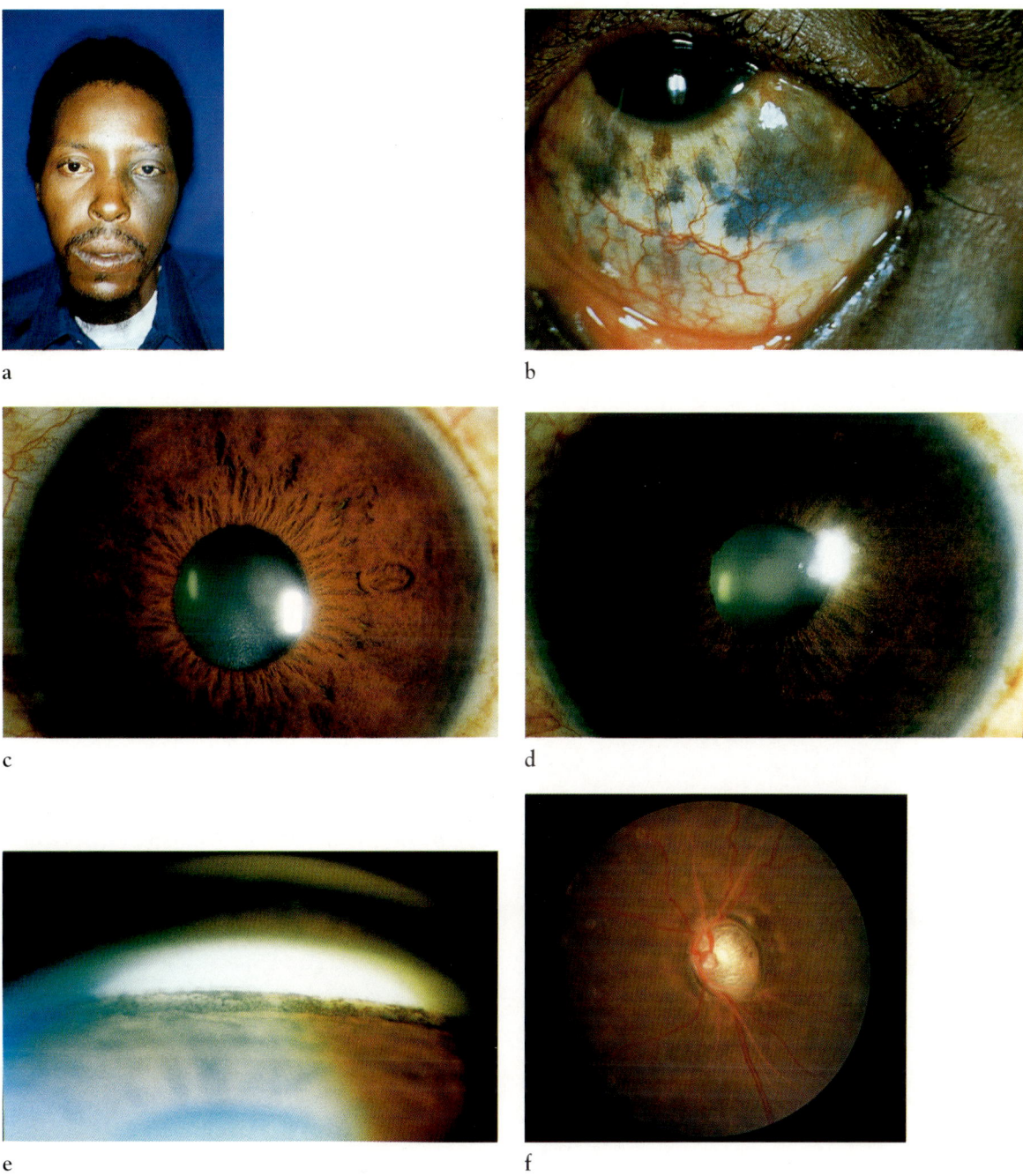

a

b

c

d

e

f

GLAUCOMAS ASSOCIATED WITH OCULAR INFLAMMATION

II36a. In most cases of acute anterior uveitis, the intraocular pressure is lower than that of the fellow eye, because of reduced aqueous production. In other cases, when the inflammation is either marked or chronic, obstruction to aqueous outflow may lead to elevated intraocular pressure and associated glaucoma. Anterior uveitis takes many forms, all of which can lead to glaucoma, and most of which are characterized by the ciliary flush of small, dilated vessels just peripheral to the limbus, as seen in this photo.

II36b. Another feature typical for nearly all forms of anterior uveitis is cell and flare of the anterior chamber, although the extent of these findings can vary considerably among the various forms of anterior uveitis. In this photo, we see a heavy flare extending from the cornea on the left to the pupil and iris on the right side of the photo.

II36c–d. Yet another clinical finding typical of most (although not all) forms of anterior uveitis is keratic precipitates, which are inflammatory deposits on the corneal endothelium. The size of the keratic precipitates can vary from extremely fine, through medium-size, to large "mutton-fat" deposits. The latter are commonly seen with chronic granulomatous uveitis, which has an especially high incidence of associated glaucoma.

II36e–f. Keratic precipitates may also be seen on the trabecular meshwork (Grant's syndrome). The ocular inflammation in this condition may otherwise be extremely mild, and the diagnosis can be missed unless careful gonioscopy is performed. The typical appearance by gonioscopy is that of gray or slightly yellow precipitates on the meshwork, with irregular peripheral anterior synechia that often attach to the precipitates (*arrows*).

(Figure II36a was provided courtesy of Gary N. Foulks, M.D.; Figure II36b was provided courtesy of L. Frank Cashwell, Jr., M.D.; Figure II36c was provided courtesy of Ruth Schirmer; Figure II36d was provided courtesy of Karim F. Damji, M.D.)

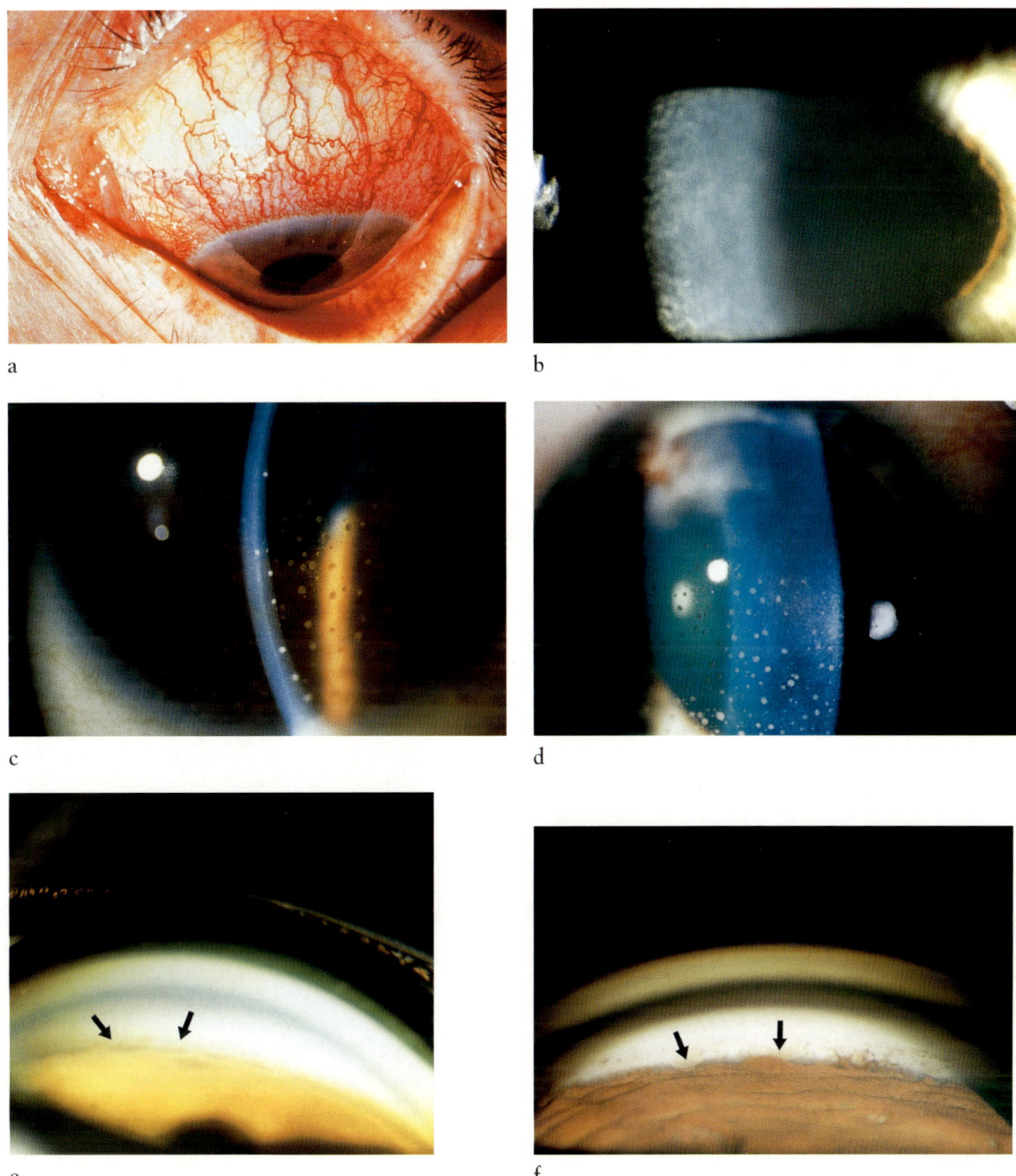

a

b

c

d

e

f

GLAUCOMAS ASSOCIATED WITH OCULAR INFLAMMATION

II37a.   Fuchs' heterochromic cyclitis is a form of chronic anterior uveitis, characterized by a uniocular, protracted course of mild inflammation, associated with heterochromia, cataracts, and occasional glaucoma. The involved eye typically has reduced iris pigmentation, as seen in the left eye of this patient.

II37b.   Slit-lamp examination of an eye with Fuchs' heterochromic cyclitis may reveal minimal aqueous flare and cell, with characteristic fine stellate keratic precipitates on the lower half of the cornea. By gonioscopy, the anterior chamber angle is open and characteristically free of synechia, although fine vessels are often seen extending onto the trabecular meshwork, as in this photo. These vessels, associated with an inflammatory membrane over the angle, may be the mechanism of glaucoma in Fuchs' heterochromic cyclitis.

II37c.   Iris nodules are seen in some patients with Fuchs' heterochromic cyclitis. These may occur along the pupillary border or may appear across the entire surface of the iris. The finding of unilateral iris nodules may be helpful in making the diagnosis of Fuchs' heterochromic cyclitis, especially in black patients, in whom the heterochromia may be less apparent.

II37d.   Another form of anterior uveitis, which may have associated iris nodules, is sarcoidosis, as seen in this photo. The nodules may involve the pupillary border (Koeppe nodules) or the stroma of the iris (Busacca nodules). These patients usually have a chronic granulomatous uveitis, with a high incidence of associated glaucoma.

II37e.   In many forms of chronic anterior uveitis, complete posterior synechial closure may develop, producing iris bombé and angle-closure glaucoma. In this photo, the cornea is to the left, and the peripheral iris has bowed forward against the peripheral cornea and anterior chamber angle, with the central iris scarred down to the lens. Such situations require a prompt iridotomy to relieve the angle-closure before peripheral anterior synechiae develop.

II37f.   Yet another typical finding in chronic anterior ocular inflammation is band keratopathy. This is a nonspecific finding, in which calcium degeneration of the cornea begins peripherally and progresses centrally to eventually form the complete band.

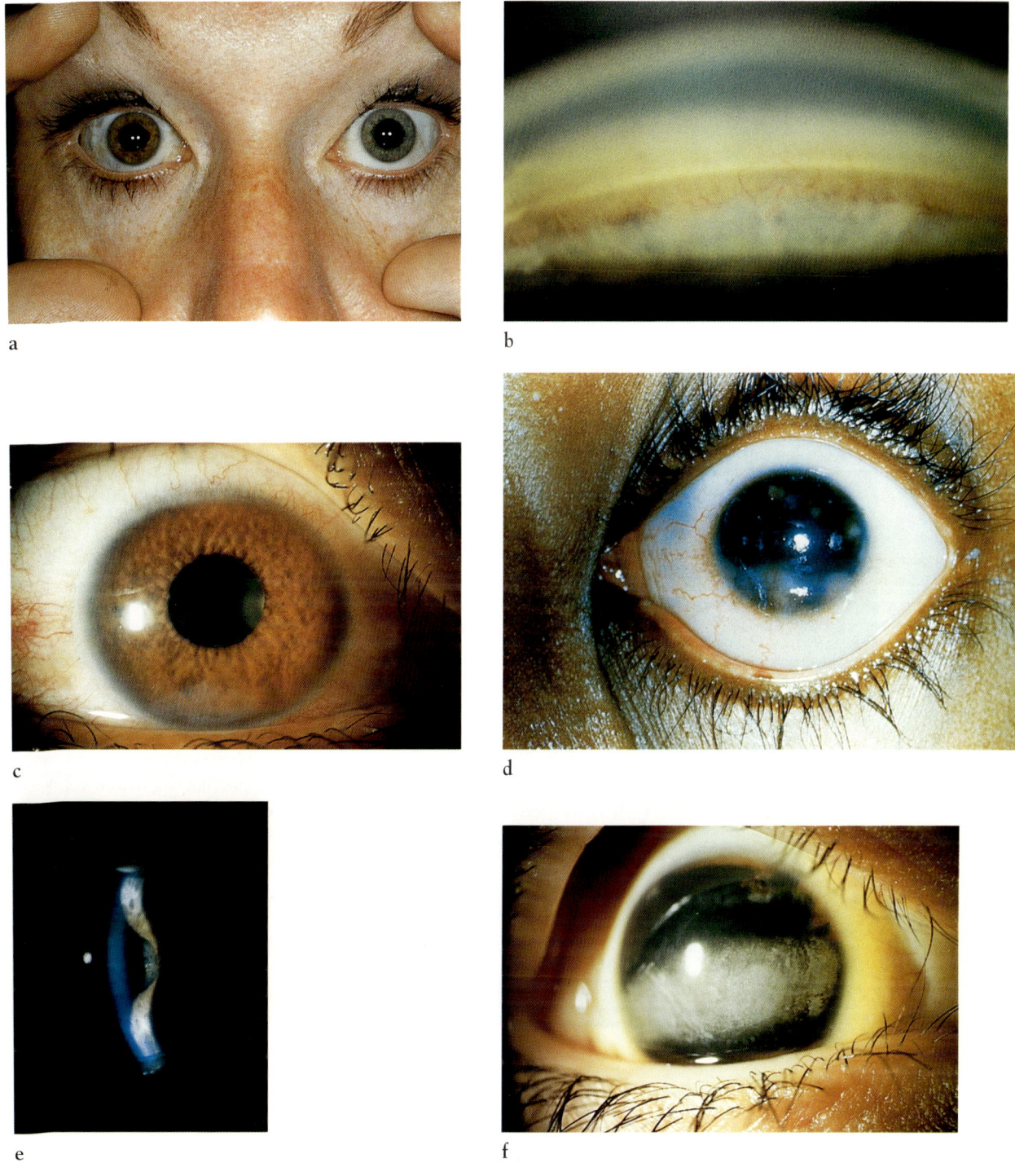

a

b

c

d

e

f

GLAUCOMAS ASSOCIATED WITH OCULAR TRAUMA

Angle Recession Glaucoma

II39a–d. Blunt injuries involving the eye are not uncommon. The initial consequence may be a hyphema, which may cause marked intraocular pressure elevation. As the blood clears, ruptures in various structures of the anterior segment may be found. The most common site of tissue disruption is in the ciliary body, which leads to the gonioscopic appearance of an irregular widening of the ciliary body band. This may be associated with glaucoma, often many years after the initial trauma, and has been referred to as angle recession glaucoma. It is not the damage to the ciliary body that causes the glaucoma, but rather the concomitant damage to the trabecular meshwork from the blunt injury. Nevertheless, it is important that angle recession be noted after trauma to indicate the risk of future glaucoma. II39a–c show the typical appearance of angle recession, in which the ciliary body band is wider in one area (*arrow*) than in the adjacent area. II39d, taken shortly after the injury, shows additional findings of a prominent scleral spur, in which the uveal tissue has been torn away, and a small hemorrhage on the wide ciliary body band.

II39e. This meridional section through the anterior chamber angle of an eye with angle recession shows the deep tear into the ciliary body with atrophy of the anterior face of the ciliary body. The trabecular meshwork, which is considerably anterior to the recessed ciliary body, is partly hyalinized and is covered on its inner aspect by an abnormal proliferation of Descemet's membrane, another mechanism of glaucoma associated with trauma.

II39f. Another form of anterior segment tissue disruption associated with blunt trauma is iridodialysis, which represents a tear in the root of the iris, as seen in this photo. While this does not lead to glaucoma, it is another indication of severe ocular trauma, indicating the risk of developing glaucoma from concomitant damage to the trabecular meshwork.

(Figure II39e was provided courtesy of Ramesh C. Tripathi, M.D., Ph.D.)

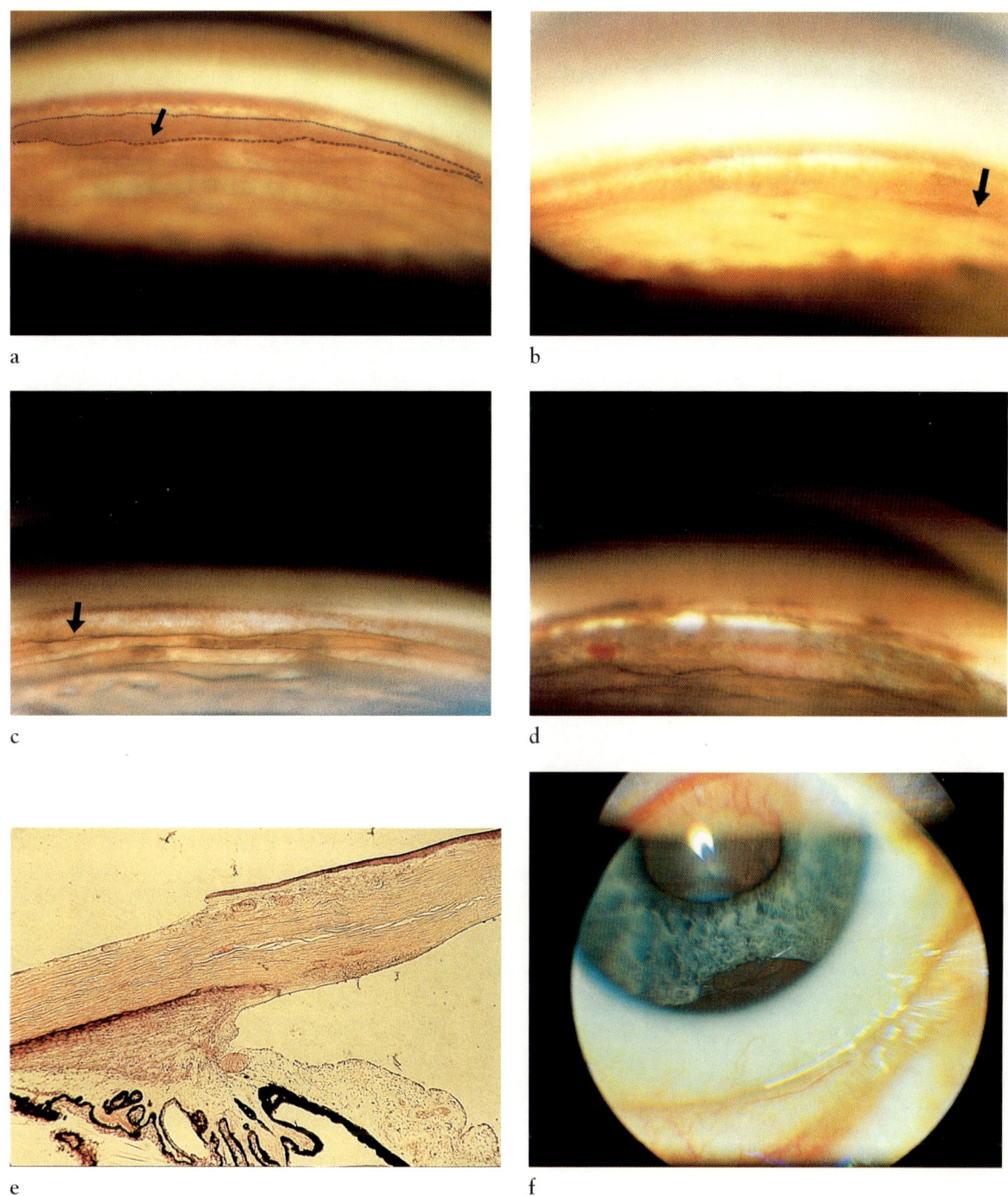

a

b

c

d

e

f

GLAUCOMAS FOLLOWING OCULAR SURGERY

II40a–b. Glaucoma can develop after cataract surgery through many mechanisms. In the aphakic eye, posterior synechiae may develop between the pupillary margin of the iris and the anterior hyaloid face, leading to iris bombe' and angle-closure glaucoma. This is apparent in II40a, in which the peripheral iris is bowed forward against the peripheral cornea, and the pupillary portion of the iris is held back against the anterior vitreous face. In some cases of glaucoma in aphakia, the intraocular pressure may be sufficient to produce corneal edema. If not relieved promptly, this can cause further endothelial damage and permanent aphakic bullous keratopathy.

II40c. Another form of angle-closure glaucoma after cataract surgery is seen with an anterior chamber intraocular lens. If the pupil is smaller than the optic and no patent iridectomy is present, the iris may be pushed forward against the back side of the intraocular lens, creating a reverse pupillary block. As seen in this photo, the peripheral iris will then bow forward around the intraocular lens, creating angle-closure glaucoma.

II40d. Another form of glaucoma associated with cataract surgery and intraocular lens implantation, especially with an anterior chamber or iris-supported lens, has been referred to as the "UGH" (uveitis, glaucoma, and hemorrhage) syndrome. These patients have recurrent bouts of uveitis and hyphema, with associated intraocular pressure elevation, as seen in this photo of an eye with an anterior chamber lens. In many cases, it is necessary to remove the intraocular lens to correct the problem.

II40e–f. Another mechanism of glaucoma after ocular surgery is associated with the use of silicone oil as a retinal tamponade in difficult vitreo-retinal procedures. The mechanism of intraocular pressure elevation in these cases may be pupillary block, which requires an inferior iridotomy, because the oil rises to the top of the eye. In other cases, the mechanism may be minute silicone oil bubbles in the anterior chamber angle. In II40e, these oil bubbles are seen to the left of the corneal reflex and on either side of the line of iris illumination. II40f is a gonioscopic view of the superior quadrant, in which a bank of silicone bubbles have accumulated, creating an "inverse pseudohypopyon."

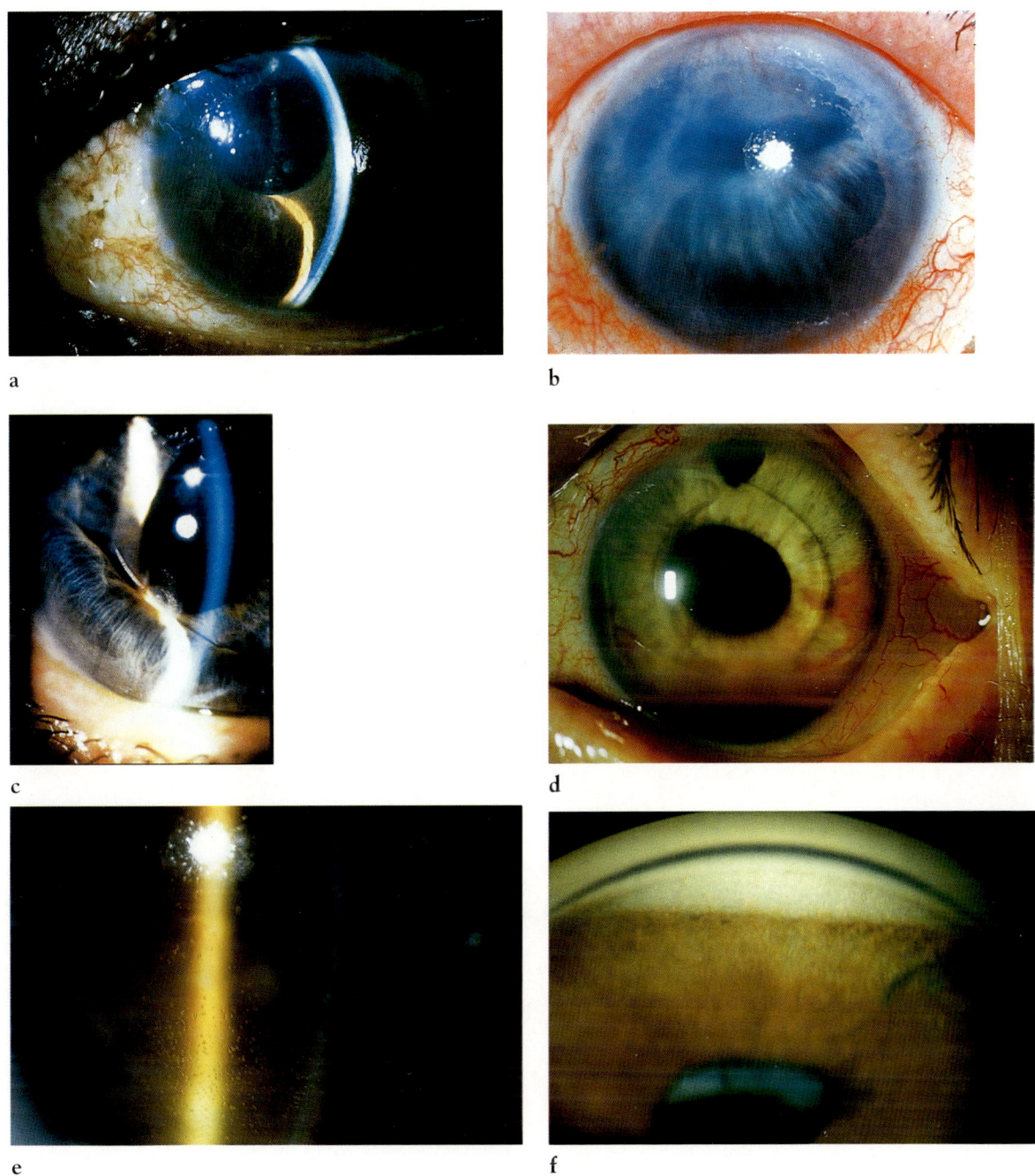

a

b

c

d

e

f

Section III

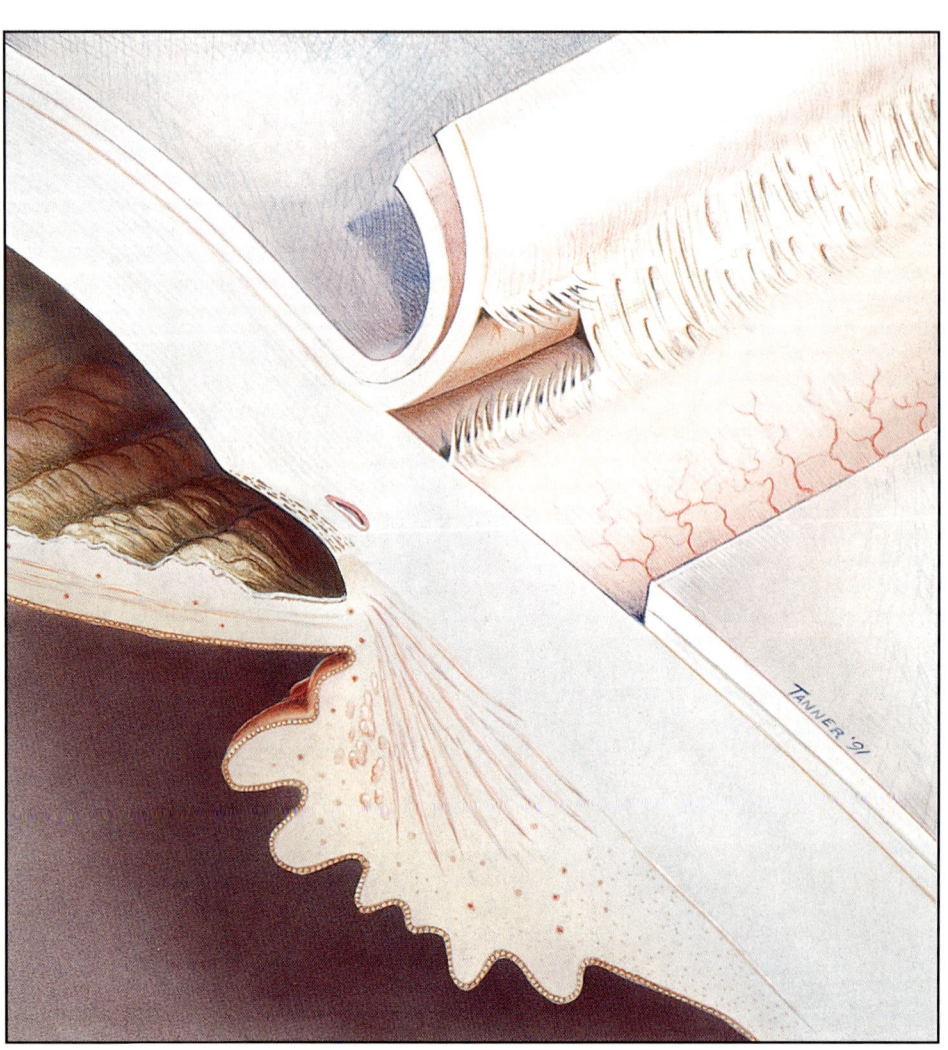

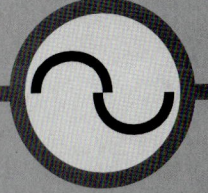

THE MANAGEMENT OF
GLAUCOMA

MEDICAL MANAGEMENT OF GLAUCOMA

Cholinergic Stimulators

III2a–b.   The cholinergic stimulators, also referred to as parasympathomimetics or miotics because of their common action on the pupil, were the first class of drugs to be introduced for the treatment of glaucoma. All the drugs in this class (which includes pilocarpine, carbachol and echothiophate iodide) share common mechanisms of action in lowering the intraocular pressure. In eyes with open-angle forms of glaucoma, the mechanism is enhanced aqueous outflow by contraction of the longitudinal portion of the ciliary muscle, as demonstrated in these two photographs. In III2a, a portion of a human autopsy eye shows the ciliary body (*large arrow*) and the anterior chamber angle (*small arrow*). Without tension on the ciliary body, the trabecular meshwork and Schlemm's canal are collapsed, and the latter structure cannot be seen in this photo. In III2b, the ciliary body is pulled posteriorly, mimicking the action of longitudinal muscle contraction, the trabecular meshwork is expanded and Schlemm's canal is open (*arrow*) because of inward, posterior displacement of the scleral spur. A similar mechanism is believed to explain the improvement in outflow facility after cholinergic stimulation in eyes with open angles.

In eyes with pupillary-block forms of glaucoma, the mechanism of improved outflow facility and reduced intraocular pressure is contraction of the sphincter muscle of the iris, which produces miosis, relieves the pupillary block and allows the anterior chamber angle to open.

III2c.   All miotics are limited by numerous ocular side effects, including miosis, induced myopia, and brow ache. The latter two side effects are both related to ciliary muscle spasm. Various efforts to minimize these side effects have included alternative delivery systems, one of which is an ocular insert that provides membrane-controlled delivery of pilocarpine (Ocusert). This photo shows the oval-shaped insert device in the inferior cul-de-sac. It can be worn in the inferior or superior cul-de-sac and typically provides constant release of the drug for 7 days, with less total drug delivery and reduced side effects compared with pilocarpine delivery in traditional drop form.

III2d.   Another side effect that was once associated with long-term pilocarpine therapy was atypical band keratopathy, characterized by calcium degeneration of the central cornea, as shown in this photo. This was found to result from the preservative, phenylmercuric nitrate, which is no longer used.

(Figures III2a and III2b were provided courtesy of David G. Campbell, M.D.)

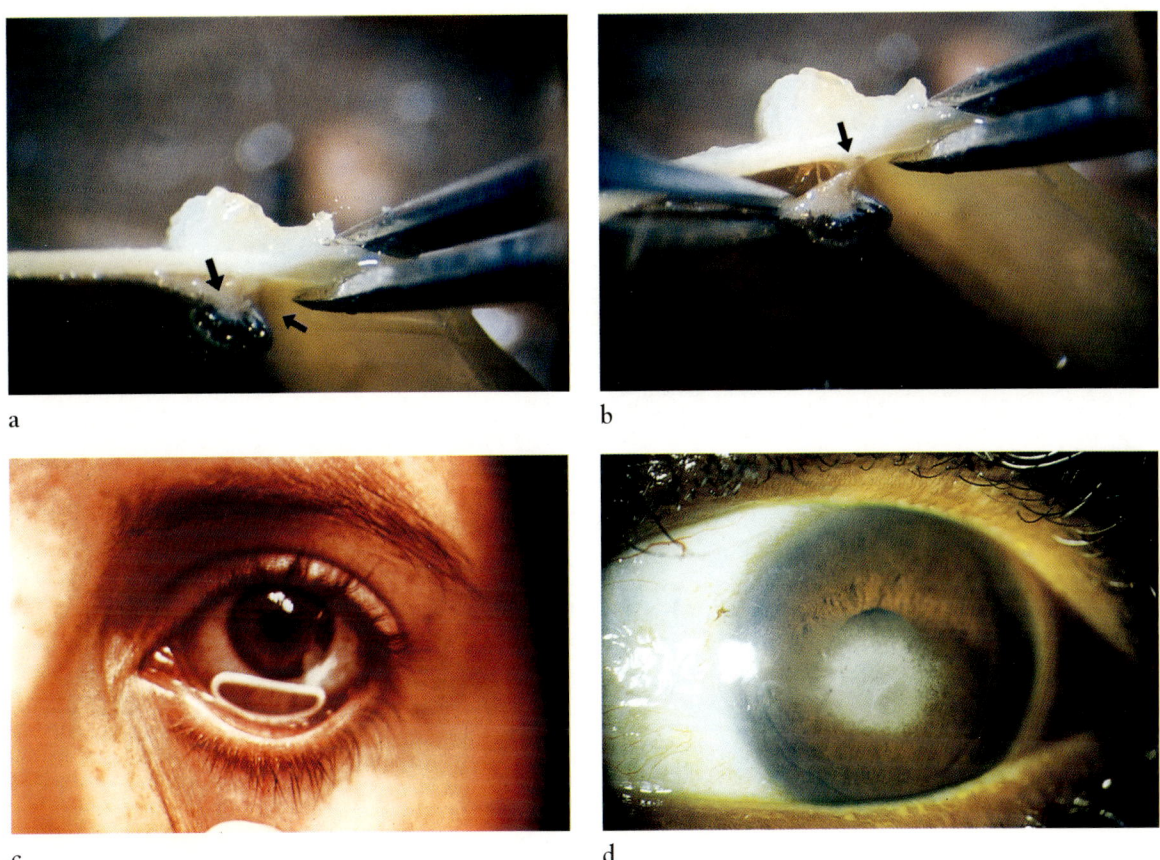

a

b

c

d

MEDICAL MANAGEMENT OF GLAUCOMA

Adrenergic Stimulators

III3a.   Epinephrine, a direct-acting alpha and beta adrenergic stimulator, or sympathomimetic, is the prototype adrenergic stimulator, although it is used less often today because of the numerous ocular side effects. This photo shows the most common ocular side effect of epinephrine, which is a diffuse conjunctival reactive hyperemia that follows the initial vasoconstrictive effect.

III3b–c.   Another common side effect of topical epinephrine therapy is the deposition of adrenochrome in the palpebral conjunctiva, the result of oxidation and polymerization of epinephrine to adrenochrome, a pigment of the melanin family. III3b shows the small, round configuration of adrenochrome deposits in the inferior palpebral conjunctiva, which is typical of the appearance in this location. III3c shows the typical appearance in the superior palpebral conjunctiva, in which the adrenochrome deposits have a "staghorn" shape.

III3d.   Another location for adrenochrome pigmentation, associated with the chronic use of topical epinephrine, is in the cornea of eyes with elevated intraocular pressure and bullous keratopathy. This has been referred to as "black cornea."

III3e–f.   Adrenochrome pigmentation may also discolor soft contact lenses, as shown in these two photos.

It should be noted that adrenochrome pigmentation is not associated with the use of dipivefrin, a prodrug of epinephrine, which is discussed further on the next page.

(Figure III3a was provided courtesy of John F. Bigger, M.D., and is reprinted with permission of Ann Ophthal, American Society of Contemporary Ophthalmology 1979;11:183. Figure III3d was provided courtesy of David Donaldson, M.D.; Figures III3b-d are reprinted with permission from Cashwell LF, Shields MB: Adrenochrome pigmentation. Arch Ophthalmol 1977;95:514–515. Copyright 1977, American Medical Association. Figures III3e–f were provided courtesy of John W. Reed, M.D., and are reprinted with permission of Ann Ophthal, American Society of Contemporary Ophthalmology 1976;8:65)

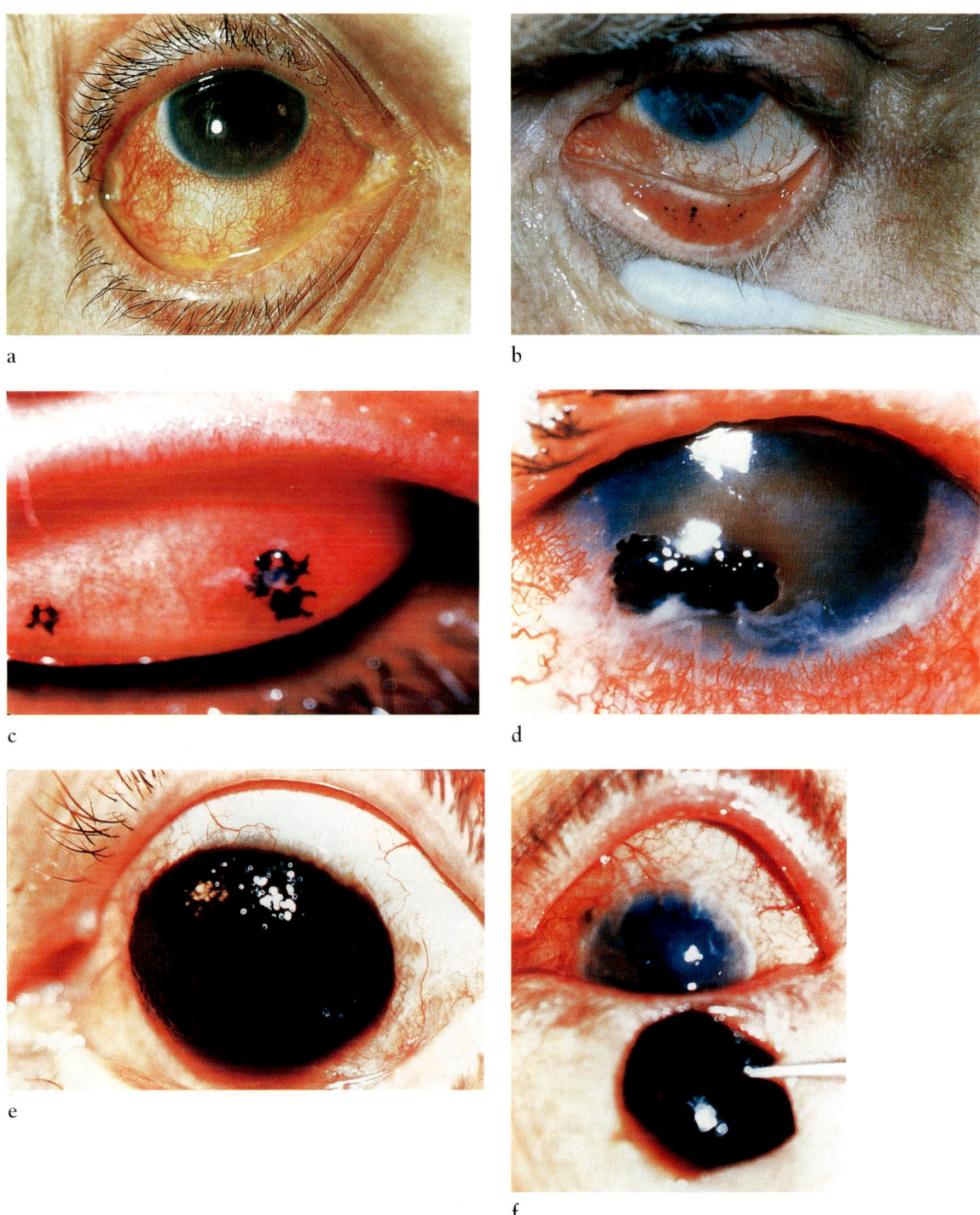

a

b

c

d

e

f

MEDICAL MANAGEMENT OF GLAUCOMA

Reactions to Topical Agents

III4a.   This photo shows the typical appearance of contact dermatitis of the lids, which can be associated with any topical medication for the long-term management of glaucoma. In many cases, this reaction is related to a preservative in the formulation, and preservative-free preparations (e.g., with timolol and pilocarpine) are available. In other cases, the active ingredient may be responsible for the reaction. Apraclonidine, an alpha$_2$-adrenergic agonist, has a particularly high incidence of contact dermatitis with chronic use.

III4b.   As noted on the previous page, reactive conjunctival hyperemia is a consistent finding with the chronic use of topical epinephrine. Dipivefrin, the prodrug of epinephrine, not only eliminates the adverse reaction of adrenochrome pigmentation, but also reduces the tendency for reactive conjunctival hyperemia. In this photo, dipivefrin was instilled in the patient's right eye (to the left in photo) and epinephrine 2% was instilled in the left eye.

It should also be noted that dipivefrin reduces the systemic reactions associated with topical epinephrine (elevated blood pressure, tachycardia, arrhythmias, headaches, tremor, nervousness, and anxiety) since it is not converted to active epinephrine until it enters the eye.

III4c–d.   The prolonged use of dipivefrin can be associated with external ocular toxicity in some patients, including large bulbar conjunctival follicles as shown in III4c (*arrow*), as well as the palpebral conjunctival follicles, as shown in III4d (*arrow*).

III4e–f.   Cicatricial pemphigoid may occur in patients on long-term topical glaucoma therapy. In most cases, the patients are on multiple glaucoma drops, and virtually all glaucoma medications have been implicated in this adverse reaction. III4e shows the linear scars of the superior conjunctiva (*arrows*), and III4f shows the foreshortening of the inferior conjunctival fornix, with linear scars (*arrows*).

(Figure III4b was provided courtesy of John F. Bigger, M.D.)

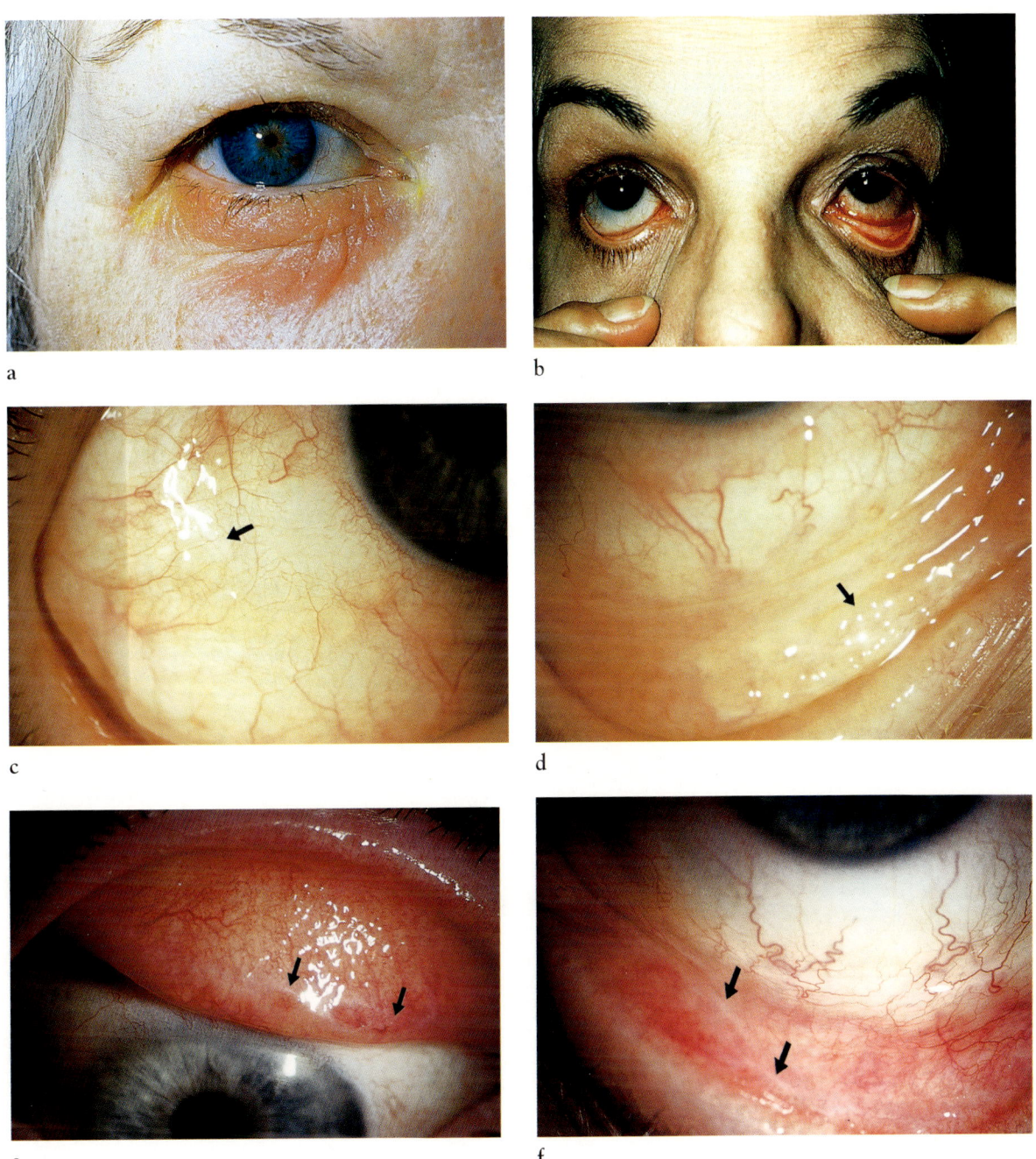

MEDICAL MANAGEMENT OF GLAUCOMA

Prostaglandins

III5a–d.   The newest class of drugs to be introduced for the chronic management of glaucoma is the prostaglandins. The first topical prostaglandin compound to be approved for the management of glaucoma is the $PGF_{2\alpha}$ isopropylester, latanoprost. In initial trials, latanoprost 0.005%, given once daily, was more effective than timolol 0.5%, given twice daily. Ocular and systemic side effects appear to be minimal with latanoprost. However, one side effect that has been observed with the medication is increased pigmentation of the iris. This side effect appears to occur only in eyes with mixed green-brown or blue/gray-brown iris color. Figures 5a and 5b depict the green-brown iris of a patient before (left) and 6 months after (right) treatment with latanoprost, while figures 5c and 5d show a blue/gray-brown iris with a typical brown ring around the pupil before (left) and 10 months after (right) latanoprost therapy.

(Reprinted with permission from Watson, P., Stjernschantz, J., the Latanoprost Study Group, Ophthalmology, 1996;103:126–137).

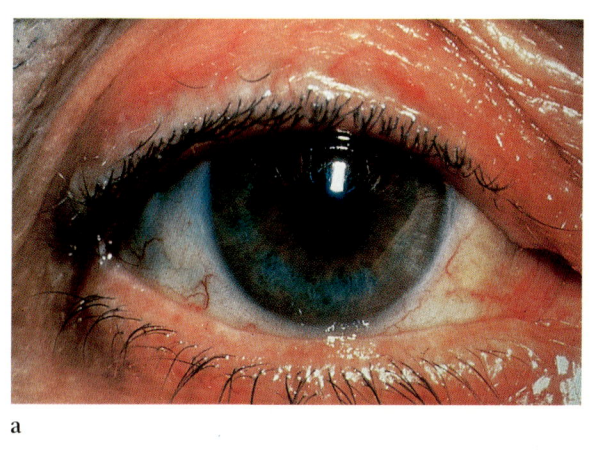

a

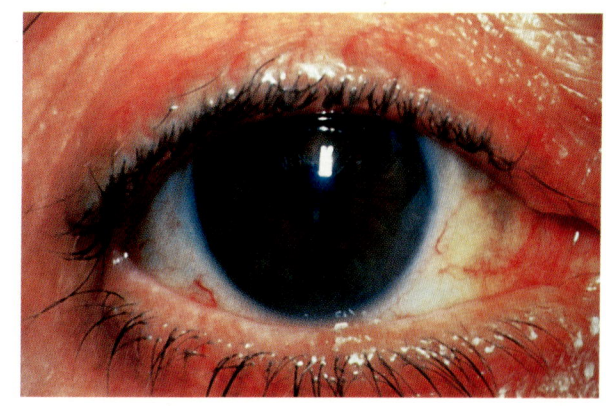

b

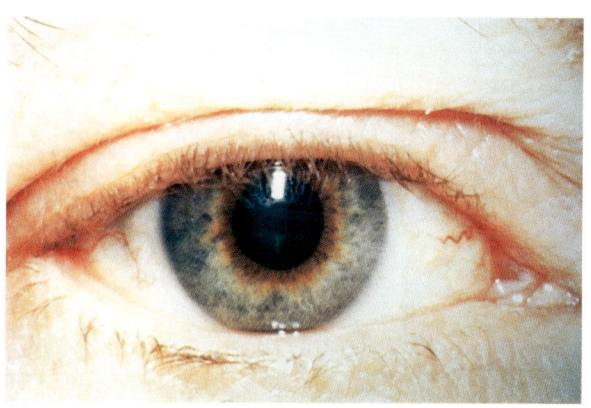

c

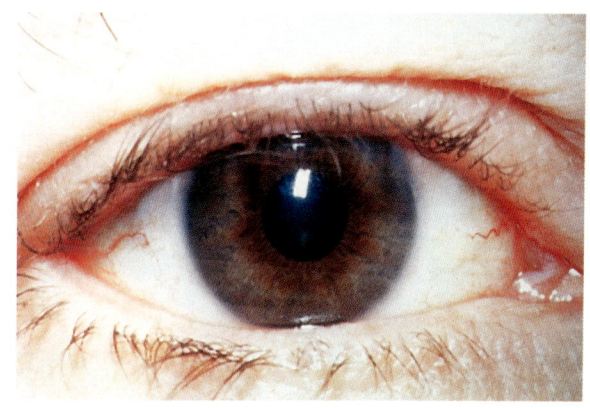

d

MEDICAL MANAGEMENT OF GLAUCOMA

Administration of Eyedrops

Several effective techniques are available for instilling eyedrops, and many patients find the technique that is most effective for them. It should not be assumed, however, that a patient knows the proper technique, and patients should be observed in the office to ensure that their technique is adequate. If the patient does not have an effective technique, he or she should be instructed in the proper administration of eyedrops. The following is one effective method.

III6a.   While looking up, the patient should pull the lower lid down to create a pocket in the inferior cul-de-sac.

III6b.   A single drop is then instilled in the inferior cul-de-sac without touching the eyedropper to ocular tissues.

III6c.   After instillation of the drop, the patient should gently close the lids for 3 to 5 minutes while placing gentle pressure over the lacrimal sac with the finger tip (nasolacrimal occlusion) to minimize loss of drug into the lacrimal drainage system.

III6d.   When instilling drops in both eyes, bilateral nasolacrimal occlusion can be performed with the thumb and index finger, as shown in this photograph.

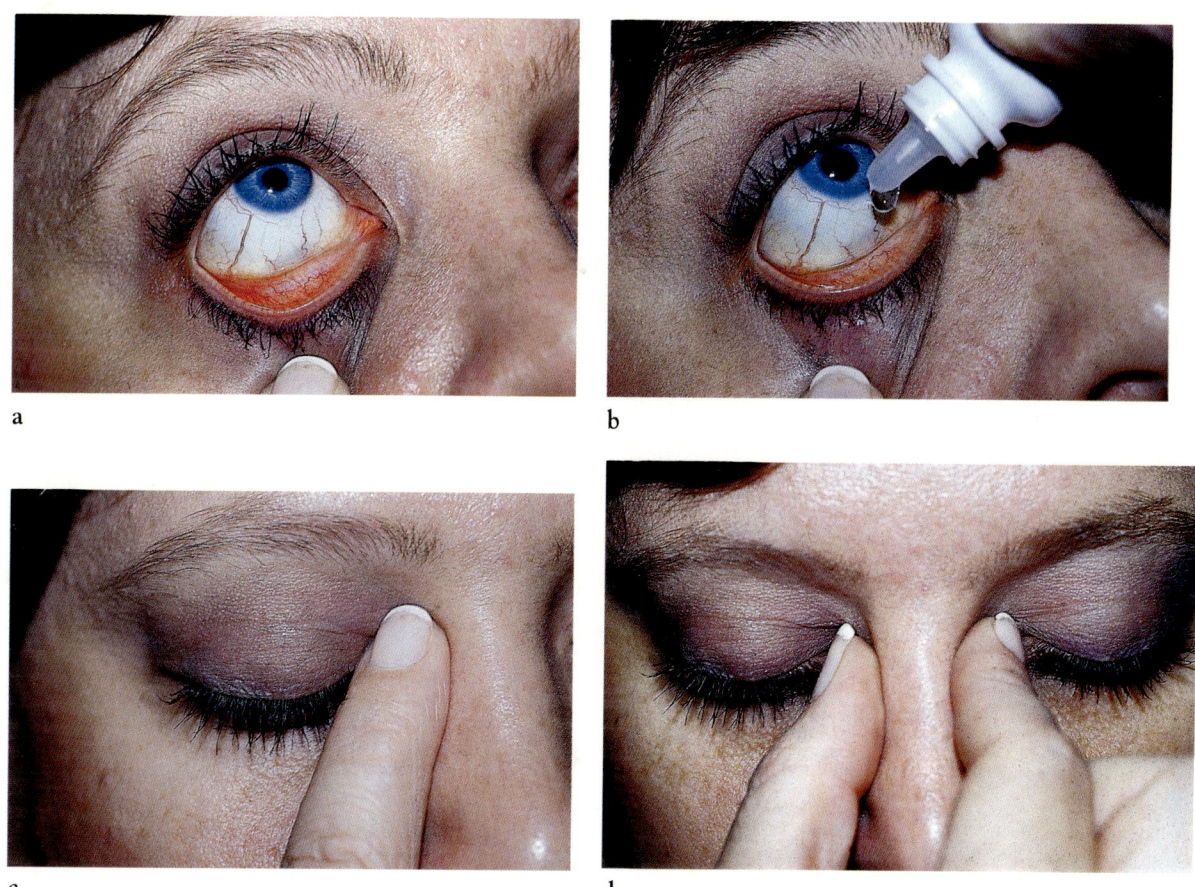

a

b

c

d

LASER TRABECULOPLASTY

III7a–b.   Several gonioprisms (contact lens with mirror for visualization of anterior chamber angle) can be used in performing laser trabeculoplasty. A commonly used lens is the standard Goldmann-type three-mirror lens, which is modified with anti-reflection coating (III7a). The Ritch trabeculoplasty laser lens (III7b) has been designed specifically for use during laser trabeculoplasty. The latter lens has two mirrors inclined at 59° for viewing the inferior quadrants and two mirrors inclined at 64° for the superior angle. Seventeen diopter plano-convex button lenses are placed over two mirrors to provide 1.4 × magnification, which reduces a 50 micron laser spot to 35 microns.

III7c.   The argon laser in either the green or blue-green wavelengths is the laser most commonly used for trabeculoplasty. In this photo, the attenuated aiming beam of the argon laser is focused on the anterior margin of the trabecular meshwork (*arrow*). This anterior placement of the laser application has been shown to reduce post-operative intraocular pressure elevation, as well as peripheral anterior synechia formation.

Alternative lasers for performing laser trabeculoplasty include the semiconductor diode laser.

III7d–f.   The typical, desirable tissue response to argon laser trabeculoplasty is a blanching of the trabecular meshwork, often associated with a small gas bubble. The bubbles are transient, but the blanch spots may persist for several days. These three photos were taken immediately after argon laser trabeculoplasty and show the blanch spots along the anterior margin of the trabecular meshwork, creating a scalloped appearance. In III7d, the blanch spots are seen best to the left of the gonioscopic photograph. In III7e, they can be faintly seen on both the right and left sides of the photograph. In III7f, which has darker trabecular meshwork pigmentation, the blanch spots are more easily seen in the entire field of view.

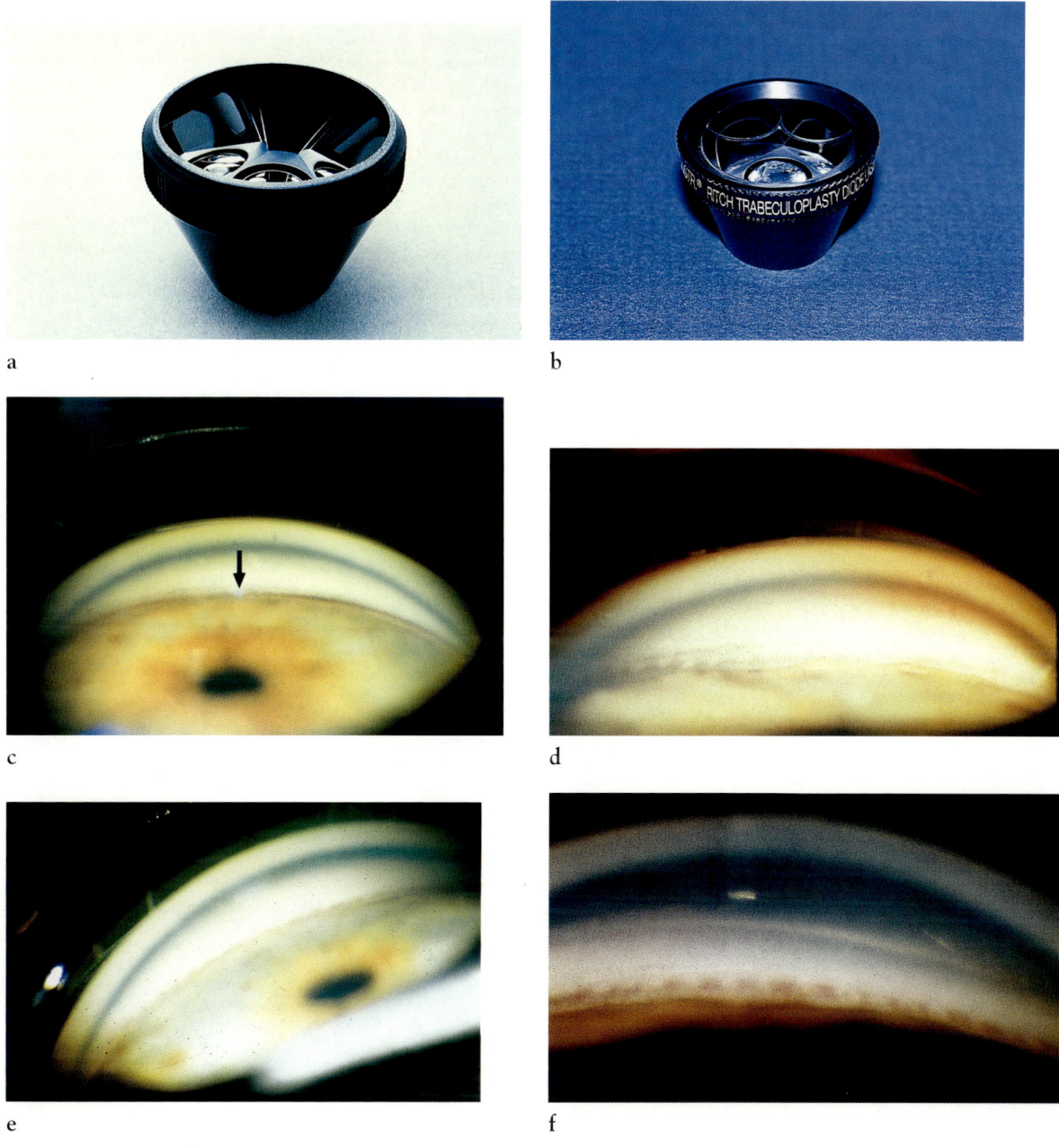

a

b

c

d

e

f

TRABECULOTOMY

Incisional trabeculotomy is an ab-externo operation for creating an opening in the trabecular meshwork to establish direct communication between the anterior chamber and Schlemm's canal. It is used most commonly in children, although success has been reported in adults.

III8a–b. A conjunctival-Tenon's capsule flap (either limbus-based or fornix-based) is first prepared. A partial-thickness, limbus-based scleral flap is then dissected beneath the conjunctival flap. The shape of the scleral flap can be triangular, as shown in III8a, or square, as shown in III8b.

III8c–d. A radial incision is then made across the sclerolimbal junction (between the gray zone and white scleral tissue) until Schlemm's canal is entered. Pushing the tissue aside with the tip of the blade during the scratch incision may help to identify the darker area of Schlemm's canal. The area should be kept dry during the scratch incision, because the sudden appearance of clear aqueous (or occasionally blood in Schlemm's canal) may also help to identify the canal.

III8e–f. Once the surgeon feels that Schlemm's canal has been entered, it is advisable to confirm the identity of the canal by threading a nylon suture into one of the cut ends of the canal. The presence of the suture in the canal can be confirmed either by gonioscopic observation or by bending the exposed portion of the suture anteriorly or posteriorly, noting whether it returns to a position parallel to the canal when released. Failure of the suture to return to the parallel position suggests that a false passage may have been created into the anterior chamber or supraciliary space.

(Figures III8a, III8c, and III8e were provided courtesy of Sharon F. Freedman, M.D.)

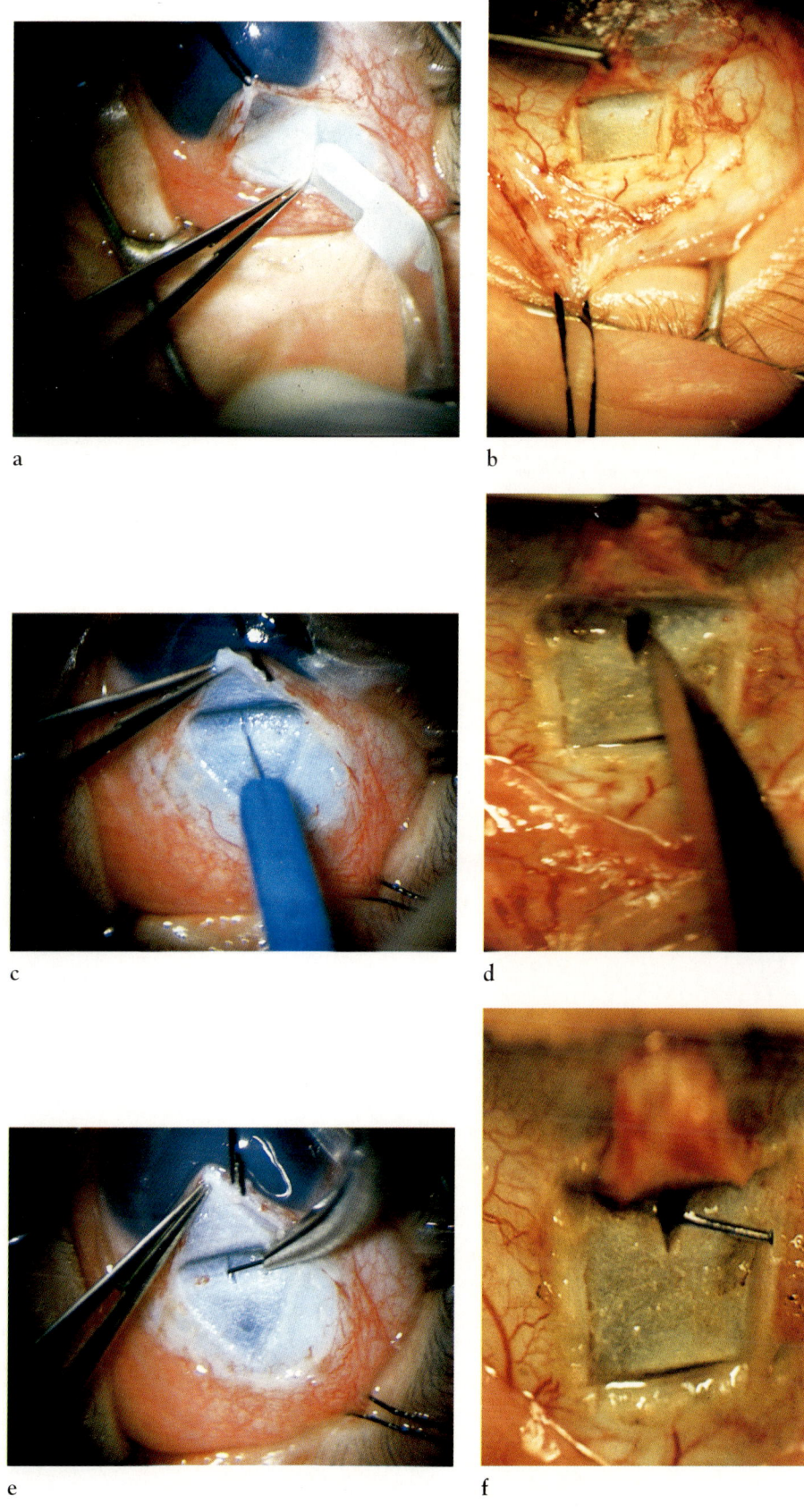

a

b

c

d

e

f

TRABECULOTOMY

III9a–b.   After confirming the location of Schlemm's canal (as discussed on the previous page), a trabeculotome is threaded into one end of Schlemm's canal. The instrument used in these two photos is a McPherson trabeculotome, which has a parallel external arm to serve as a guide for the position of the internal arm.

III9c–e.   The internal arm of the trabeculotome is advanced in Schlemm's canal until resistance is met. The trabeculotome is then rotated into the anterior chamber, which tears through the trabecular meshwork and any other barriers to aqueous flow between the anterior chamber and Schlemm's canal. The same procedure is then performed on the other side of the radial incision.

III9f.   Having completed the trabeculotomy on both sides of the radial incision, the scleral flap is then closed tightly, as shown in this photo. The conjunctival flap is then closed with a running suture. Postoperative care typically includes the use of topical antibiotics and steroids. A low dose of pilocarpine may also be helpful by keeping the cut edges of the trabecular meshwork separated, and the pupil can be dilated once daily with phenylephrine to avoid posterior synechiae.

(Figures III9a, III9c, III9d, and III9f were provided courtesy of Sharon F. Freedman, M.D.)

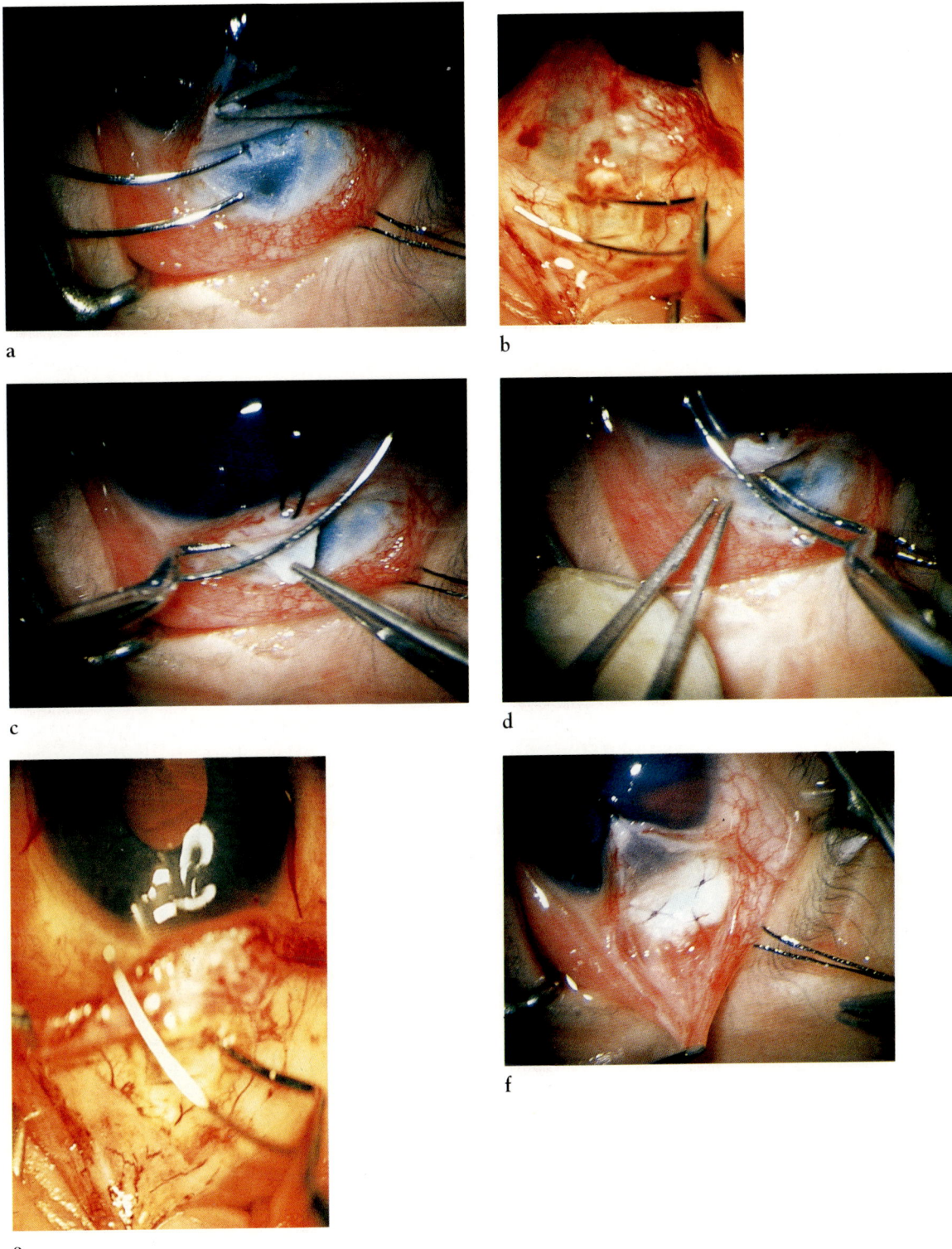

a

b

c

d

e

f

GONIOTOMY

Goniotomy is a time-honored operation for several forms of childhood glaucoma. It differs from trabeculotomy in that it uses an ab-interno approach and incises only the internal obstructive tissue in the anterior chamber angle, rather than the full thickness of the trabecular meshwork.

III10a.   A Barkan surgical goniolens is placed on the cornea with a bridge of viscous solution, such as methylcellulose. The lens should be placed over the nasal cornea, leaving 2 to 3 mm of temporal cornea exposed for the knife entry.

III10b.   A Barkan goniotomy knife, or similar knife, penetrates the cornea near the limbus at the 10 o'clock position in the right eye or 4 o'clock position in the left eye. The blade is then passed across the anterior chamber to a point in the chamber angle 180° from the site of entry. Note the fixation of the globe in this photo, which is essential for accurate placement and incision with the blade.

III10c–d.   Using the tip of the goniotomy blade, the angle tissue is incised behind Schwalbe's line, or just before the high insertion of the iris. The intent is to incise only the abnormal layer of tissue in front of the trabecular meshwork, and this is best judged by observing a white line develop as the cut edge of the tissue retracts posteriorly, which is seen in both photos (*arrows*). The incision is typically extended for approximately one-third of the angle circumference.

The goniotomy knife is then withdrawn, taking care not to injure adjacent ocular structures. The anterior chamber is then deepened with air or a balanced salt solution. Postoperative management consists of topical antibiotics, a miotic, and topical steroids.

III10e–f.   These light microscopic photographs show the appearance of the anterior chamber angle in congenital glaucoma before and after a goniotomy. In III10e, condensed tissue can be seen extending from the peripheral iris to the anterior trabecular meshwork, pulling the peripheral iris toward the meshwork. This condensed tissue is the target for incision by goniotomy. III10f shows the eye of a child who died shortly after a goniotomy procedure. The condensed tissue has been excised (*arrow*), allowing the peripheral iris to fall away from the trabecular meshwork.

(Figures III10a–d were provided courtesy of Sharon F. Freedman, M.D.; Figures III10e–f were provided courtesy of David S. Walton, M.D.)

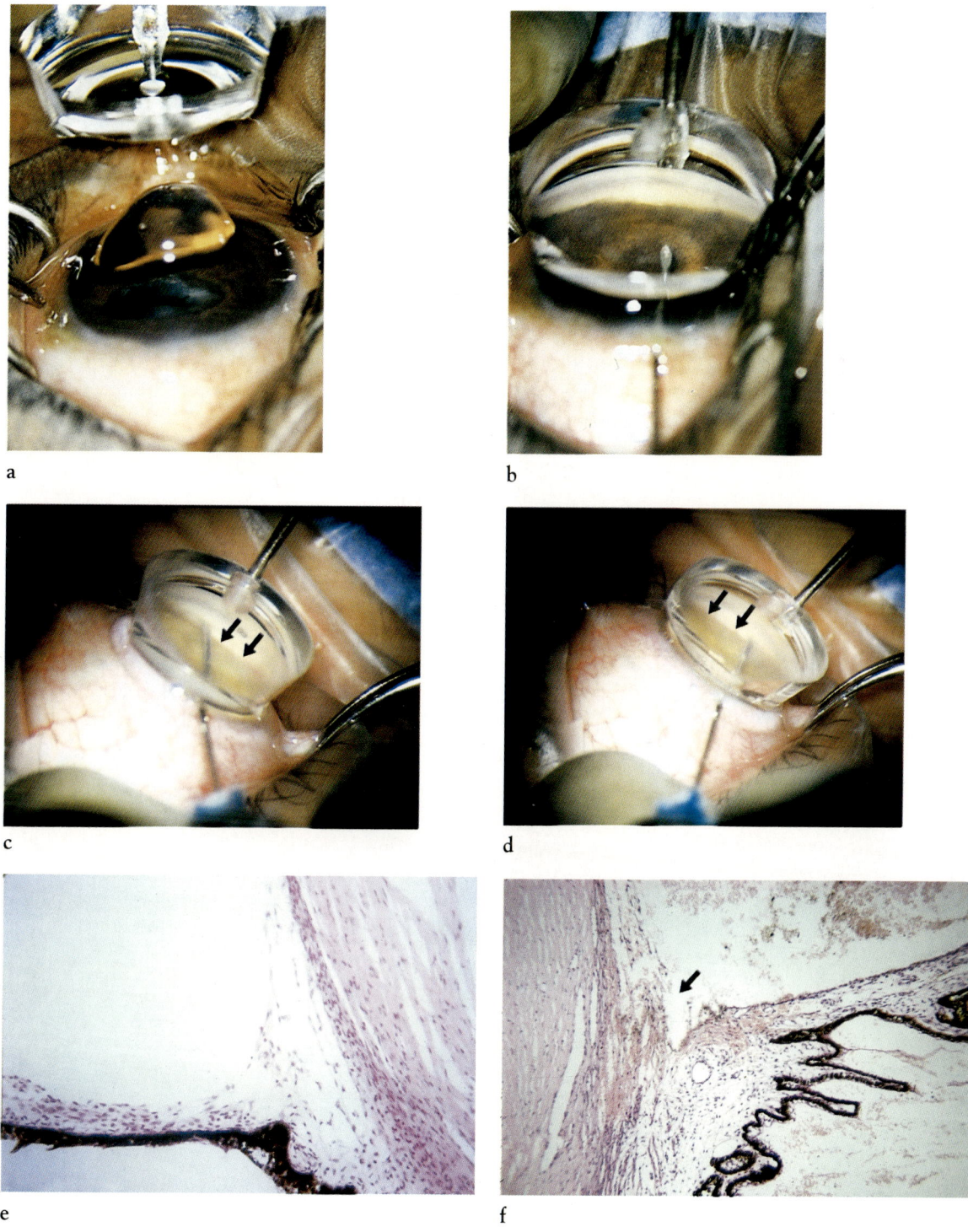

a

b

c

d

e

f

LASER IRIDOTOMY

III11a. A laser iridotomy is best performed with a contact lens, such as the Abraham iridotomy lens in this photo. The lens has a 66 diopter plano-convex button bonded to the front of the lens, which doubles the laser beam diameter at the level of the cornea, while reducing it to approximately one-half the original size on the iris. These changes in the diameter of the laser beam reduce the power density at the cornea to one-fourth the original level, while increasing it on the iris by a factor of four.

III11b. This photo shows the magnification of the iris, achieved with the Abraham iridotomy lens. This and similar lenses are available for use with either argon or neodymium:YAG lasers.

III11c–d. These two photos demonstrate the creation of a crater in the stroma of a medium brown iris using argon laser. The location of the iridotomy has been moved centrally to take advantage of the increased iris pigmentation for improved laser absorption. Standard settings for this stage of the argon laser iridotomy are 0.1 to 0.2 second duration, 50 microns spot size, and 700 to 1500 (average 1000) milliwatts. The first few applications may produce gas bubbles, as shown in III11c. The bubbles will usually float away from the treatment site, but can be dislodged by subsequent laser applications, if necessary. The stromal crater is then enlarged to approximately 500 microns in diameter with a cluster of several contiguous laser burns. Penetration of iris stroma to the pigment epithelium is usually indicated by a cloud of pigment, as shown in III11d.
  When treating either a dark brown, thick iris, or a light blue, thin iris, the duration of exposure for the first stage of argon laser iridotomy should be changed to 0.02 to 0.05 seconds for the brown iris and 0.5 seconds for the blue iris.

III11e–f. Once the stromal crater has been completed in stage 1 of argon laser iridotomy, the settings should be changed for elimination of pigment epithelium, as stage 2 of the procedure. Typical settings for this stage are 0.1 to 0.2 second duration, 50 to 100 microns, and approximately 500 milliwatts. These settings are used for irides of all colors, since the pigment epithelial layer is similar in all eyes. The lower intensity burns are needed for this stage of the procedure to avoid dislodging adjacent pigment epithelium, creating a so-called "cascade phenomenon," which causes further obstruction of the iridotomy. In III11e, pigment epithelium can be seen obstructing the iridotomy, most of which has been eliminated in III11f.

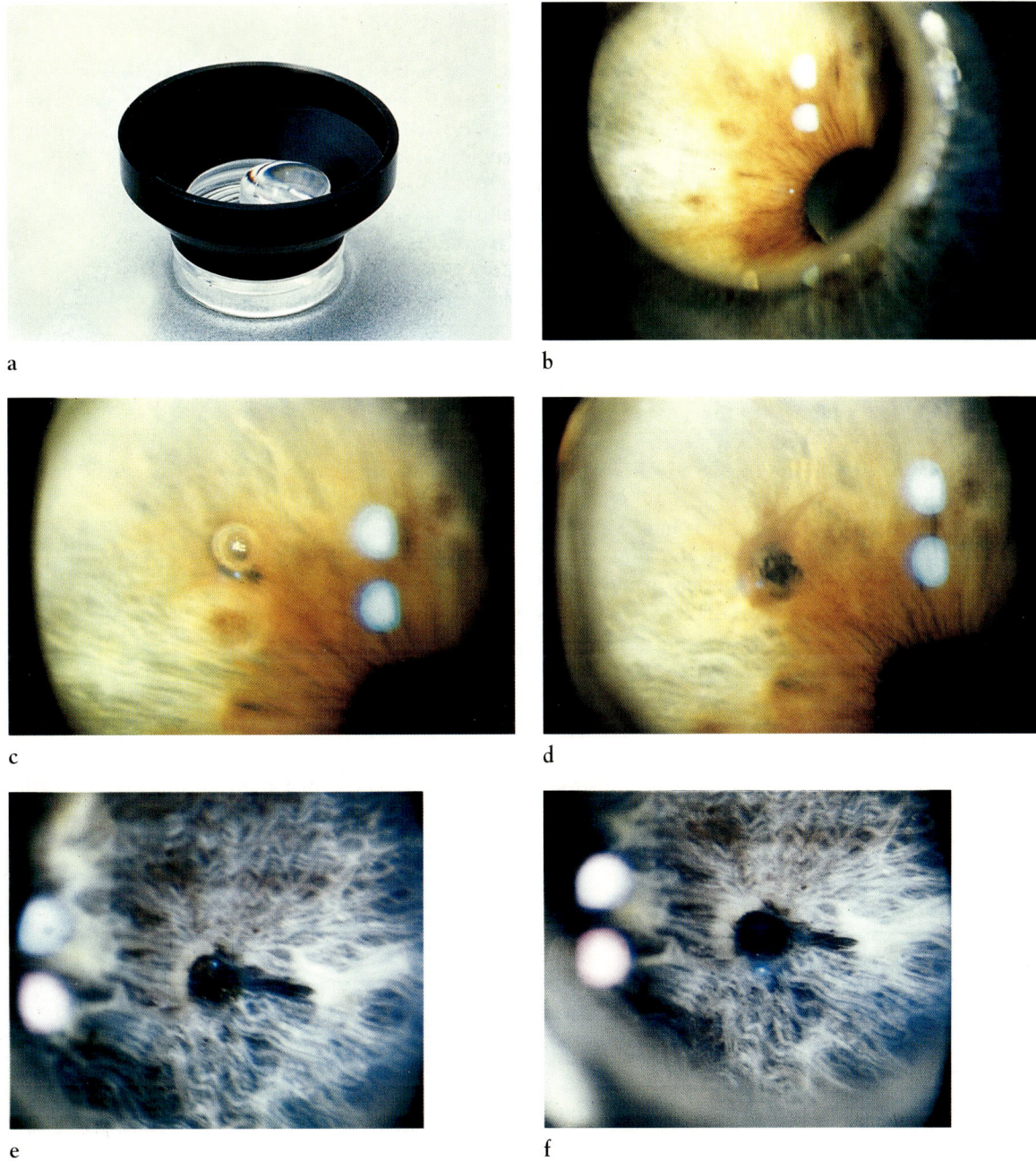

a

b

c

d

e

f

TRABECULECTOMY

Bridle Sutures

Adequate surgical exposure is a critical first step in a successful glaucoma filtering procedure. This involves the selection of a lid speculum that will not only maintain good separation of the lids, but will also elevate the lids slightly from the globe. Equally important in obtaining good surgical exposure is the bridle suture. The two most common types of bridle sutures used in glaucoma filtering surgery are the clear corneal suture and the superior rectus suture.

III14a–b.   Placement of a clear corneal bridle suture can be performed with a 6-0 silk suture on a tapered, cutting needle. The needle should be passed as deeply as possible into the stroma, without entering the anterior chamber. A placement that is too superficial may allow the suture to pull through the cornea. The width of the corneal bite should be 3 to 5 mm.

III14c.   The clear corneal bridle suture is then attached to the surgical drape of the cheek, using either a hemostat or tape. As seen in this photo, excellent exposure can be achieved with the clear corneal bridle suture. A disadvantage, however, is that it may cause distortion of the cornea and shallowing of the anterior chamber during the surgical procedure.

III14d.   Placement of a superior rectus bridle suture is usually performed with a 4-0 silk suture on a noncutting needle. With the eye turned down, the muscle is first grasped with forceps just posterior to the site of insertion through the closed conjunctiva. The muscle is then pulled away from the globe, and the needle is passed directly beneath the tips of the forceps. The bridle suture should then be pulled over the forehead to confirm that it has engaged the rectus muscle. Failure to incorporate the muscle into the suture bite will only cause stretching of the conjunctiva without adequate downward rotation of the eyeball. Once proper placement of the bridle suture has been confirmed, it is then attached to the head of the drape with a clamp or tape. The advantage of this bridle suture, compared with the clear corneal suture, is that it is farther away from the surgical site. Disadvantages, however, include possible subconjunctival bleeding and holes in the conjunctiva, which might leak postoperatively, although both are rare.

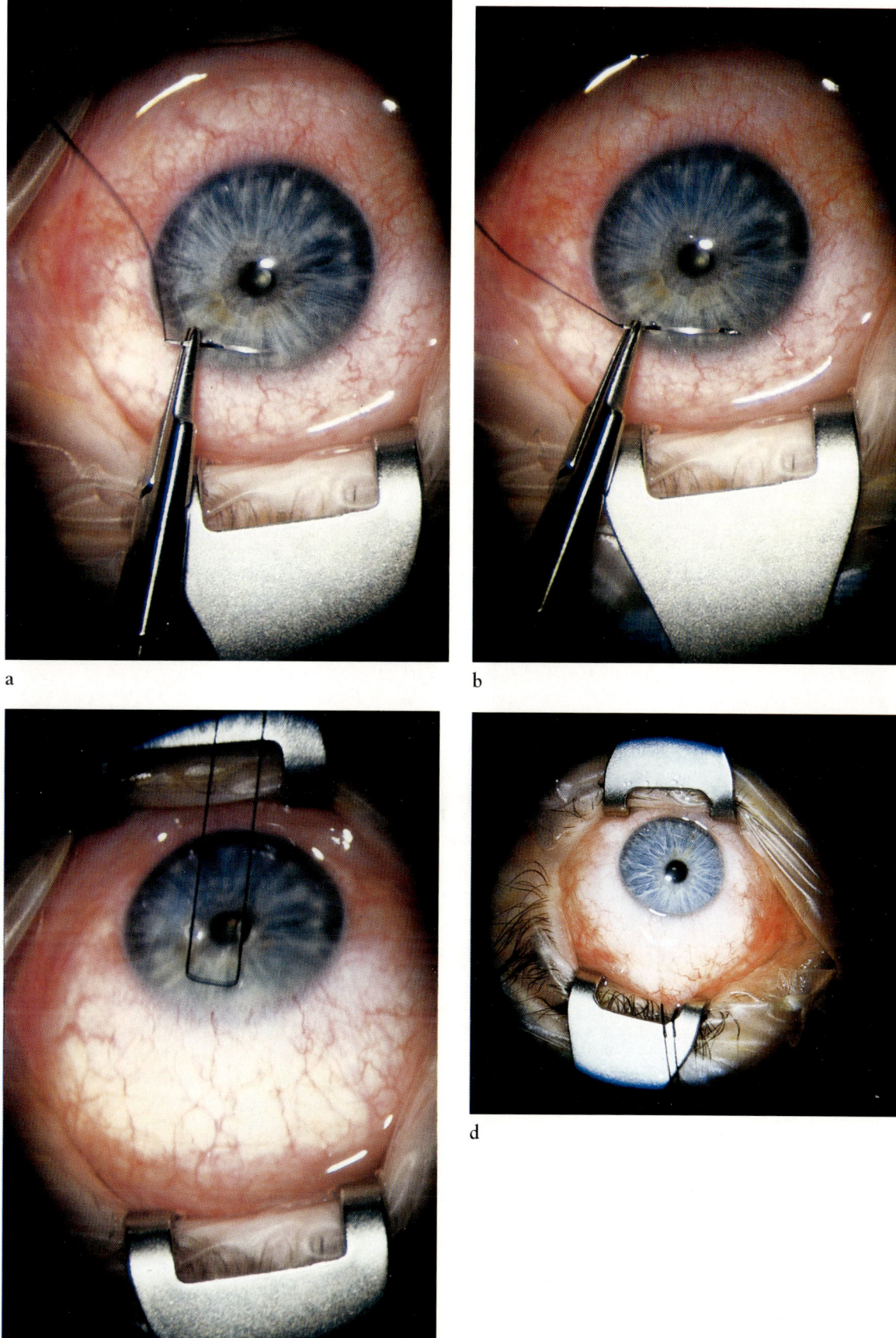

a

b

c

d

TRABECULECTOMY

Conjunctival-Tenon's Capsule Flap

The conjunctival flap in a trabeculectomy can either be limbus-based or fornix-based. Both techniques have advocates among glaucoma surgeons, and neither technique has proven superiority over the other. My personal preference is the limbus-based flap, which will be shown in this series of surgical photographs. This is not to say, however, that excellent results cannot be obtained with the fornix-based flap.

III15a. Conjunctiva is first incised approximately 8 mm behind the limbus. Surgeons also differ in their preferred location for the trabeculectomy as an initial procedure. Some place it at the 12 o'clock position, while others may prefer the temporal or nasal superior quadrant. If phacoemulsification is anticipated in the future (which is a potential for any phakic eye), it may be advisable to place the trabeculectomy in such a way that the surgeon's preferred site for phacoemulsification remains available. This point may be less important now with the popularity of clear cornea phacoemulsification. In any case, the conjunctival incision should be extended circumferentially for approximately 2 clock hours in the desired surgical site.

III15b. After the conjunctival incision is completed, Tenon's capsule should now be grasped and incised to the same extent as the overlying conjunctival incision. Care must be taken during the incision on Tenon's capsule to avoid underlying anterior ciliary arteries, which can produce brisk bleeding. This intraoperative complication is best avoided by pulling the Tenon's capsule well away from the sclera during the incision.

III15c. Having completed the incision through both conjunctiva and Tenon's capsule, the latter structure is then dissected from episclera to the limbus. This should be performed with blunt dissection whenever possible. In this photo, a blunt dissecting instrument has been created by filing the edge of a surgical blade. The side of the scissor blade may work equally well. Note that a surgical sponge is being used to retract the conjunctival-Tenon's capsule flap. It is advisable to minimize the manipulation of these structures with forceps to avoid the risk of tearing the tissue.

III15d. After the dissection of the conjunctival-Tenon's capsule flap is completed, it is advisable to confirm that the dissection has been carried all the way to the limbus. In this photo, the confirmation is accomplished by pulling the flap over the blunt dissecting blade and noting that the latter is adjacent to the limbus. Failure to adequately extend the dissection to the limbus may cause the subsequent placement of the drainage fistula to be too posterior, over uveal tissue.

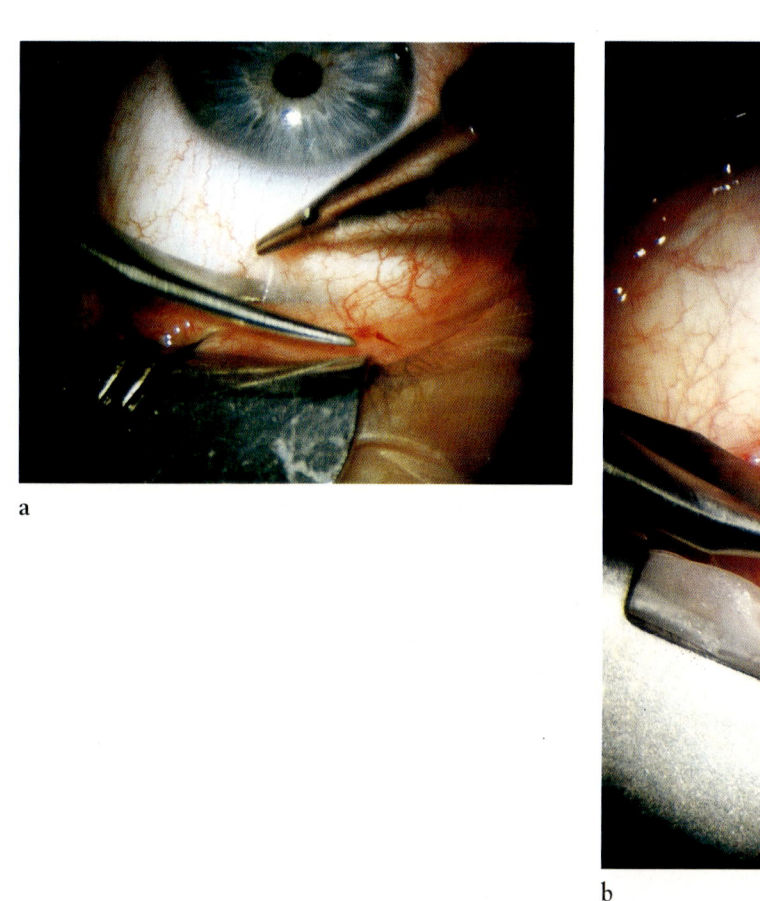

a

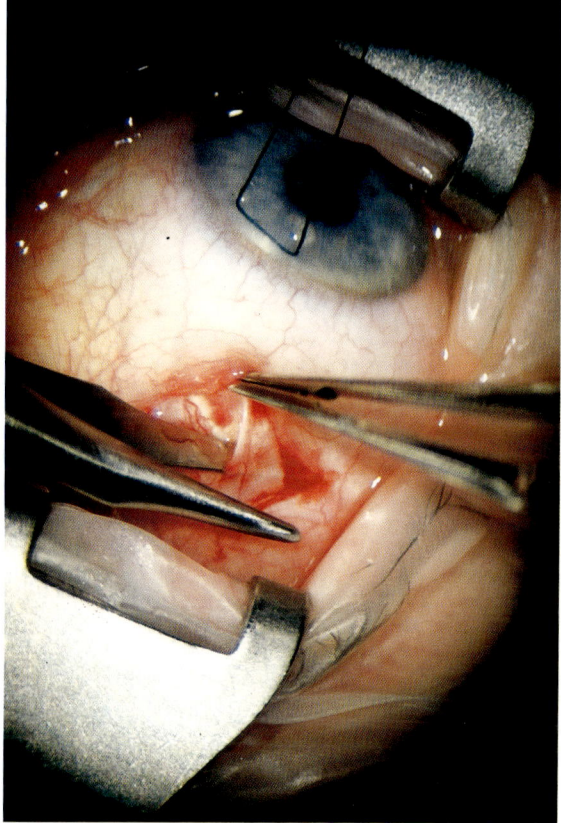

b

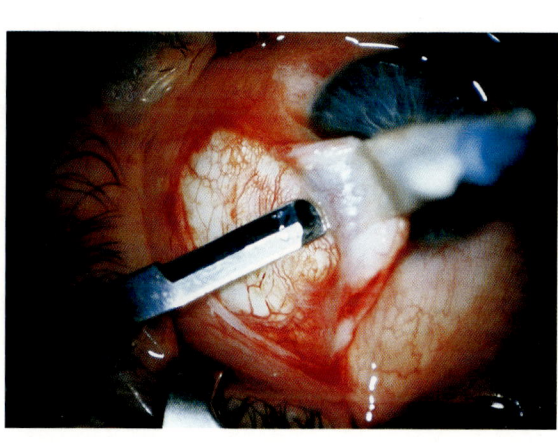

c

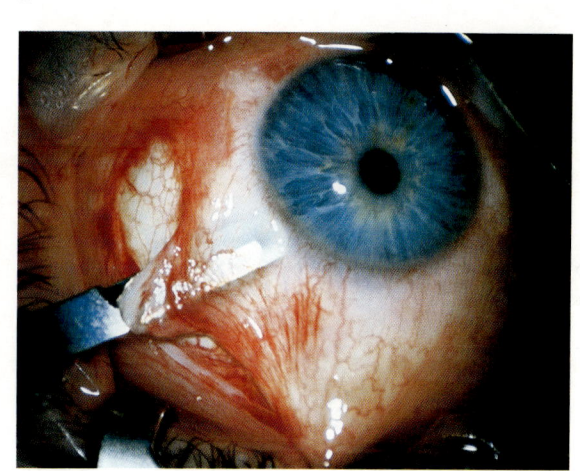

d

TRABECULECTOMY

Tenonectomy

Another aspect of the trabeculectomy procedure in which surgeons have differences of opinion involves whether to remove Tenon's capsule from the conjunctival flap. No clear evidence is available that this improves the long-term success rate with trabeculectomy. Furthermore, with the use of antimetabolites, many surgeons prefer to leave Tenon's capsule intact to provide a thicker filtering bleb and tighter wound closure. One advantage to tenonectomy, however, especially in the patient with a thick capsule, is a better view of the scleral sutures, in the event that postoperative laser suture lysis is required. In any case, Tenon's capsule can be removed in two ways: total tenonectomy or partial tenonectomy.

III16a–c. In performing a total tenonectomy, conjunctiva is first dissected from the underlying Tenon's capsule. Because these two structures are more tightly adherent than is the case between Tenon's capsule and episclera, sharp dissection with scissors is required. The technique involves clipping tissue strands where necessary and bluntly dissecting wherever possible by spreading the scissor blades. This technique runs a high risk of button-holing the conjunctiva, which can be minimized by always observing the tips of the blades beneath the conjunctiva, as show in III16a. Also note that non-toothed conjunctival forceps are being used to grasp the conjunctiva, again to avoid tearing that tissue.

Once the dissection of conjunctiva has been extended to the limbus, the conjunctiva is then reflected over the cornea with a moist sponge and the Tenon's capsule is incised adjacent to the limbus, as shown in III16b. Tenon's capsule is then bluntly dissected posteriorly and excised near the initial incision of the conjunctiva, as shown in III16c.

III16d–f. In performing partial tenonectomy, the surgeon bluntly dissects Tenon's capsule from episclera, as described on the previous page. The capsule is then grasped with two forceps and stretched posteriorly, as shown in III16d. The portion of Tenon's capsule that can be stretched away from the conjunctival flap is then excised along the margin of the conjunctival flap, as shown in III16e–f.

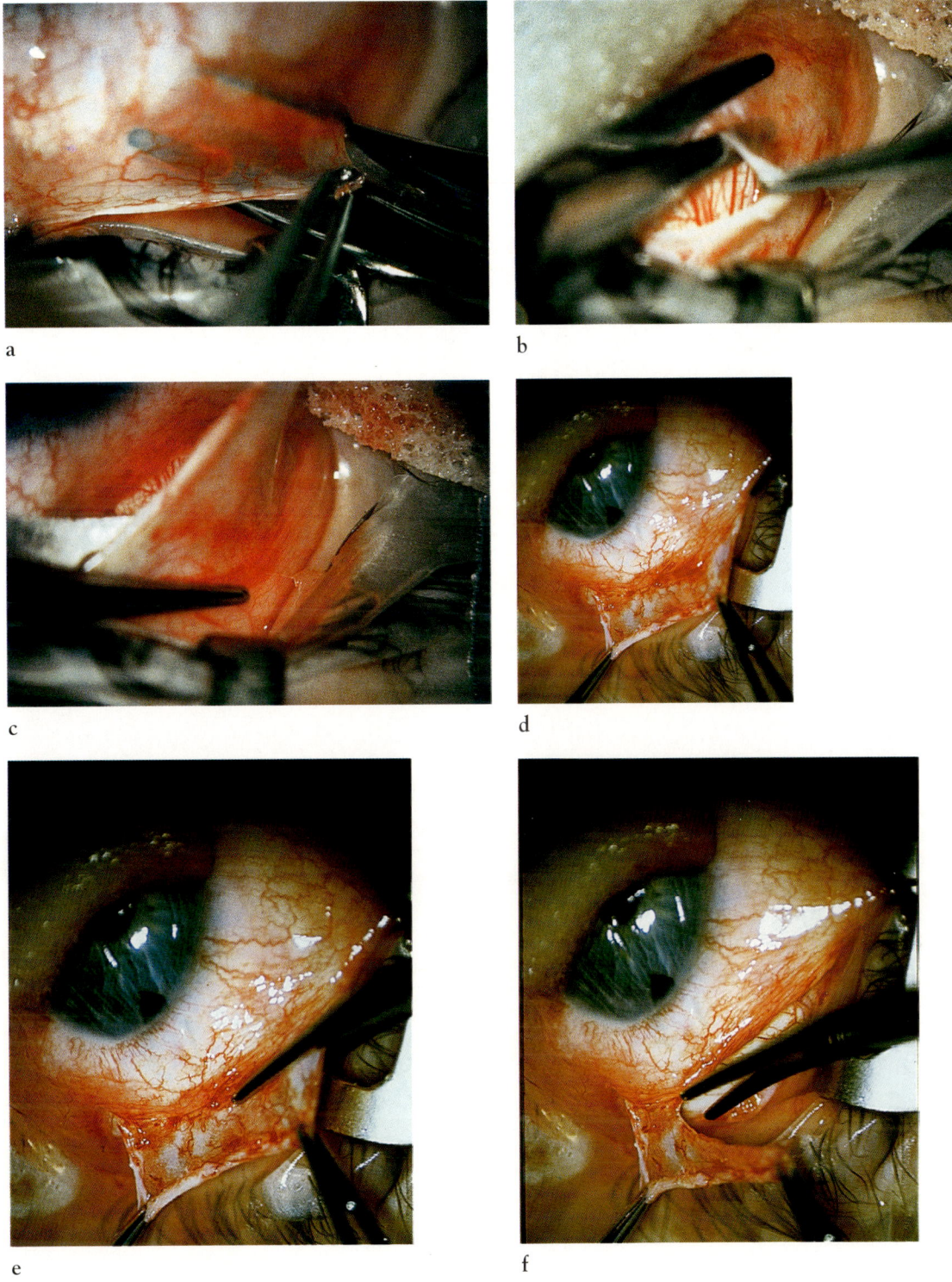

a

b

c

d

e

f

TRABECULECTOMY

Application of Antimetabolite

The leading cause of failure with any glaucoma filtering procedure is excessive scarring of the conjunctival bleb. The concept of pharmacologic modulation of wound healing, therefore, may be the most significant advance in glaucoma filtering surgery since it was introduced at the beginning of this century. The antimetabolites currently in use for this purpose, however, are also associated with significant postoperative complications, and the optimum protocol and indications for these adjunctive drugs have yet to be established. Nevertheless, they do provide a significant improvement in long-term pressure control, especially in high-risk patients, and are now commonly used in many trabeculectomy procedures.

The antimetabolites that have been used most commonly are 5-fluorouracil, which can be given either intraoperatively or postoperatively by subconjunctival injection, and mitomycin-C, which is administered intraoperatively as described below.

III17a.   A variety of vehicles have been used for delivering mitomycin-C during the trabeculectomy procedure. An instrument wipe (Merocel) can be used for this purpose, as shown in this photo. It can be cut to approximately 5 × 7 mm or to fit the required surgical area.

III17b.   Several drops of mitomycin-C are then placed on the sponge. Concentrations of mitomycin-C, as used by different surgeons, range from 0.2 to 0.5 mg/ml.

III17c–e.   The saturated sponge is then placed beneath the conjunctival-Tenon's capsule flap. Note in III17e that Tenon's capsule is pulled over the sponge, but the free margin of the conjunctival flap is allowed to retract slightly, which may help to avoid postoperative wound leak. The duration of exposure also varies among surgeons, with ranges of 1 to 5 minutes. Some surgeons titrate the time exposure according to the individual patient's risk for postoperative fibrosis.

III17f.   After removing the mitomycin-C sponge, the surgeon grasps Tenon's capsule with two forceps, and the assistant irrigates the exposed tissues with approximately 30 cc of balanced salt solution.

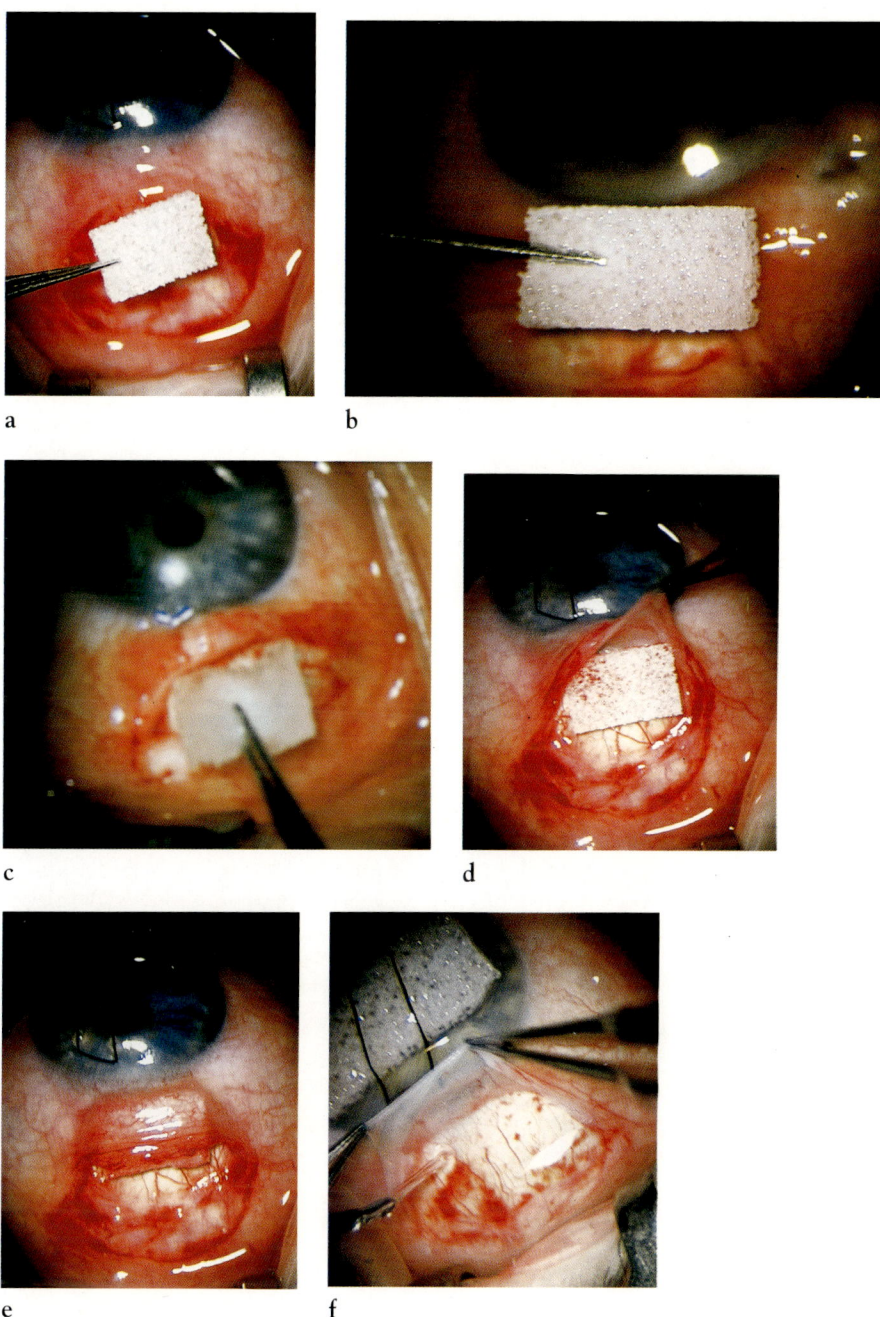

a

b

c

d

e

f

TRABECULECTOMY

Preparation of Scleral Flap

III18a. Hemostasis should be maintained throughout the trabeculectomy procedure. The cautery, however, should be minimal and gentle to avoid shrinkage or charring of tissues. One useful cautery instrument to achieve these goals is a 23-gage, tapered, blunt-tipped bipolar cautery unit, as shown in this photo.

III18b. The bipolar cautery unit is used to outline the area of the scleral flap. Although a square flap of approximately 5 × 5 mm is being used in this series, a triangular flap or several other shapes work equally well.

III18c–d. In order to achieve tight closure of the scleral flap, it is desirable to have sharp, clean margins. This is best accomplished with a diamond blade, as shown in these photos. Note that a surgical sponge is being used to gently retract the conjunctival-Tenon's capsule flap to avoid damage to these structures that might occur with the use of forceps. The sponge can also be used to stabilize the globe during the outlining of the scleral flap, since the diamond blade cuts with minimal resistance.

III18e. It is also advisable to create a thick scleral flap of approximately two-thirds scleral thickness in order to achieve tight wound closure. A helpful technique in maintaining a constant plane of dissection during the development of the scleral flap is to put tension on the flap with the forceps and sweep the edge of the blade across the fibers that are tented up between the two layers.

III18f. As in preparing the conjunctival-Tenon's capsule flap, it is important to ensure that the dissection of the scleral flap has extended to the limbus. This is best confirmed by noting at least 1 mm of gray zone, as noted in the anterior margin of the bed of scleral dissection in this photograph. The junction between the gray and white zones represents the location of scleral spur.

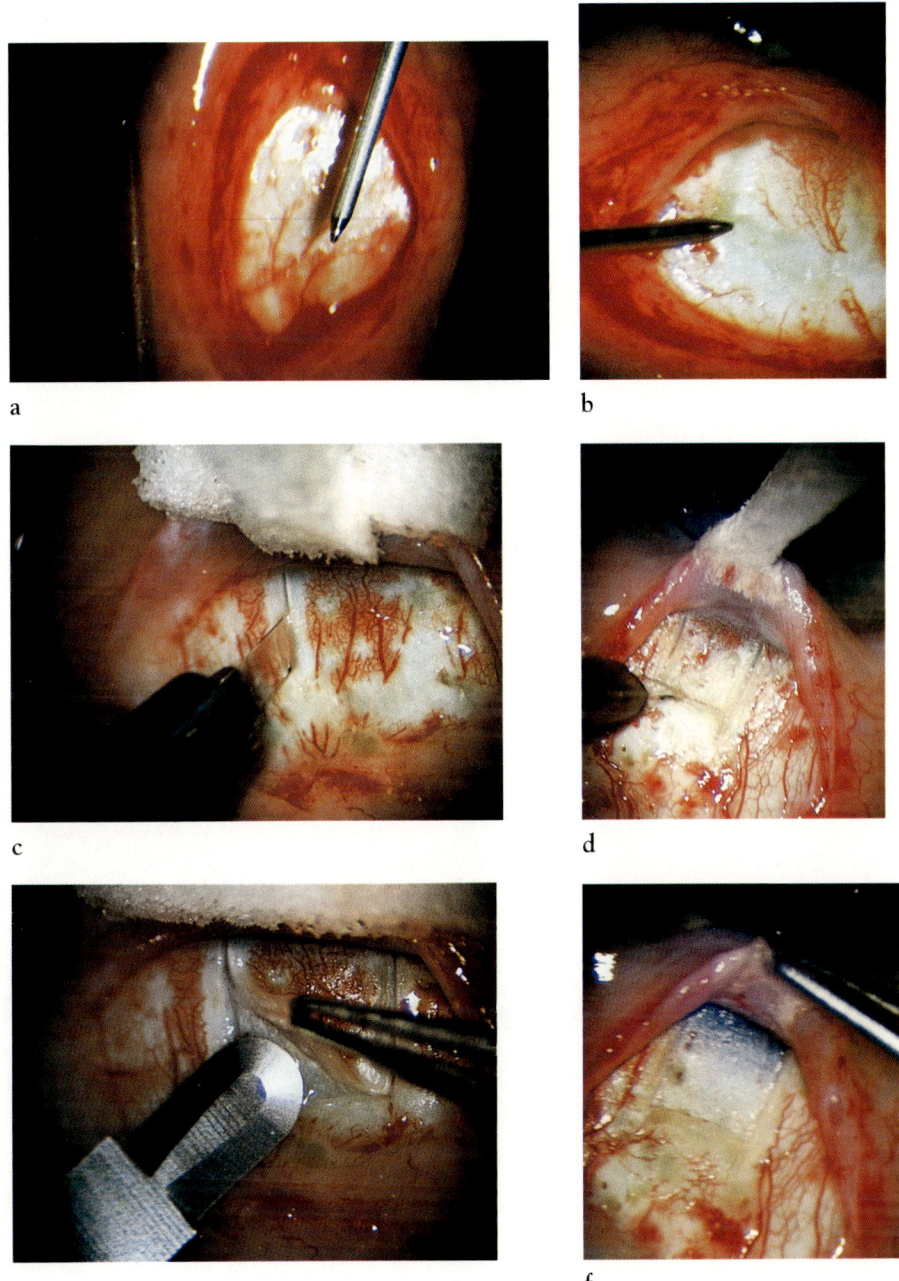

a

b

c

d

e

f

TRABECULECTOMY

Creation of the Fistula

III19a.   Before beginning creation of the fistula beneath the scleral flap, a paracentesis is made at the limbus in the inferior temporal quadrant for the purpose of injecting balanced salt solution into the anterior chamber later in the operation. This can be performed at the beginning of the operation. If antimetabolites are used, however, it may be advisable to wait until after that stage of the operation.

III19b.   The first step in creating the surgical fistula beneath the scleral flap is to incise the anterior border of the fistula, just posterior to the hinge of the scleral flap, with a sharp, pointed blade as shown in this photo. The blade is held parallel to the limbus with the cutting edge up, to minimize the risk of damaging the lens. The incision is extended to within approximately 0.5 mm of either side of the scleral flap.

III19c.   Radial incisions are then made with scissors on either side of the initial incision, approximately 0.5 mm from the edge of the bed of scleral dissection. These incisions should be carried to the junction between the gray and white ones.

III19d.   The three initial incisions have now created a flap of deep limbal tissue, which can be reflected to expose the trabecular meshwork and scleral spur (*arrow*).

III19e–f.   The fistula is then completed by cutting along the scleral spur under direct visualization, as shown in III19e. III19f shows the excised block of deep limbal tissue, which contains the trabecular meshwork (*arrow*).

An alternative technique for creation of the scleral flap, preferred by many glaucoma surgeons, is to use a sclerectomy punch to excise tissue from the posterior margin of the initial limbal incision.

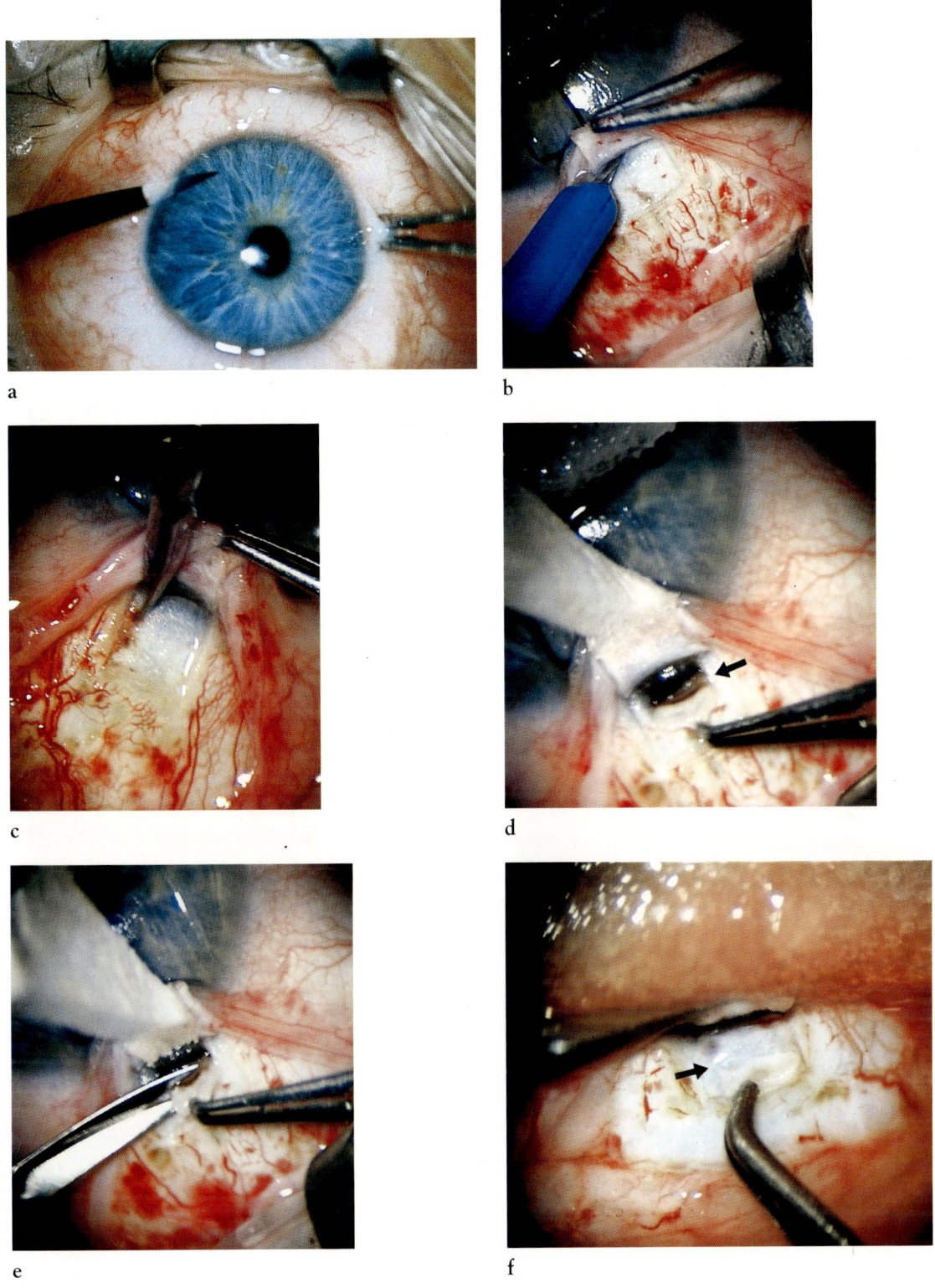

a

b

c

d

e

f

TRABECULECTOMY

Peripheral Iridectomy

III20a–b.   An important intraoperative technique to avoid obstruction of the fistula by iris postoperatively is to create a large peripheral iridectomy. This is accomplished by grasping the peripheral iris with forceps, pulling it through the fistula, and excising it near the fistula with a single cut of the scissors.

III20c.   After cutting the peripheral iridectomy, the edges of the iris may remain trapped in the fistula. The iris should be gently reposited into the anterior chamber either by stroking over the cornea from peripheral to central with a blunt instrument, such as a muscle hook, or by gently irrigating balanced salt solution through the fistula. This should be done until the pupil is round and the peripheral iridectomy can clearly be seen through the peripheral cornea.

III20d.   Another structure that may obstruct the fistula postoperatively is the ciliary processes. If the tips of these structures are visible through the peripheral iridectomy, it is possible to apply light bipolar cautery, as shown in this photo, which causes the processes to retract and minimizes the risk of postoperative obstruction of the fistula.

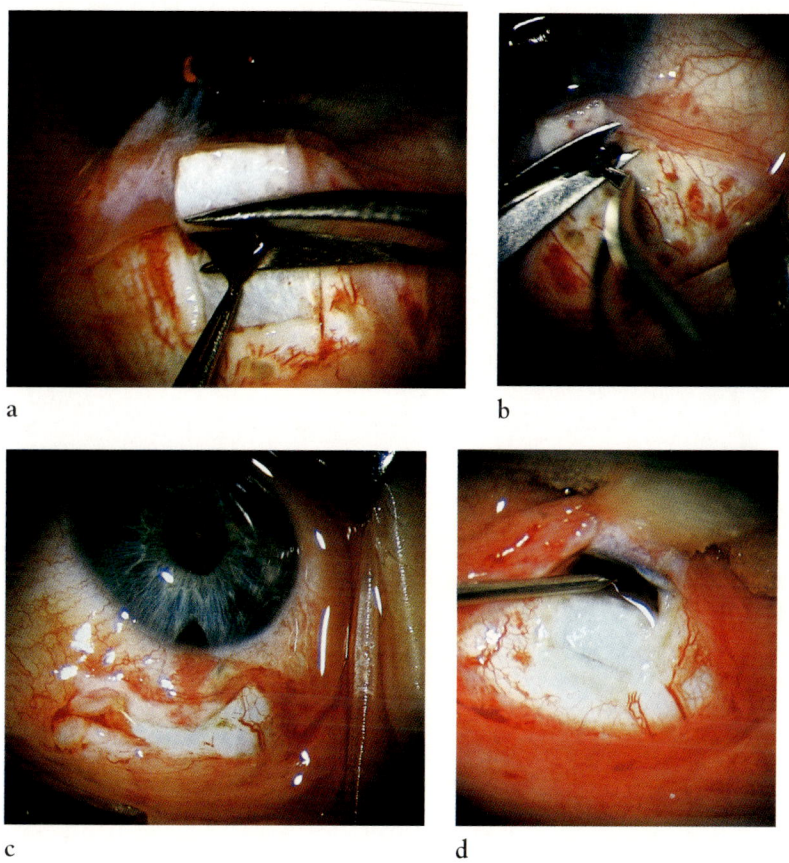

a

b

c

d

TRABECULECTOMY

Closure of Scleral Flap

III21a.   Tight closure of the scleral flap is desirable, especially with the adjunctive use of antimetabolites, to avoid the postoperative complications of hypotony and flat anterior chamber. In this case, five 10-0 nylon sutures are used to achieve tight closure of the scleral flap.

III21b.   As shown in this photo, two of the five sutures are placed at the two posterior corners of the scleral flap. The other three are placed along the three sides. It is important to notice, however, that the two sutures on the lateral sides are fairly close to the limbus, where flow of aqueous is most likely to occur. These two sutures, therefore, provide the main control of aqueous flow and are the sutures most likely to be cut with the laser if flow is not adequate postoperatively.

III21c.   It is advisable to place all five sutures and then inspect beneath the scleral flap before tying the sutures. The main reason for this technique is that bleeding may occur on the posterior side of the scleral flap during placement of the sutures, and this is more difficult to approach if the flap has already been partially closed.

III21d–e.   After the surgeon inspects beneath the scleral flap to ensure that the fistula is patent and no bleeding is present, he or she then ties the five sutures, as shown in III21d, and rotates them to bury each knot, as shown in III21e.

III21f.   After the the scleral flap is closed, balanced salt solution is then injected through the previously prepared paracentesis to test the closure of the scleral flap. During this procedure, it is desirable to see the anterior chamber deepen and the eye become firm before the balanced salt solution slowly oozes around the margins of the scleral flap. If the flow around the flap margins is too brisk, and the anterior chamber tends to flatten, additional sutures must be placed in the flap. Less often a suture may need to be loosened, if there is no flow around the margins of the scleral flap.

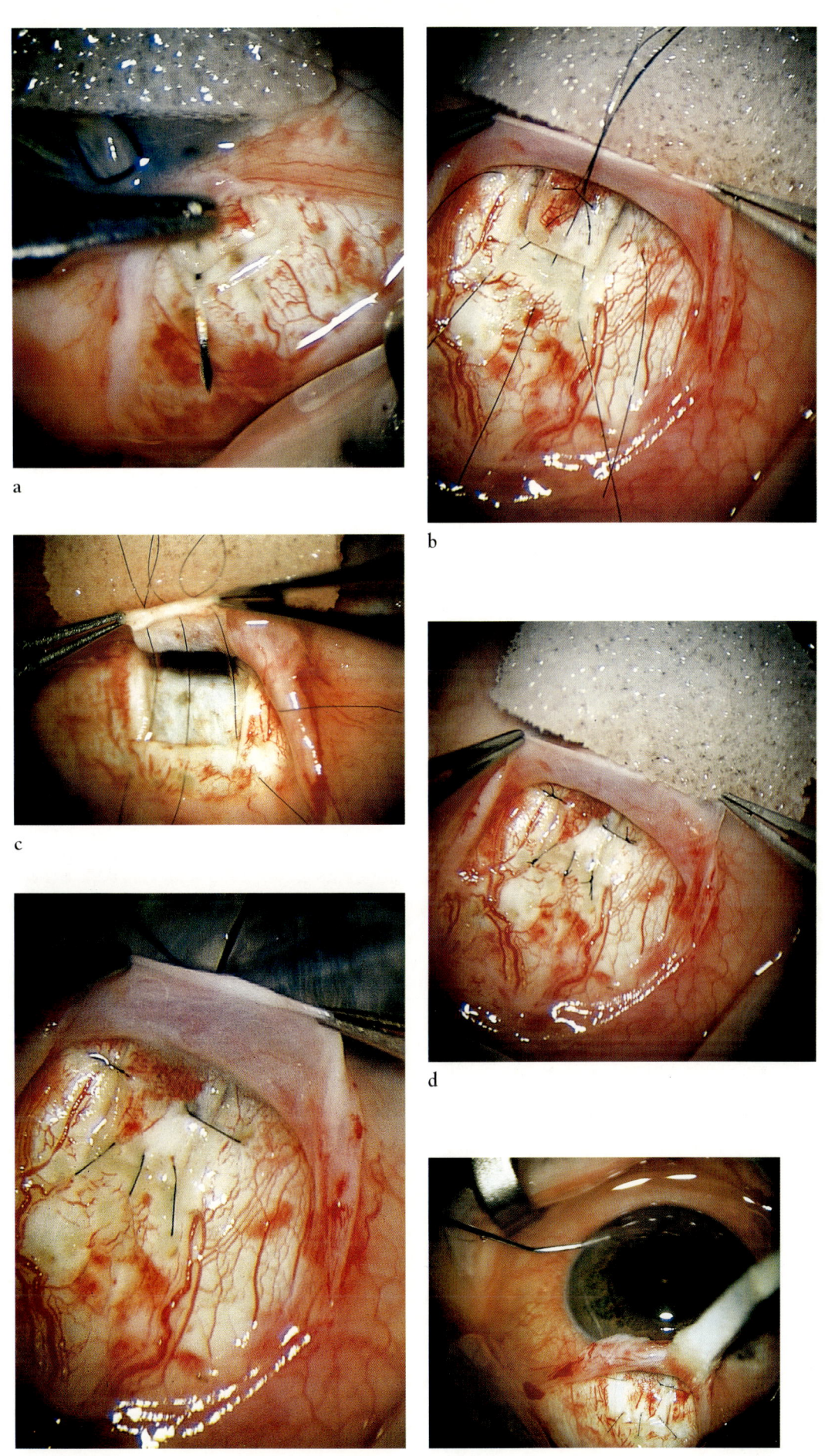

a

b

c

d

e

f

LIBRARY
POST GRADUATE CENTRE
KETTERING GENERAL HOSPITAL

TRABECULECTOMY

Releasable Sutures

As noted on previous pages, an effort should be made to maintain tight closure of the scleral flap. It is better to be faced with an elevated intraocular pressure that can be corrected by releasing a suture in the scleral flap in the early postoperative course than to be faced with hypotony and a flat anterior chamber. One technique for releasing sutures in the scleral flap postoperatively is the use of laser suture lysis. In some cases, however, this may be difficult because of either a thick Tenon's capsule, which prevents a good view of the suture, or the lack of a readily available laser unit. In these cases, a releasable suture may be preferable. A number of different techniques for releasable sutures have been described. The technique shown here was developed by Murray A. Johnstone, M.D.

III22a. A double-armed 10-0 or 9-0 nylon suture on cutting needles is passed from peripheral cornea, beneath the conjunctival flap, and out on the scleral side just behind the hinge of the conjunctival flap on either side of the scleral flap.

III22b. The two arms of the nylon suture should be adjacent to the lateral margins of the scleral flap. To ensure a proper relationship between the sutures and the margin of the flap, it may be easier to prepare the scleral flap after placing the two arms of the suture.

III22c. After completing the trabeculectomy procedure in the same manner as described on the previous pages, a second nylon suture is passed through the two posterior corners of the scleral flap and the adjacent scleral. The suture is then tied loosely (*arrow*), so that the scleral flap can elevate approximately 0.5 mm from the scleral bed.

III22d. One arm of the initial, double-armed suture is then passed beneath the posterior portion of the second suture (*arrow*).

III22e. By putting tension on the two arms of the initial suture and tying them tightly, tension is also placed on the second suture, which pulls the scleral flap closed posteriorly. The x-shaped arrangement between the two sutures also tamponades the rest of the scleral flap.

III22f. This postoperative view shows the corneal portion of the first suture (*arrow*), which becomes buried beneath epithelium. It is usually removed 1 to 2 months postoperatively, or sooner, if necessary.

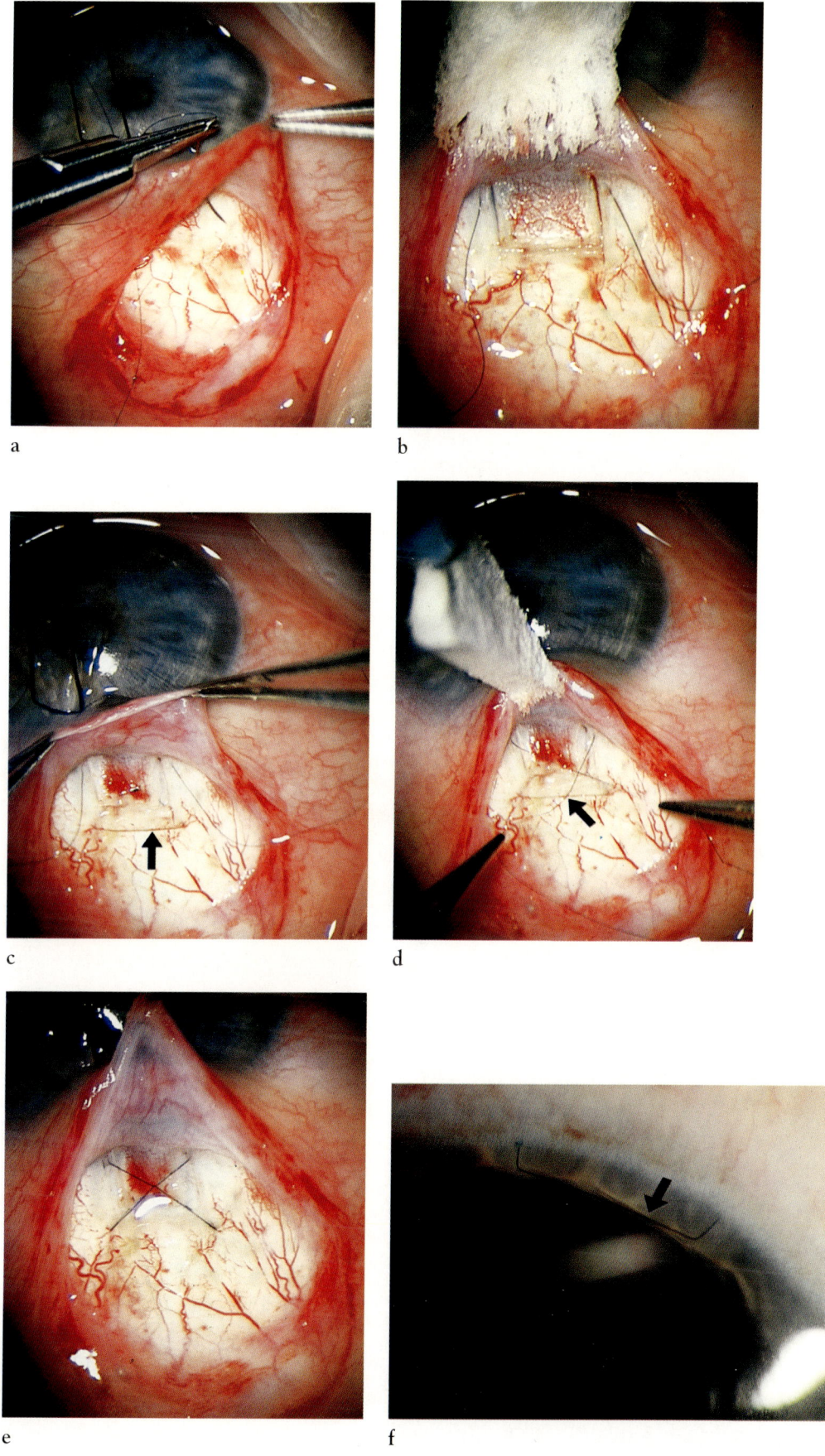

a

b

c

d

e

f

TRABECULECTOMY

Closure of Conjunctival Flap

III23a. Tight closure of the conjunctival-Tenon's capsule flap is also critical to avoid wound leak that can lead to hypotony, flat anterior chamber, and loss of the filtering bleb. A useful suture for this stage of the operation is a 10-0 absorbable suture, such as polyglycolic acid or polyglactin, on a tapered, wire needle. In this case, a double, running closure is being used, with closure of Tenon's capsule, shown in this figure.

III23b. After Tenon's capsule is closed, the conjunctival flap is now closed with the same absorbable suture. Closure of the conjunctiva is the most critical of these two layers. It is advisable to take a fairly generous bite of conjunctiva from the posterior side of the wound to bunch the tissue up between each bite, which tends to promote water-tight closure.

III23c. After the conjunctival flap is closed (*arrow*), the incision line should have a "beaded appearance" because of the bunching up of conjunctival tissue between each suture bite.

III23d. Balanced salt solution is again injected into the anterior chamber via the paracentesis. The purpose of this technique is to ensure that the fistula is patent, as evidenced by the elevation of the conjunctival flap, and that the conjunctival closure is watertight, as evidenced by the retention of the elevated bleb and deep anterior chamber.

III23e–f. After injecting balanced salt into the anterior chamber and observing elevation of the filtering bleb, it is also advisable to carefully inspect the margin of the conjunctival flap to ensure watertight closure. Some surgeons prefer to use fluorescein to detect small leaks, although close inspection under the operating microscope is usually sufficient to detect any significant leaks, which may require additional suturing.

At the end of the procedure, the eye is dressed with atropine and antibiotic-steroid ointments. Postoperative management also includes the use of antibiotics, steroids, and atropine.

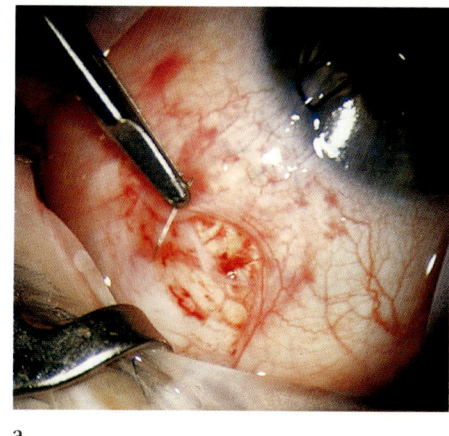

a

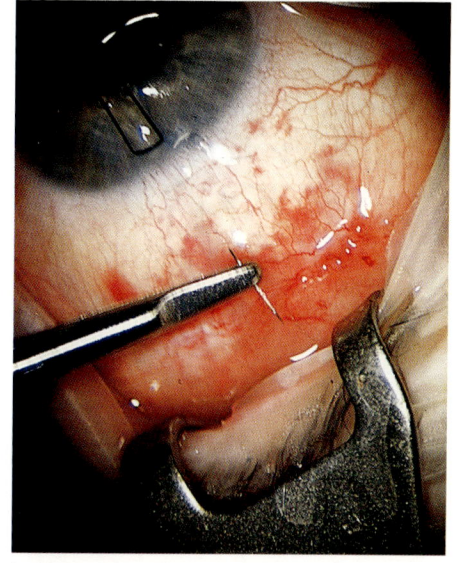

b

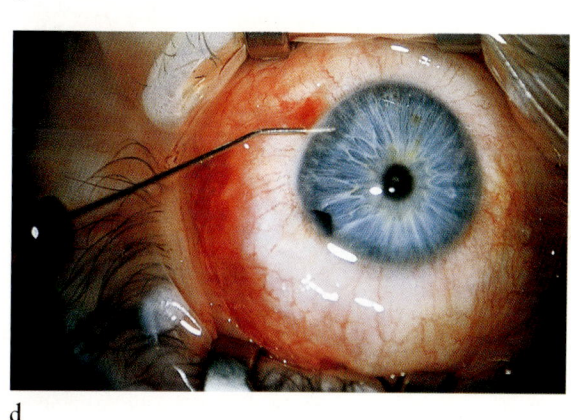

d

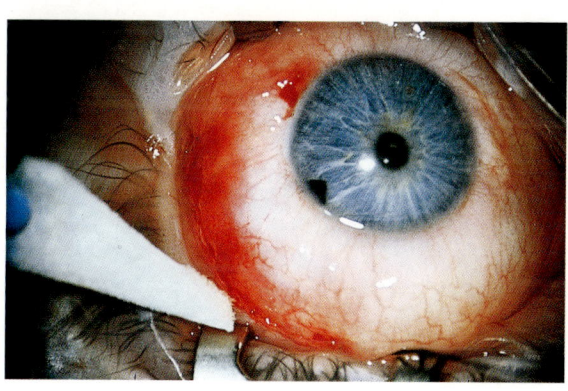

c

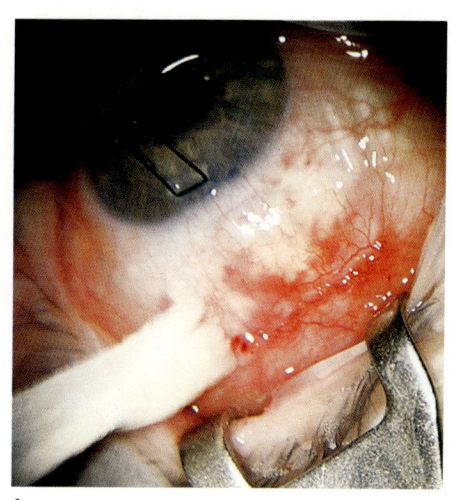

e

f

TRABECULECTOMY

Laser Sclerostomies

An alternative to the use of scissors or a sclerectomy punch in creating the fistula for a glaucoma filtering procedure is to use laser energy to create a sclerostomy. This can be done from either an ab-interno or ab-externo approach.

III24a. With internal laser sclerostomy, the conjunctiva near the limbus in the intended surgical site is first elevated with a subconjunctival injection, such as balanced salt solution. A small incision is then made at the limbus approximately 180° from the intended surgical site. As shown in this photo, the laser probe is then inserted through the incision, passed across the anterior chamber, and positioned at the site of the intended fistula. Laser energy is then used to create the full-thickness fistula beneath the elevated subconjunctival space.

III24b. This gonioscopic view in an eye after internal laser sclerostomy shows the patent sclerostomy (*arrow*). Note also the cauterized peripheral iris adjacent to the fistula. Several lasers, including argon, neodymium:YAG, and semiconductor diode, have been evaluated for internal laser sclerostomy, which is still under investigation.

III24c–d. With ab-externo laser sclerostomy, a Holmium laser probe is most commonly used. In III24c, the conjunctiva has been elevated at the limbus with the injection of a viscoelastic, and an incision several millimeters from the limbus is created with a 30-gauge needle, marked with Rose Bengal. The laser probe is then inserted through the needle hole. III24d shows the placement of the laser probe with the tip at the limbus in the site of the intended sclerostomy. The Holmium laser probe emits the laser energy at a right angle to the shaft of the probe, which allows creation of a full-thickness sclerostomy with the probe positioned as shown in this photo.

III24e. This gonioscopic view of an eye after ab-externo Holmium laser sclerostomy shows the properly placed sclerostomy site anterior to the trabecular meshwork (*arrow*). Pigment in this African-American patient clearly demarcates the extent of the sclerostomy opening, which is approximately 750 microns in length internally.

III24f. This light microscopic photo shows the full-thickness sclerostomy (*arrow*) and the adjacent scleral damage in a rabbit eye after ab-externo Holmium laser sclerostomy.

(Figures III24a and III24b were provided courtesy of Eve J. Higginbotham, M.D.; Figures III24c and III24e were provided courtesy of Wayne F. March, M.D.; Fig III24d reprinted with permission from Iwach A, Hoskins HD, Jr: Laser sclerostomy for management of glaucoma. Curr Opinion in Ophthalmol 1993;4:85–92. Fig III24f reprinted with permission from Hoskins HD, Jr: Subconjunctival THC: YAG laser sclerostomy ab externo in the rabbit. Ophthalmic Surg 1990;21(8):589–592.)

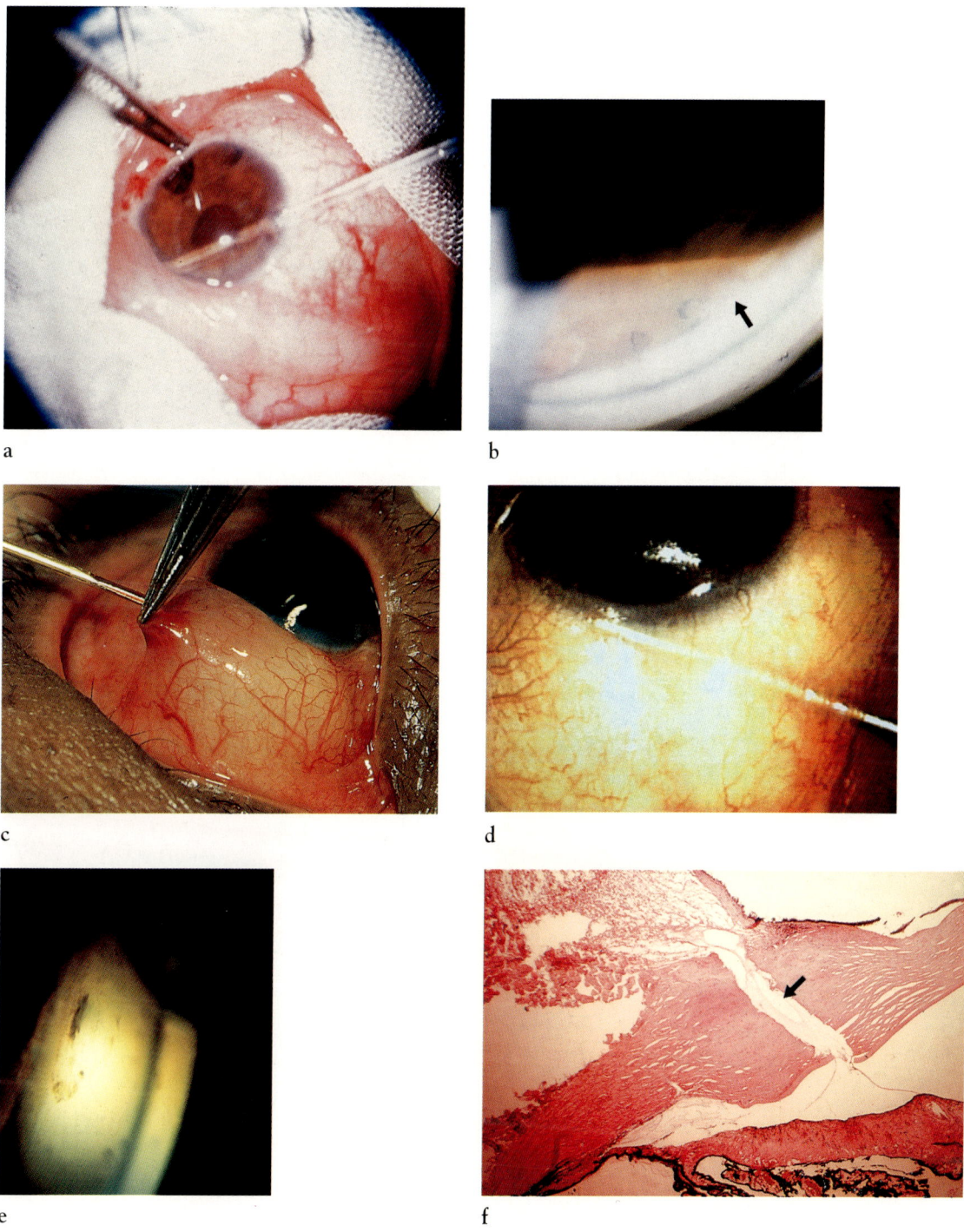

a

b

c

d

e

f

TRABECULECTOMY

Glaucoma Filtering Blebs

With some rare exceptions, all successful glaucoma filtering procedures will have a "filtering bleb," or elevation of the conjunctiva near the site of the fistula. The blebs may vary considerably in appearance, with some being low, diffuse, and partially vascularized, while others are more elevated, circumscribed, and avascular. A few types of blebs are shown on this page, and others will be demonstrated subsequently under Complications of Filtering Surgery.

III25a–b.   These two photos show the successful filtering blebs in the right (III25a) and left (III25b) eyes of the same patient. Mitomycin-C was used in this patient because of bilateral pseudophakia. Note the elevated, circumscribed appearance of the bleb in the right eye, which was photographed 3 months after surgery, and the more diffuse appearance of the bleb in the left eye, which was photographed 9 months postoperatively.

III25c.   Mitomycin-C was also used in the creation of this filtering procedure. The filtering bleb, however, is excessively avascular and thin-walled, which is a potential complication with the adjunctive use of antimetabolites, which will be discussed under Complications of Filtering Surgery.

III25d.   This filtering bleb was created in an inferior quadrant, because of scarring in the superior quadrants. This location, however, is now known to be associated with a high incidence of endophthalmitis, and preferred procedures in such cases include a drainage implant device or a cyclodestructive procedure.

III25e–f.   These two filtering blebs were created with ab externo Holmium laser sclerostomy. III25e was obtained 18 months after surgery, and III25f was taken 2 years postoperatively. Note the visualization of the sclerostomy beneath the filtering bleb in III25f.

(Figures III25e and III25f were provided courtesy of Wayne F. March, M.D.)

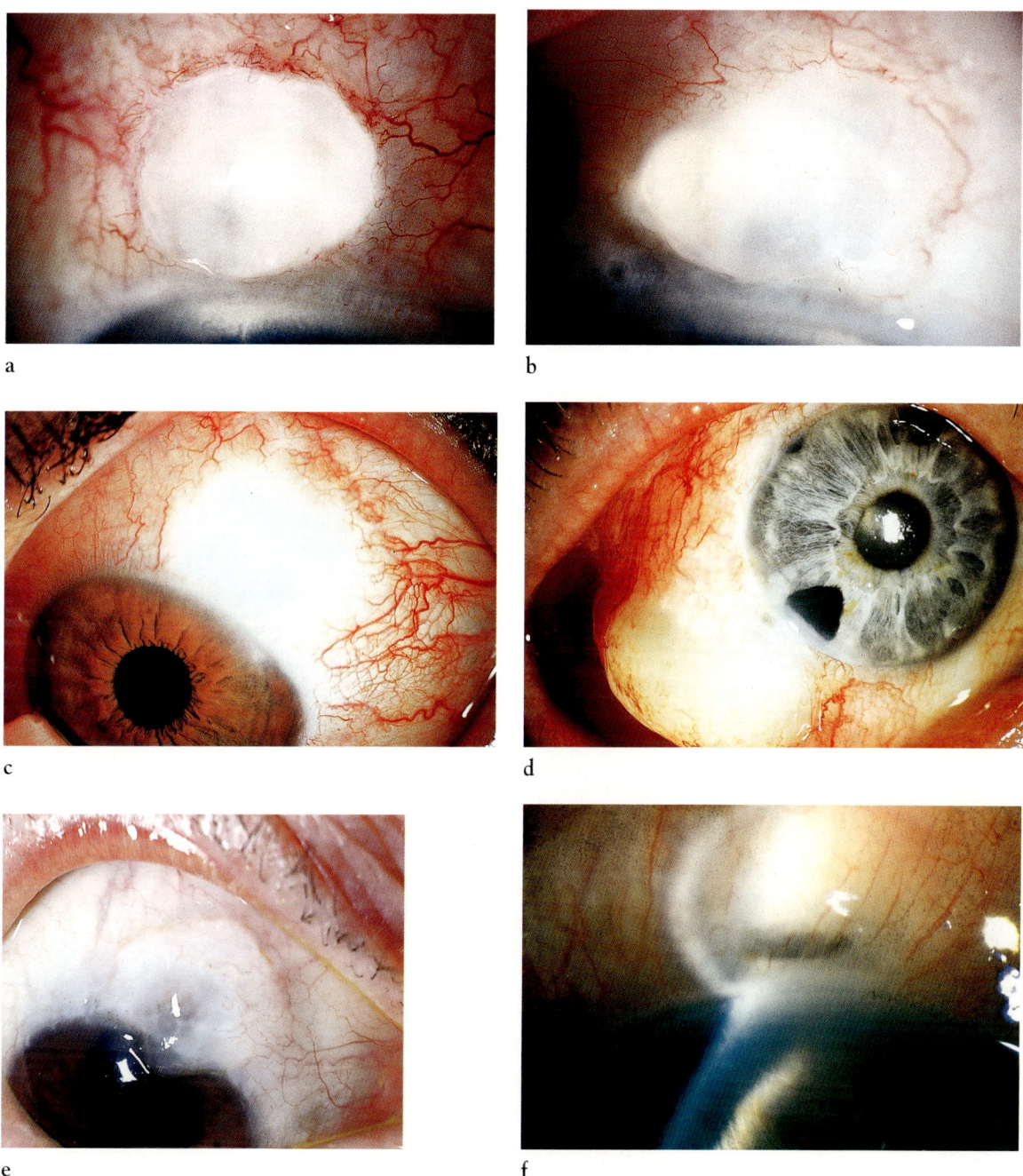

COMPLICATIONS OF FILTERING SURGERY

Shallow/Flat Anterior Chamber

III26a.   A common early postoperative complication of glaucoma filtering surgery is a shallow or flat anterior chamber. When associated with a low intraocular pressure, this usually indicates an overfiltering bleb or a wound leak. Management depends upon the degree of anterior chamber loss. If a narrow space exists between the cornea and lens and a gentle touch between cornea and peripheral iris, with no corneal decompensation, as shown in this photo, conservative management is indicated. Most of these eyes will undergo spontaneous deepening of the anterior chamber during the first 2 postoperative weeks. If central lens-cornea touch, with corneal decompensation, occurs, immediate intervention is indicated, as discussed on this and subsequent pages.

III26b–c.   If the anterior chamber is shallow, but the intraocular pressure is elevated, three possibilities must be considered: malignant glaucoma, delayed suprachoroidal hemorrhage, and pupillary block. The first two are characterized by a forward shift of the lens-iris diaphragm, as shown in III26b, while pupillary block is characterized by a deeper central anterior chamber with forward bowing of the peripheral iris (iris bombé), as shown in III26c.

III26d–g.   If the anterior chamber is flat and the intraocular pressure is low because of either an overfiltering bleb or bleb leakage, pressure patching with focal tamponade is often the first step in the management of the problem. A fusiform-shaped cotton ball is placed over the upper lid in the location corresponding to the surgical fistula (III26d). An oval gauze pad is folded and placed beneath the brow (III26d) and a second oval pad is placed over the first pad and the brow. Tape is then stretched tightly from the forehead to the cheek to press the pads against the eye (III26f). When properly applied, the tension created by the tape should create folds in the forehead and cheek. This patch should only be left on during the daytime, because the eye will rotate up during sleep, placing the tamponade over the cornea.

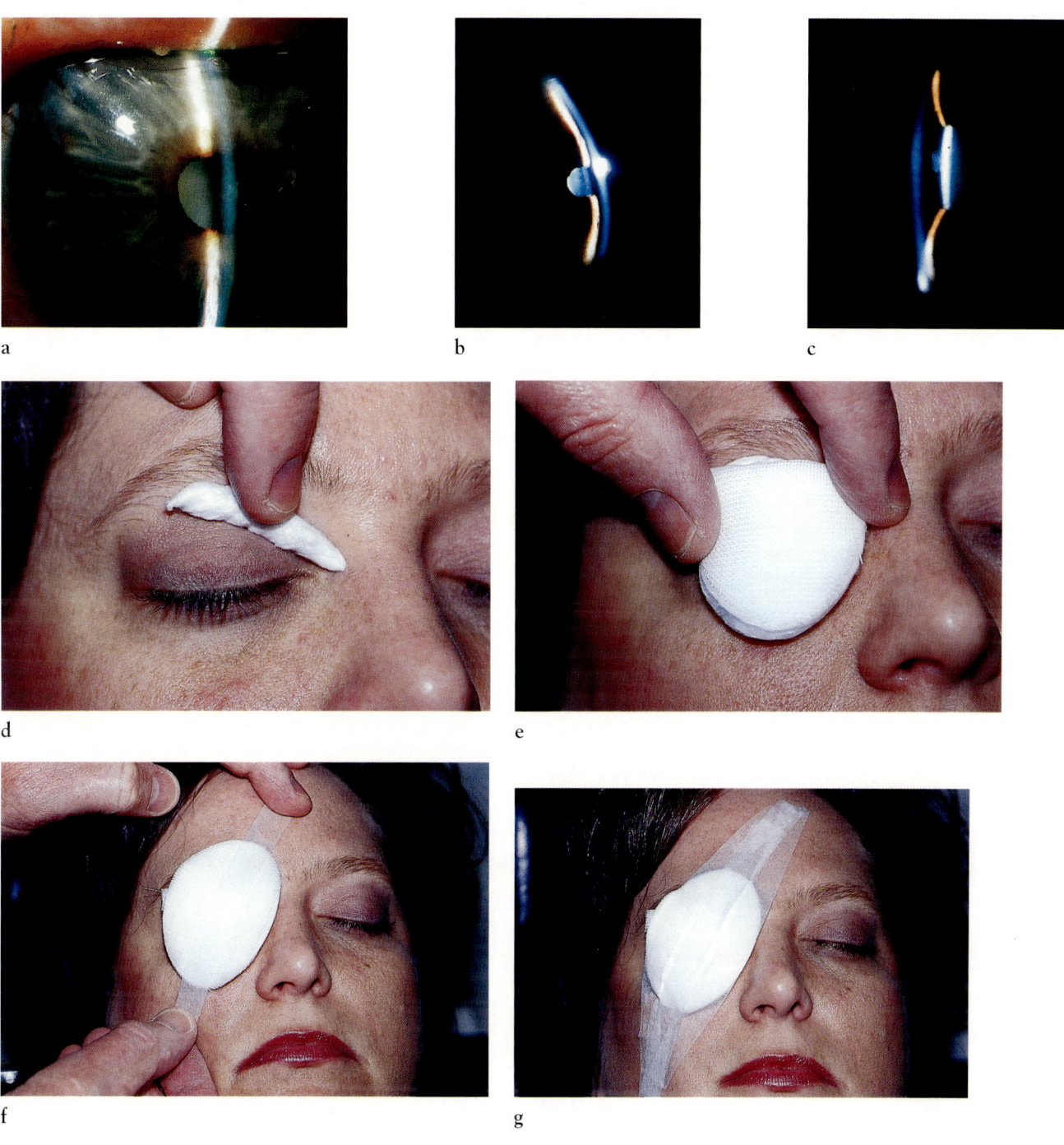

a

b

c

d

e

f

g

COMPLICATIONS OF FILTERING SURGERY

Shallow/Flat Anterior Chamber

III27a–b. When pressure patching alone is inadequate to correct an overfiltering or leaking bleb, the next step may be to use a scleral shell, such as the Simmons shell, developed by Dr. Richard J. Simmons. As shown in these two photos, the shell is thickened in one peripheral quadrant (outlined in black) to provide tamponade over the surgical site. Two rows of holes are also provided for placing and positioning the shell.

III27c. This photo shows the proper placement of the Simmons shell with the area of tamponade over the surgical site. Once the shell is properly positioned, a pressure patch is applied, as described on the previous page.

III27d. One problem with the shell is the tendency for rotation, in which case the tamponade may no longer cover the surgical site. One solution to this problem, as first suggested by Dr. Robert Ritch, is to attach a silk suture through one of the holes in the shell and tape the suture to the skin just temporal to the eye.

III27e–f. It is advisable to examine the patient on a daily basis, while he or she is wearing the Simmons shell. The pressure patch is removed, but the shell is left in place, and the patient is examined at the slit lamp to evaluate the change in anterior chamber depth and to ensure that the shell is properly positioned. The pressure patch is then reapplied; this is usually continued for 3 days, or until the anterior chamber is deep and any leaking site has closed.

(All photographs on this page were provided courtesy of Richard J. Simmons, M.D.) Figure III27d reprinted with permission from Joiner DW, Liebmann JM, Ritch R: A modification of the use of the glaucoma tamponade shell. Ophthal Surv 1989; 20(6):441–442.

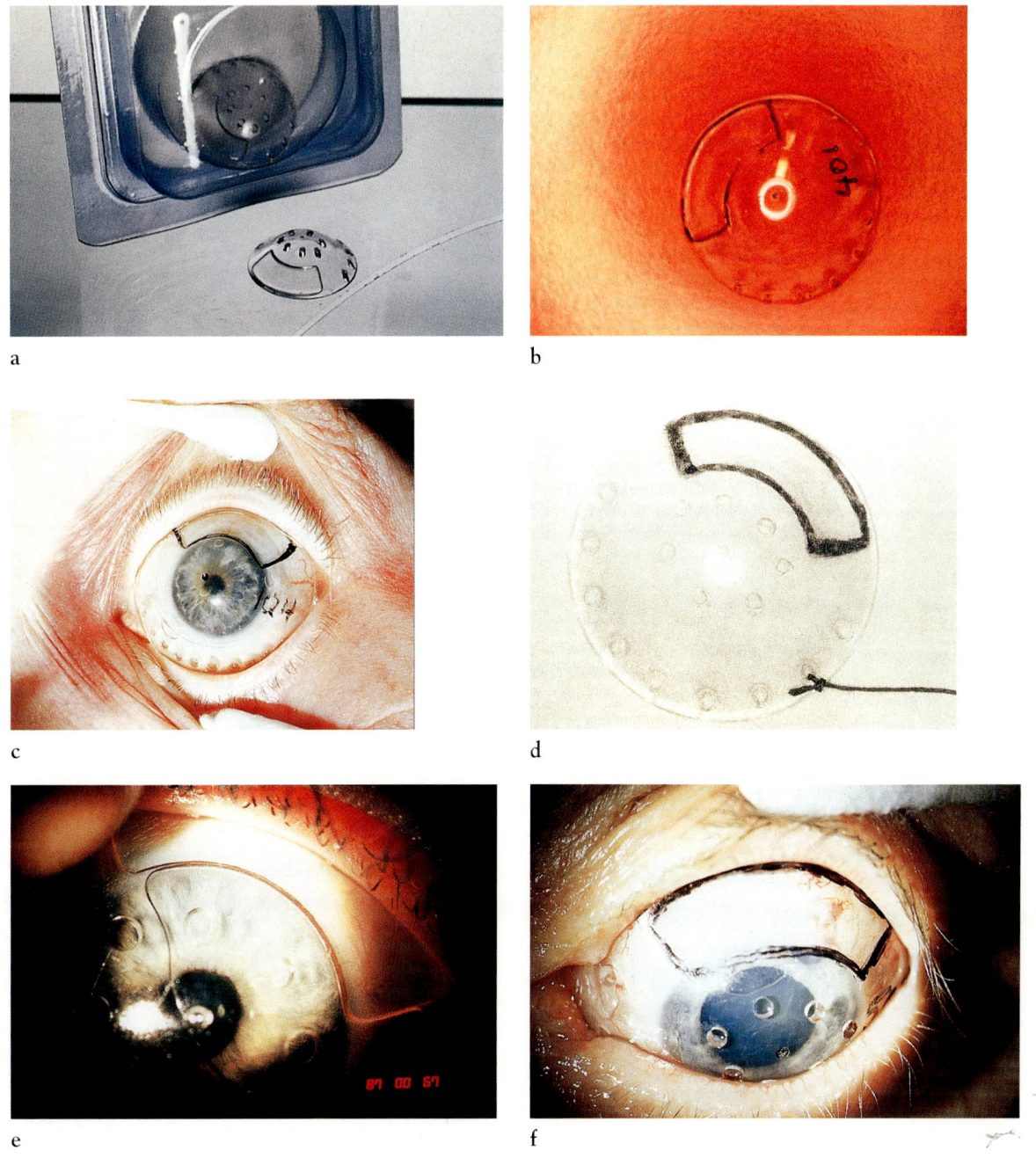

a

b

c

d

e

f

COMPLICATIONS OF FILTERING SURGERY

Malignant Glaucoma

III28a.   As previously noted, if the anterior chamber is shallow or flat and the intraocular pressure is elevated during the early postoperative period, malignant (ciliary block) glaucoma must be considered. The condition is initially managed medically with atropine and aqueous supressants. If the condition persists beyond approximately 3 days, however, surgical intervention is indicated. One surgical approach, especially in the phakic eye, is posterior sclerotomy and air injection, the steps of which are shown on this and the following page.

III28b.   The first step in the posterior sclerotomy and air injection is to create a paracentesis, usually in the inferior temporal quadrant.

III28c.   A distance of 3.5 mm is then measured from the limbus and marked. This is usually performed in the inferior temporal or inferior nasal quadrant.

III28d.   A tapered blade, such as a Wheeler knife, is used to enter the vitreous cavity at the measured 3.5 mm distance from the limbus. A distance of 10 mm is first measured from the tip of the blade and marked with a surgical marking pen.

III28e.   The tapered blade is then inserted through conjunctiva, sclera, and pars plana into the vitreous cavity. Care is taken to aim the tip of the blade toward the optic nerve and not allow the blade to go beyond the measured 10 mm.

III28f.   The tapered blade is then turned, to separate the edges of the wound and allow release of aqueous, which can be seen in this photo.

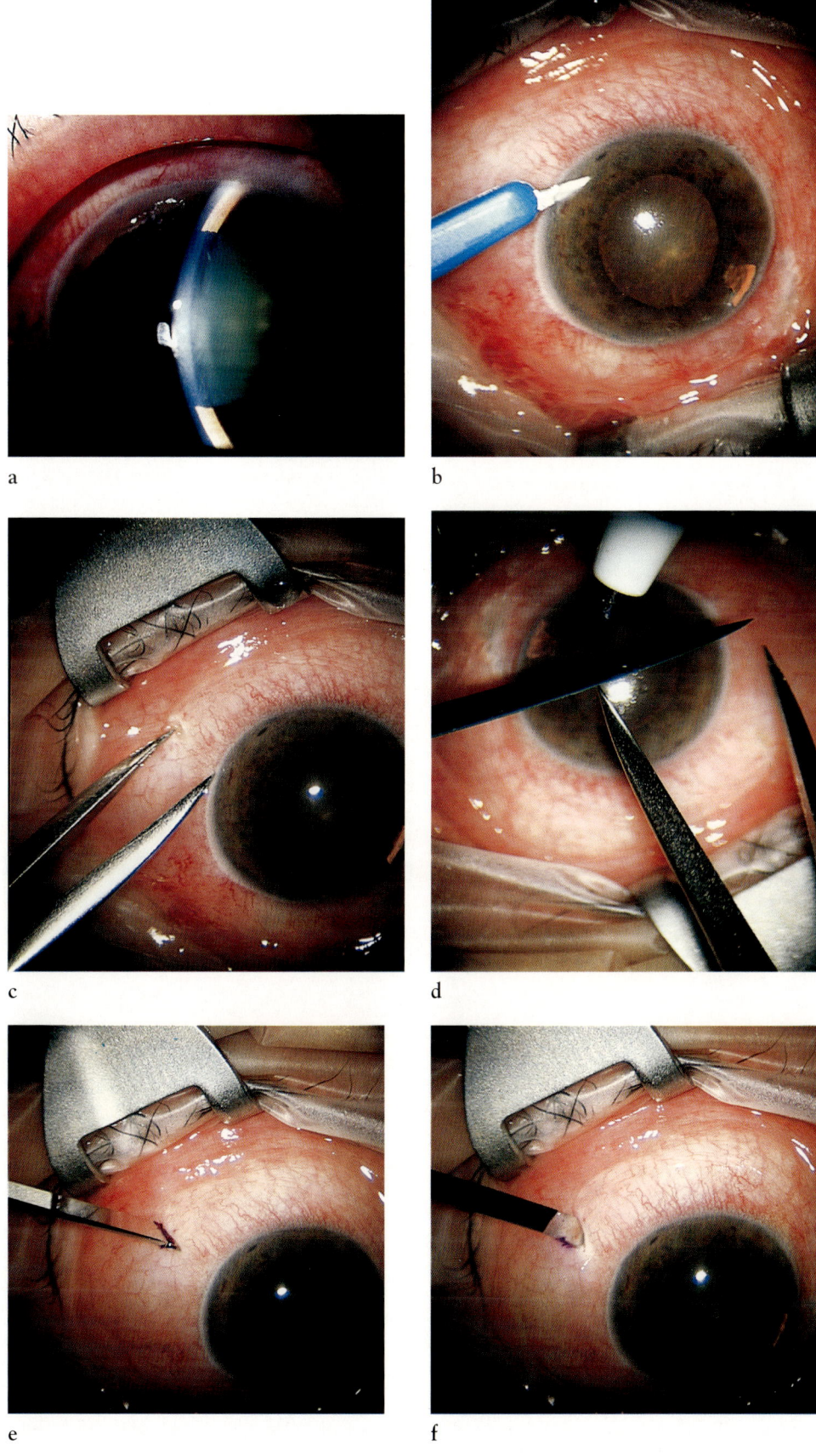

COMPLICATIONS OF FILTERING SURGERY

Malignant Glaucoma

III29a.   The next step in the posterior sclerotomy and air injection for malignant glaucoma (following the steps noted on the previous page) is to measure 10 to 12 mm on an 18-gage blunt needle.

III29b.   The blunt needle is then inserted through the previously prepared pars plana incision, again aiming toward the optic nerve, and not allowing the needle to go beyond the measured 10 to 12 mm.

III29c.   With the blunt needle in place, gentle aspiration is performed, watching for clear fluid to enter the syringe. If resistance is met, a slight reflux of the syringe is allowed, and the tip of the needle is repositioned in an attempt to locate pockets of aqueous within the vitreous cavity. With the aspiration of the pockets of aqueous, the anterior chamber and cornea will often collapse, as shown in this photo.

III29d.   Air is then injected into the anterior chamber via the previously prepared paracentesis. As much air as possible should be injected into the anterior chamber to force the lens posteriorly, thereby breaking the ciliary block between the equator of the lens and the ciliary processes.

III29e.   At the completion of the posterior sclerotomy and air injection procedure, the anterior chamber is deep with the large air bubble.

III29f.   This slit-lamp view shows the eye of the same patient as in III28a, one day after posterior sclerotomy and air injection for malignant glaucoma. A large air bubble is still present in the deep anterior chamber angle.

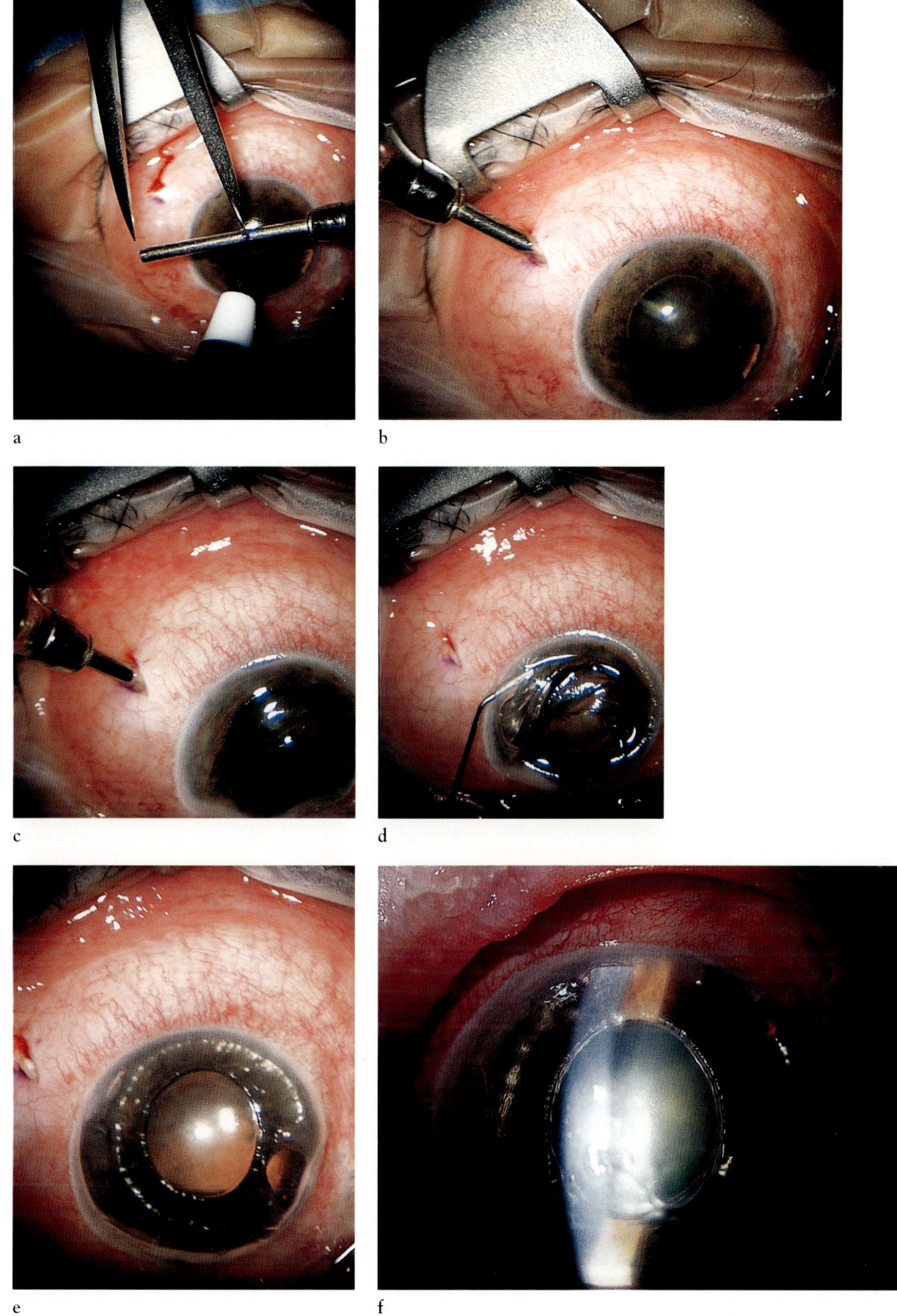

a

b

c

d

e

f

COMPLICATIONS OF FILTERING SURGERY

The Failing Bleb

III30a.   The typical appearance of a failing filtering bleb is a flat, heavily vascularized conjunctiva in the site of the filtering surgery. The anterior chamber is typically deep and the pressure is elevated. The first step in the management of such a complication is to perform gonioscopy to ensure that the fistula is unobstructed internally. If the fistula is patent (which is usually the case), the next step should be digital pressure, as described on this page. Additional measures may include laser suture lysis or the removal of a releasable suture.

III30b.   Pharmacologic measures are also indicated for the failing bleb. Increasing the steroid therapy, such as prednisolone 1% every 2 hours, may prove helpful. In addition, the postoperative use of 5-fluorouracil may help to reverse the failing bleb. The usual protocol is 5 mg (e.g., 0.1 cc of 50 mg/ml) for 5 to 10 injections over the first 2 to 3 postoperative weeks. The injections are usually made in an inferior quadrant, although some surgeons prefer to place them closer to the filtering site. In either case, the injections can be made at the slit lamp, as shown in this photo.

III30c.   As noted above, one of the first steps in the management of a failing bleb is digital pressure. This should first be performed by the physician, as shown in this figure. The patient is instructed to look up, and firm, steady, pressure is applied to the eye inferiorly through the lower lid with the two index fingers. Alternatively, the procedure can be performed at the slit lamp, in which the patient is instructed to look down and the pressure is applied in a superior quadrant, near the filtering site, through the upper lid, with one finger. Another technique is to apply pressure with a cotton-tipped applicator directly to the conjunctiva adjacent to the edge of the scleral flap.

III30d.   In some cases, digital pressure by the physician in the office on one or two occasions is sufficient to re-establish function of the filtering bleb. If the bleb continues to show signs of failure on followup visits, however, it may be advisable to instruct the patient in digital pressure at home. The patient should be told to first wash the hands and trim the finger nails. The patient then looks up and places his or her index fingers against the inferior quadrant of the scleral through the lower lid. Firm pressure should be applied for 10 to 15 seconds, and this is usually repeated 4 times each day, until the bleb is well established or it is judged that the digital pressure is having no effect.

(Figure III30b was provided courtesy of R. Rand Allingham, M.D.)

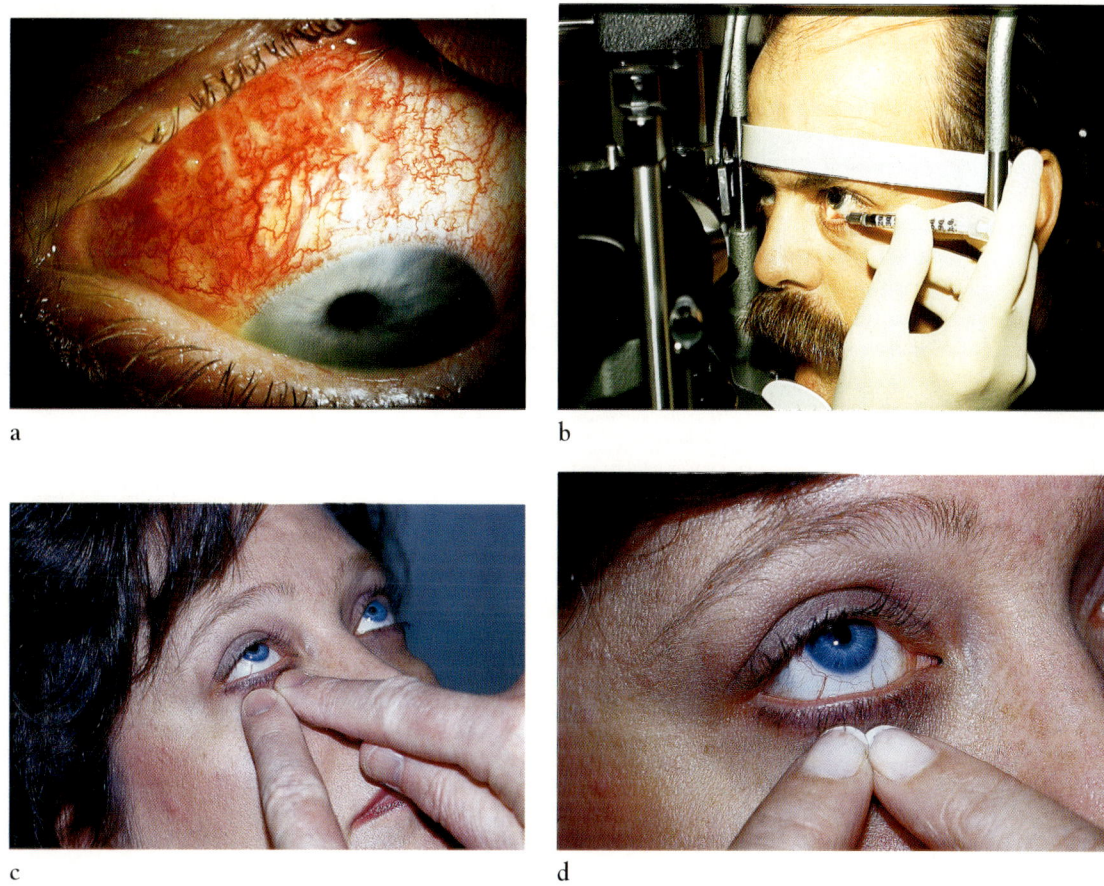

a

b

c

d

COMPLICATIONS OF FILTERING SURGERY

The Encapsulated Bleb

III31a. Some patients may present, usually a month or more after filtering surgery, with a deep anterior chamber, elevated intraocular pressure, and a filtering bleb that is elevated, but that has a tense, smooth-domed appearance with large vessels and clear conjunctiva between the vessels. This has been referred to as an encapsulated bleb. It is caused by a thick layer of connective tissue just beneath the conjunctiva, which can usually be seen by moving the conjunctiva at the slit lamp (with a finger against the upper lid) and noting the rigid, vascularized tissue beneath the conjunctiva, which does not move.

III31b. The appropriate management for the encapsulated bleb is to resume anti-glaucoma medication, since most of these blebs will begin to function over the course of the next 2 to 3 months. If the pressure cannot be controlled medically, however, surgical intervention is indicated. One technique is called needling, in which a needle is passed beneath the conjunctiva and is used as a knife to cut an opening in the connective tissue layer. If this is not effective, a more definitive approach is surgical revision of the encapsulated bleb, as shown in the following series of photos. An incision is first made through conjunctiva several mms behind the encapsulated bleb.

III31c. The conjunctiva is then carefully dissected from the underlying layer of connective tissue. This dissection can be performed bluntly, in part, by spreading the scissors, although areas of firmer scarring require sharp dissection with the scissors. It is important to see the tips of the scissors beneath the conjunctiva, as shown in this photograph, to avoid button-holing the conjunctiva.

III31d. After the dome of dense connective tissue has been unroofed, it is surrounded with a layer of cautery, as shown in this photo, before incision.

III31e. In this photo, the layer of dense connective tissue is being excised with scissors, and the triangular-shaped scleral flap from the original procedure can now be seen. It is usually not necessary to manipulate the scleral flap, because flow around the flap is typically present beneath the layer of connective tissue.

III31f. After the layer of dense connective tissue is removed, the conjunctival flap is again approximated with a running fine, absorbable suture.

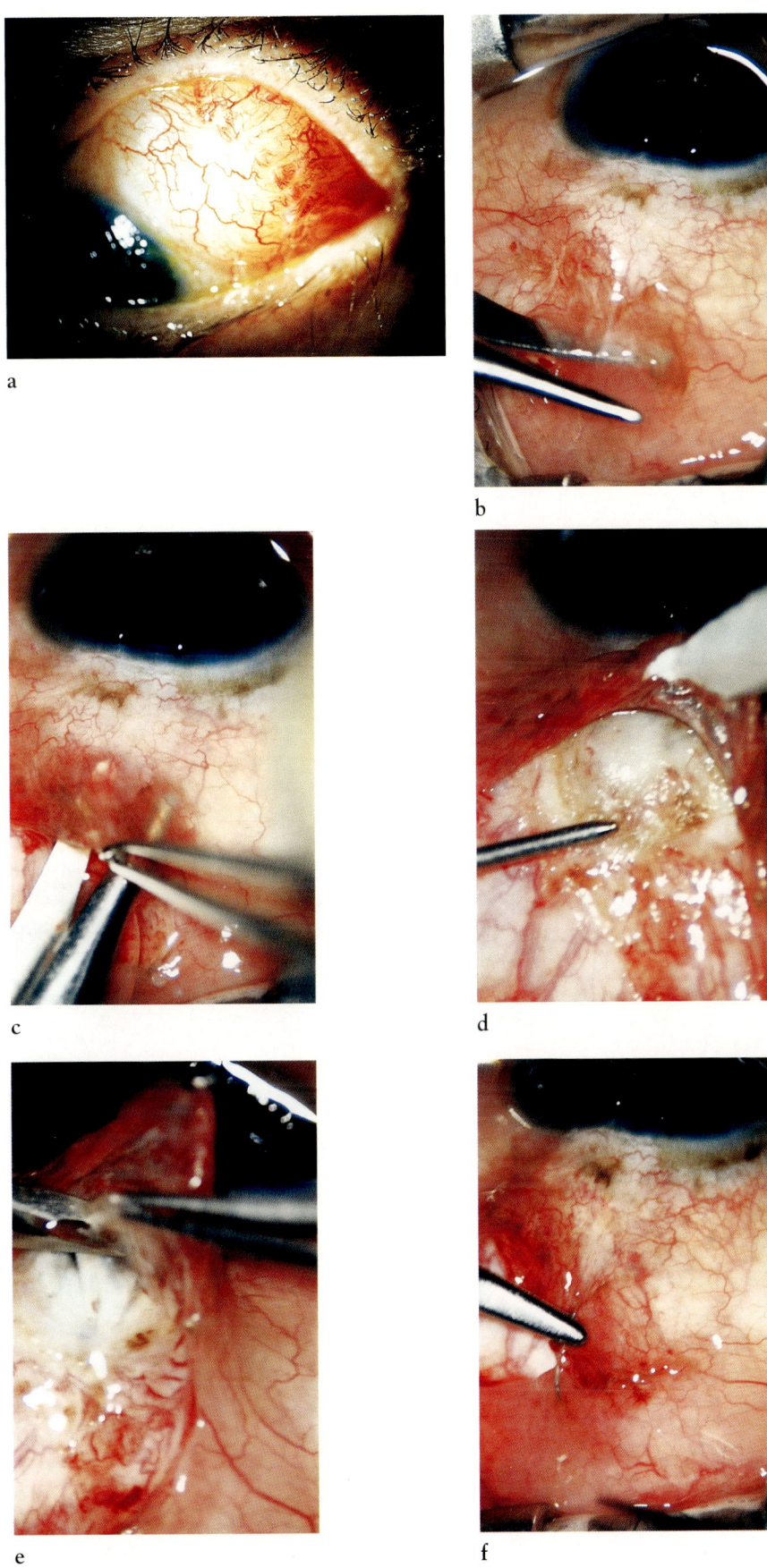

COMPLICATIONS OF FILTERING SURGERY

Leaking/Overfiltering Bleb

III32a.   Leakage of a filtering bleb, which is usually associated with a shallow to flat anterior chamber and low intraocular pressure, can occur either in the early or late postoperative period. In this photograph, an avascular, thin-walled filtering bleb was found to be leaking near the limbus.

III32b.   Leakage from the filtering bleb can be clearly documented with the use of the Seidel test, in which fluorescein is applied to the area in question and observed at the slit lamp with a cobalt blue light. Leaking aqueous will be seen as bright yellow fluid flowing from the leaking site, as seen in this photo.

III32c.   In some cases, the shallow anterior chamber and low intraocular pressure may be caused by an over-filtering bleb. This may result from extension of the filtering bleb from the surgical site, as shown in this photo, in which the filtering bleb in the superior nasal quadrant has extended inferiorly into the inferior nasal quadrant. In many cases, these will resolve spontaneously or with pressure patching. In other cases, trichloroacetic acid application may help to flatten the extended portion of the bleb.

III32d.   In other cases, the overfiltering bleb may be caused by a localized, but excessively thin bleb. This has become an especially common problem since the advent of adjunctive mitomycin-C with a trabeculectomy procedure. This photo shows the typical appearance of a filtering bleb after trabeculectomy with mitomycin-C, showing the markedly avascular, thin-walled conjunctiva.

III32e–f.   The hypotony associated with an overfiltering bleb can create many complications, including a characteristic maculopathy, with marked reduction in visual acuity. In some cases, the only effective method for reversing this complication is to excise the thin-walled bleb and replace it with healthy conjunctiva from above, which is shown later in this section. III32e shows such an eye in which the bleb was removed, and III32f shows the tissue that was excised, with thin-irregular epithelium over loose connective tissue.

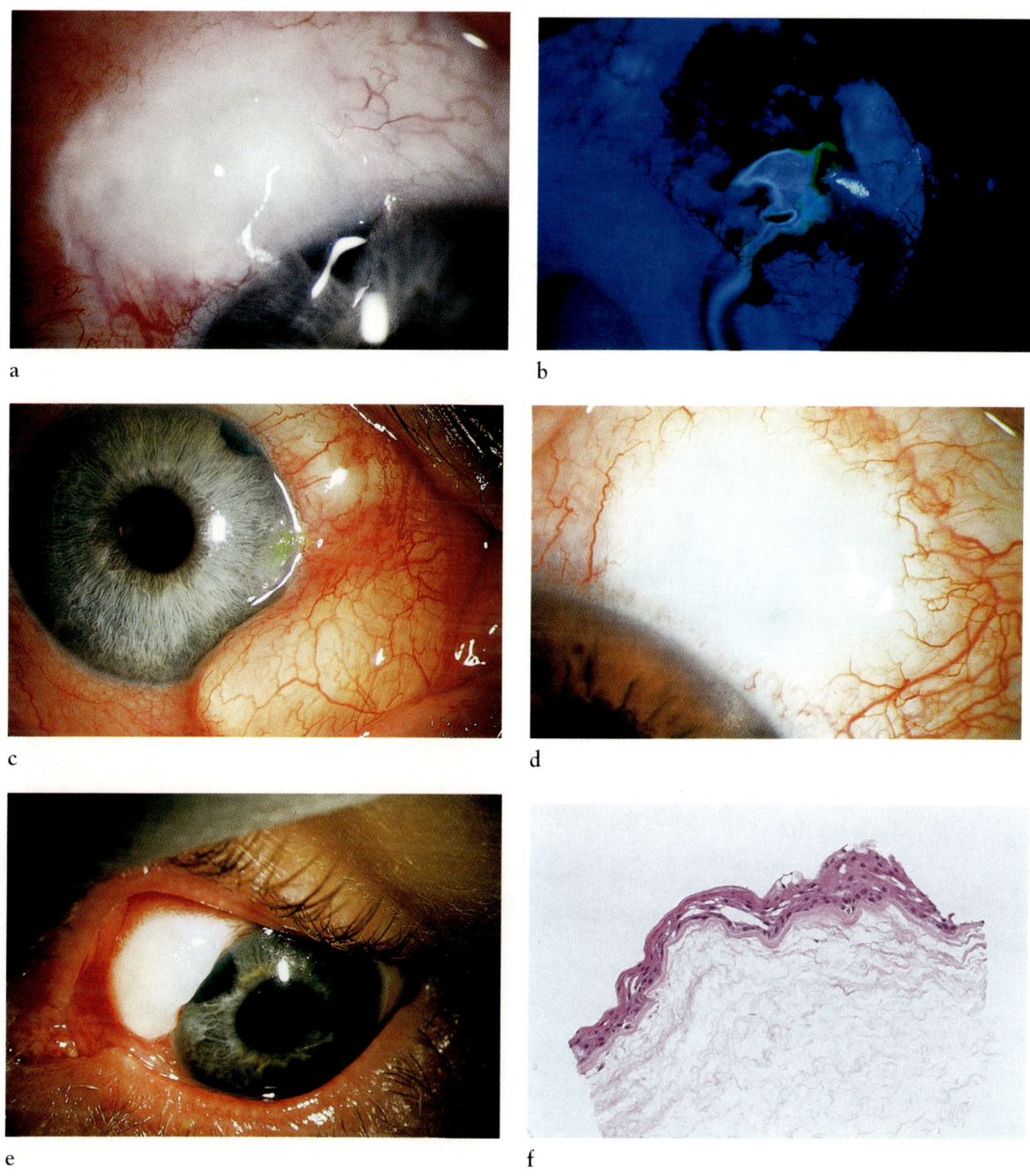

a

b

c

d

e

f

COMPLICATIONS OF FILTERING SURGERY

Leaking/Overfiltering Bleb

III33a–b.   Several methods have been developed to manage the leaking or overfiltering bleb, especially after the adjunctive use of mitomycin-C. One procedure, which was developed by Dr. James B. Wise, is the injection of autologous blood into the filtering bleb. The blood is first withdrawn from a vein in the patient's arm or hand and the needle is then changed to a 30 gauge. With the patient at the slit lamp or under an operating microscope in a minor room, the needle is passed beneath the conjunctiva, adjacent to the bleb, then into the bleb, and the bleb is filled with the blood, as shown in these two photographs. One complication of the procedure is the extension of the blood into the anterior chamber, which can be minimized by injecting viscoelastic into the anterior chamber.

III33c–f.   An alternative to autologous blood injection for the overfiltering bleb is a laser procedure developed by Dr. Mary G. Lynch. The procedure involves the use of the Microruptor II neodymium:YAG laser. III33c shows a filtering bleb before the procedure. At the laser slit lamp, using settings of 3 joules and 20 milliseconds duration, a series of 30 to 70 spots are applied around and throughout the entire depth of the bleb. III33d shows the appearance of the eye immediately after the procedure. Note the relative flattening of the bleb, compared with the preoperative photo. III33e shows the same eye one day postoperatively, and III33f shows the eye one month after the laser surgery. Note the reduction in the size of the bleb and the increased pigment in the base of the bleb.

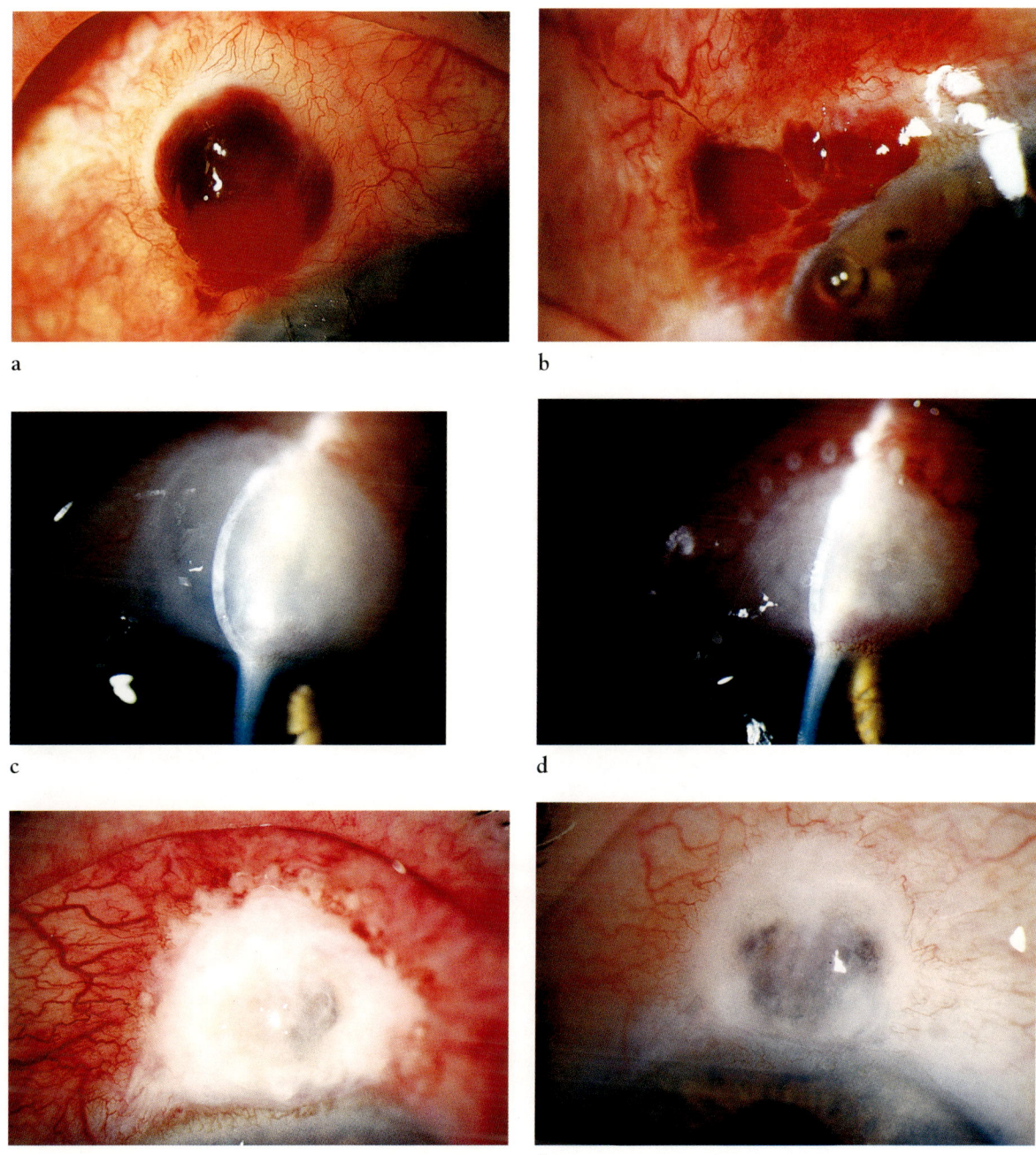

a

b

c

d

e

f

COMPLICATIONS OF FILTERING SURGERY

Late Complications

III34a.   This photo shows a dellen (*arrow*), which is a thinning of the peripheral cornea because of a disturbance of the tear film as a result of the adjacent, elevated filtering bleb. This may occur in either the early or late postoperative period and can usually be managed with ocular lubricants.

III34b.   At any time during the postoperative course, the filtering bleb may become thin and begin to leak with loss of the anterior chamber, as shown in this photo.

III34c.   Another leaking filtering bleb in the late postoperative period. The photo shows an extremely thin-walled outpatching of the bleb near the limbus at the lower portion of the slit beam.

III34d.   In addition to the complications of a flat anterior chamber and hypotony, the leaking filtering bleb also increases the risk of endophthalmitis. This usually begins with infection in the filtering bleb, as shown in this photo, which is referred to as blebitis. At this stage, anterior chamber reaction may also occur, but the vitreous is clear. If the infection is not treated promptly, however, it can progress to fulminate endophthalmitis.

III34e–f.   In most cases of leaking filtering blebs in the late postoperative course, especially if they have been associated with blebitis or endophthalmitis, it is necessary to revise the filtering bleb by the technique shown on the next page. III34e shows the appearance of the bleb after revision of the eye in III34c, and III34f shows the postoperative appearance after bleb revision in the patient in III34d, after the infection was successfully treated.

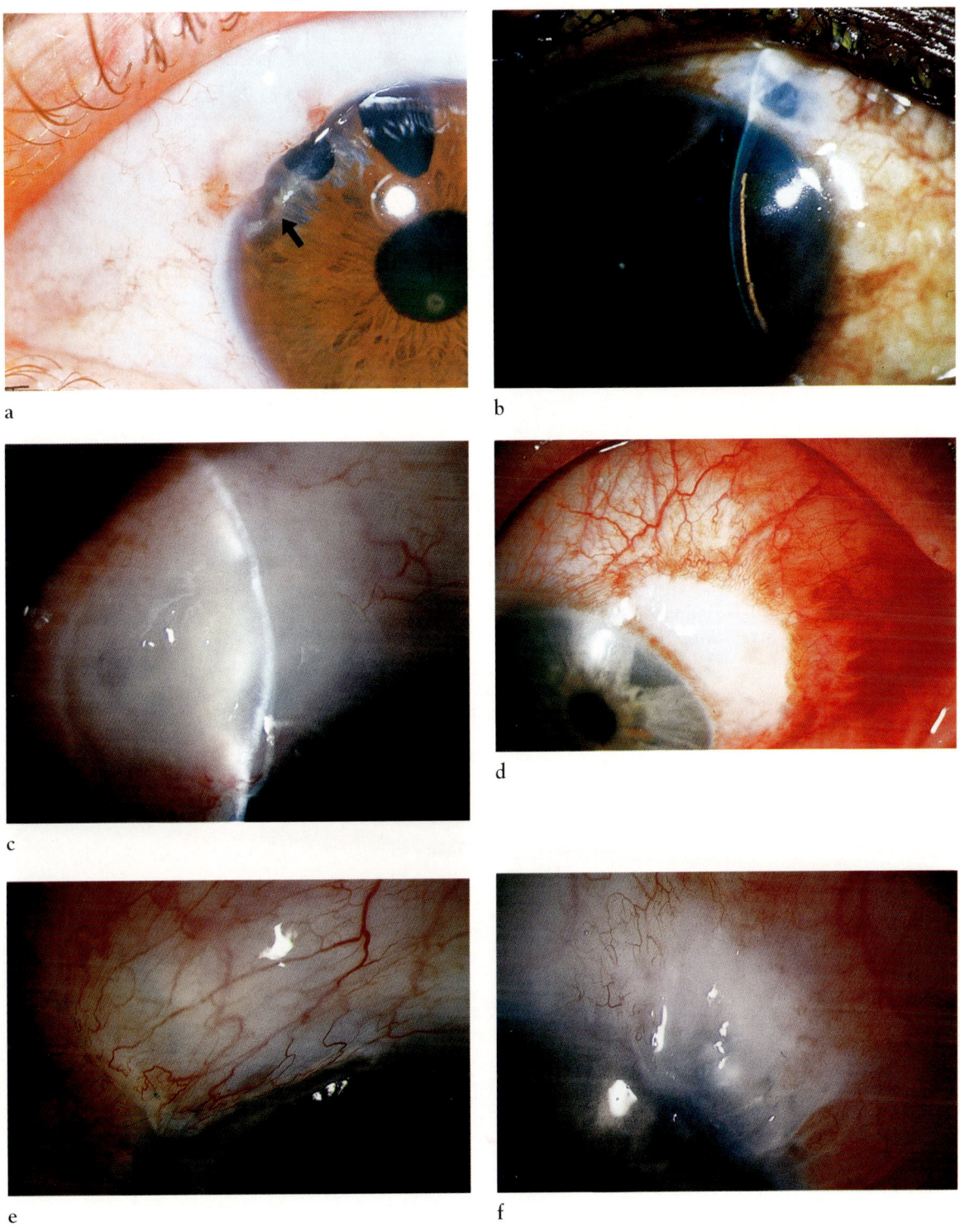

COMPLICATIONS OF FILTERING SURGERY

Bleb Revision

As noted on the previous pages, it is occasionally necessary to repair a leaking or overfiltering bleb by excising the thin-walled tissue and replacing it with healthy conjunctiva. The following surgical steps show one technique by which this can be accomplished.

III35a.   The thin-walled, avascular filtering bleb is first outlined with a knife.

III35b.   The thin-walled bleb is next dissected from the underlying scleral with scissors.

III35c.   After the thin-walled bleb has been dissected to the limbus, it is excised at the limbus with scissors. Cautery is then applied as needed.

III35d.   Conjunctiva behind the surgical site is then undermined with blunt-tipped scissors. It is preferable to undermine only conjunctiva, rather than including Tenon's capsule, since the conjunctiva alone will stretch better than when combined with Tenon's.

III35e.   Because the previous, leaking filtering bleb was large, it was necessary to rotate adjacent conjunctiva from the side of the defect to fill it in.

III35f.   The new conjunctival flap is secured at the limbus with a running suture of fine, absorbable material, and the margins of the remaining radial defect are also approximated with a running suture. The postoperative appearance of this case is shown in III34e.

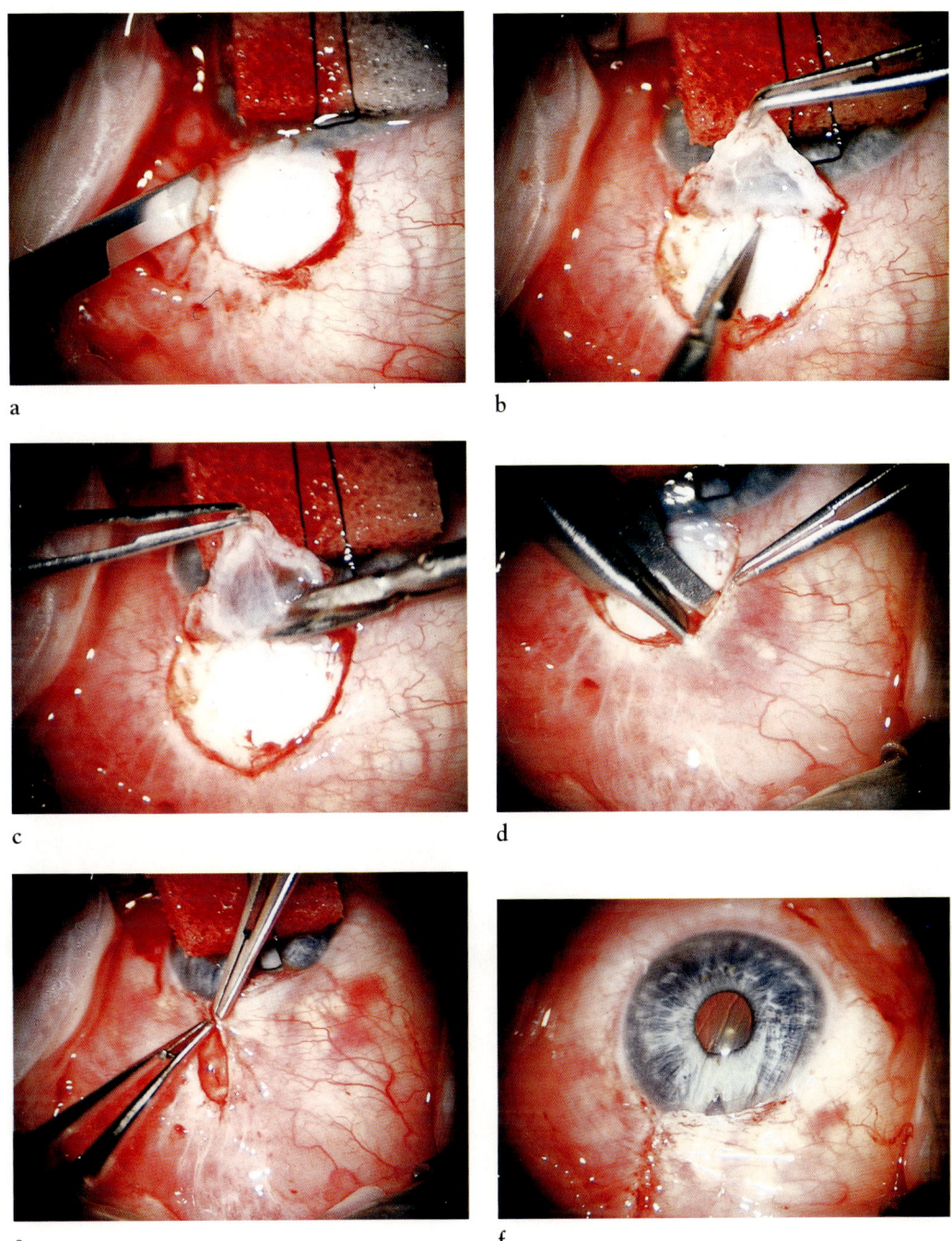

a

b

c

d

e

f

COMPLICATIONS OF FILTERING SURGERY

Overhanging Blebs

III36a–b.   Another late complication of glaucoma filtering surgery that was more common with the full-thickness procedures is an extension of the bleb over the cornea. In some extreme cases, the over-hanging bleb can approach the visual axis, interfering with visual acuity. If the bleb is interfering with vision or is otherwise symptomatic, it can be surgically removed by bluntly dissecting the bleb from the cornea and excising it near the limbus. In some cases, the remaining tissue is sufficiently firm to allow suturing of the filtering bleb back to the limbus, as shown in this preoperative (III36a) and postoperative (III36b) case.

III36c–d.   In other cases of overhanging filtering blebs, the tissue may be too thin to allow suturing at the limbus. In such cases, it is necessary to excise the entire bleb and bring down healthy conjunctiva, similar to the approach described on the previous page. This is shown in these preoperative (III36c) and postoperative (III36d) photos.

III36d–f.   These light microscopic photographs show the overhanging filtering bleb that was excised from the eye in III36c–d. The higher magnification in III36f shows a markedly attenuated epithelium covering hydropic corneal stroma. It is postulated that the mechanism of formation of the overhanging bleb involves aqueous humor dissection between corneal epithelium and stroma, leading to abnormal hydration of the superficial lamellae.

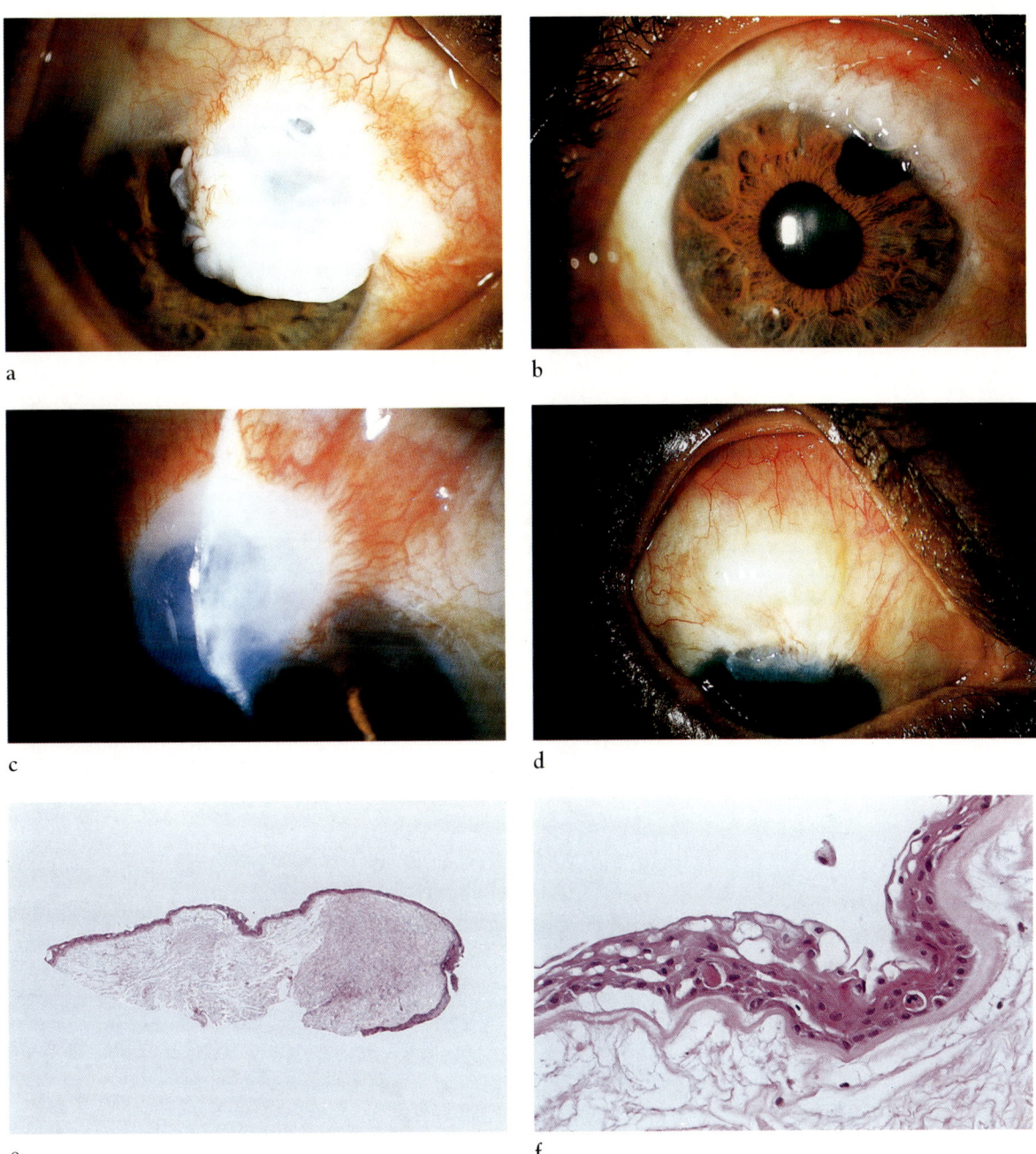

a

b

c

d

e

f

DRAINAGE IMPLANT SURGERY

Implant Devices

When standard techniques of glaucoma filtering surgery are inadequate, usually because of excessive conjunctival scarring in the superior quadrants, an alternative approach to improve aqueous outflow is one of several glaucoma drainage implant procedures. All modern drainage implant devices have the same basic design, which consists of a plastic tube that extends from the anterior chamber (or, in some cases, the vitreous cavity) to a plate, disc or encircling eliminant beneath conjunctiva and Tenon's capsule. The devices differ primarily according to the size and shape of the external component and to whether they contain a pressure-regulating valve. Several of the more commonly used drainage implant devices are shown on this page.

III37a.   Glaucoma drainage implant devices (left to right): 1) Krupin eye valve with disc; 2) Baerveldt implant; 3) Ahmed glaucoma valve; 4) double-plate Molteno implant; and 5) single-plate Molteno implant. The Krupin and Ahmed implants represent drainage devices with pressure-regulating valves, while the Baerveldt and Molteno have unobstructed drainage tubes.

III37b.   This photograph shows further detail of the double-plate and single-plate Molteno implants. In both designs, the plate consists of thin acrylic with a diameter of 13 mm and an area of 135 mm^2 attached to a silicone tube. In the double-plate implant, a second tube connects the two plates, giving an increased surface area of 270 mm^2. The plates have a thickened rim, which is perforated to allow suturing to the sclera.

III37c.   A common early postoperative complication associated with unobstructed, open drainage tubes is hypotony, because of excessive filtration. The dual-chamber Molteno implant, as shown in this photograph, was design to address that problem. The V-shaped "pressure ridge" on the upper surface of the plate encases an area of 10.5 mm^2 around the opening of the silicone tube, which helps to regulate the flow of aqueous into the main bleb cavity during the early postoperative period.

III37d.   Another approach to avoiding the early postoperative complication of excessive drainage and hypotony is the inclusion of a one-way valve in the implant design. This concept was first incorporated into the Krupin-Denver valve, which has undergone several modifications to the current Krupin eye valve with disc, as shown in this photograph. The valve-effect is created by making slits in the closed external end of the Silastic tube and is manometrically calibrated to open at pressures between 10 and 12 mm Hg and close between 8 and 10 mm Hg.

(Figure III37a was provided courtesy by Donald S. Minckler, M.D.; Figures III37b and III37c were provided courtesy of Jeffrey Freedman, M.D., Ph.D.; Figure III37d was provided courtesy of Theodore Krupin, M.D.)

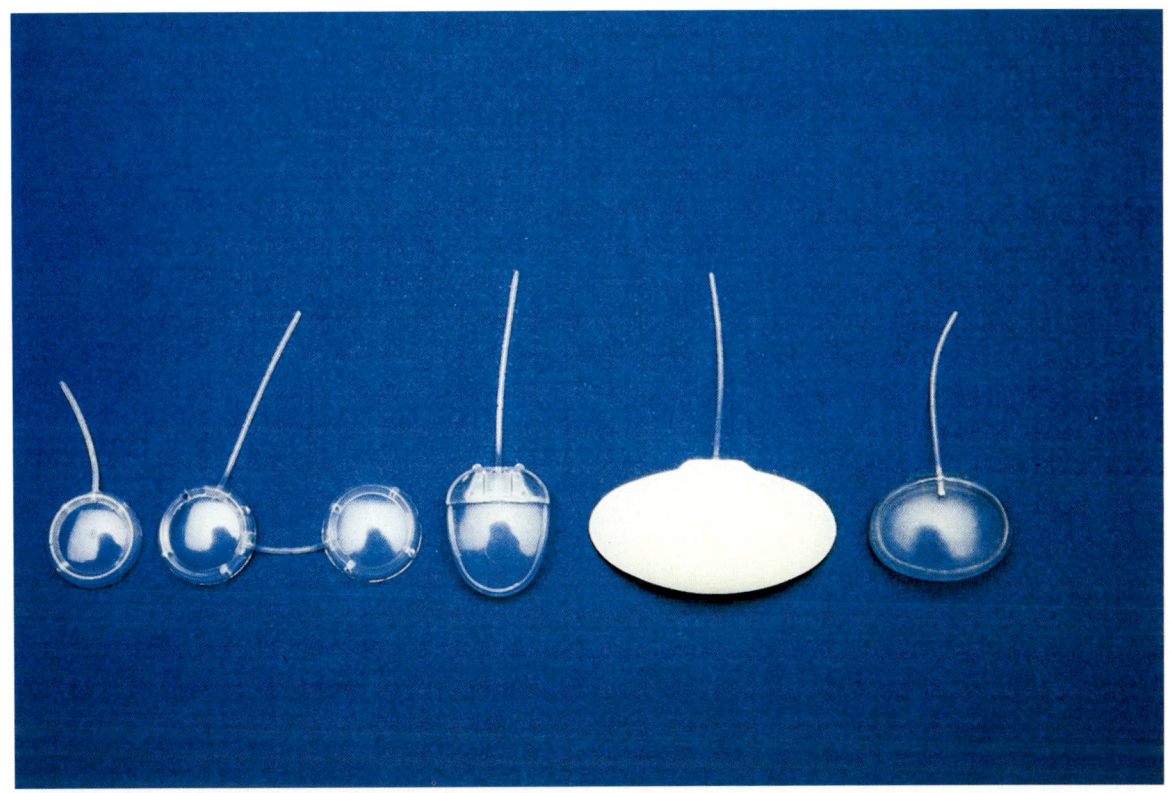

a

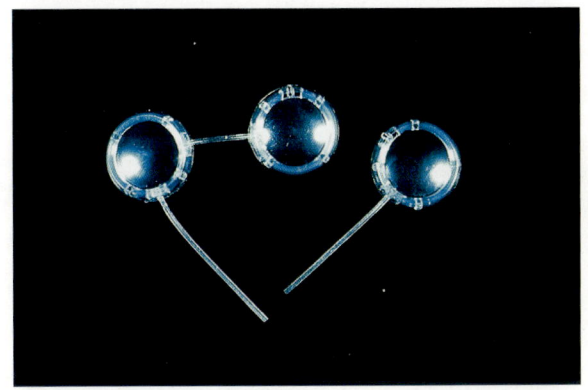

b

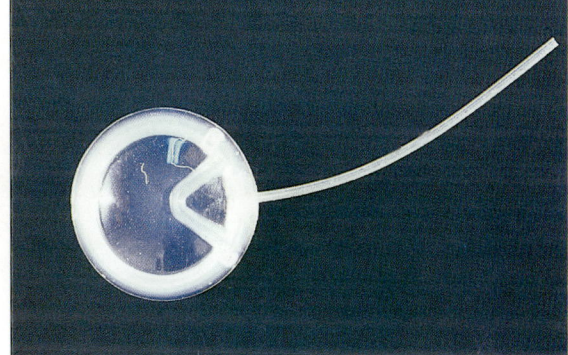

c

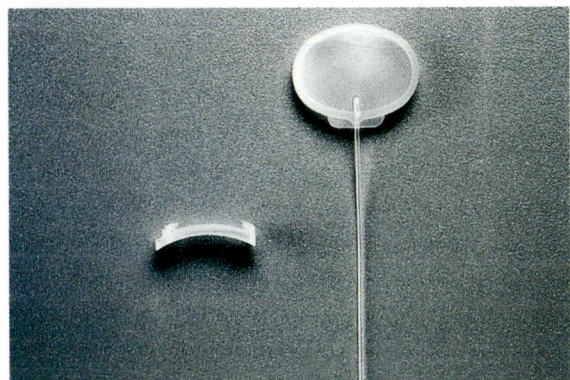

d

DRAINAGE IMPLANT SURGERY

Technique of Molteno Implantation

III38a. A dual-chamber Molteno implant is being used for the drainage implant procedure in this series of photographs. The plate is seen in this photo, with preplaced sutures through the perforations in the thickened rim.

III38b. A fornix-based conjunctival flap is created in a superior quadrant (the supero-temporal quadrant is preferred whenever possible). Blunt dissection must be carried posteriorly between the two rectus muscles to or beyond the equator of the globe. The plate is then tucked into sub-Tenon's posteriorly and sutured to the sclera with the anterior border 9 to 10 mm from the limbus.

III38c. Before inserting the silicone tube into the anterior chamber, the tube is cut bevel up to permit its extension for 2 to 3 mm into the anterior chamber. The purpose of the bevel-up cut of the tube is to prevent iris incarceration.

III38d. A 22-gauge needle is used to create a limbal passage into the anterior chamber for the tube. The angle at which the needle enters the anterior chamber is critical, because it is important that the tube vault between cornea and iris, without touching either structure. The yellow structure above the needle is preserved donor sclera, which has been sutured to the eye at one end of the rectangle and flapped back to allow insertion of the tube.

III38e. After inserting the silicone tube into the anterior chamber, the rectangle of donor sclera is approximated to cover the externalized portion of the tube adjacent to the limbus. The structure that is seen extending further into the anterior chamber is a suture, which has been threaded into the silicone tube to serve as a stent during the early postoperative period to reduce the risk of excessive filtration and hypotony.

III38f. The conjunctival flap is approximated at the limbus. The tip of the silicone tube can be seen in the anterior chamber. Subconjunctival steroids and antibiotics are usually injected at the completion of the procedure in a quadrant away from the surgical site. The basic postoperative management is the same as that described previously for filtering surgery.

(All figures on this page were provided courtesy of Jeffrey Freedman, M.D., Ph.D.)

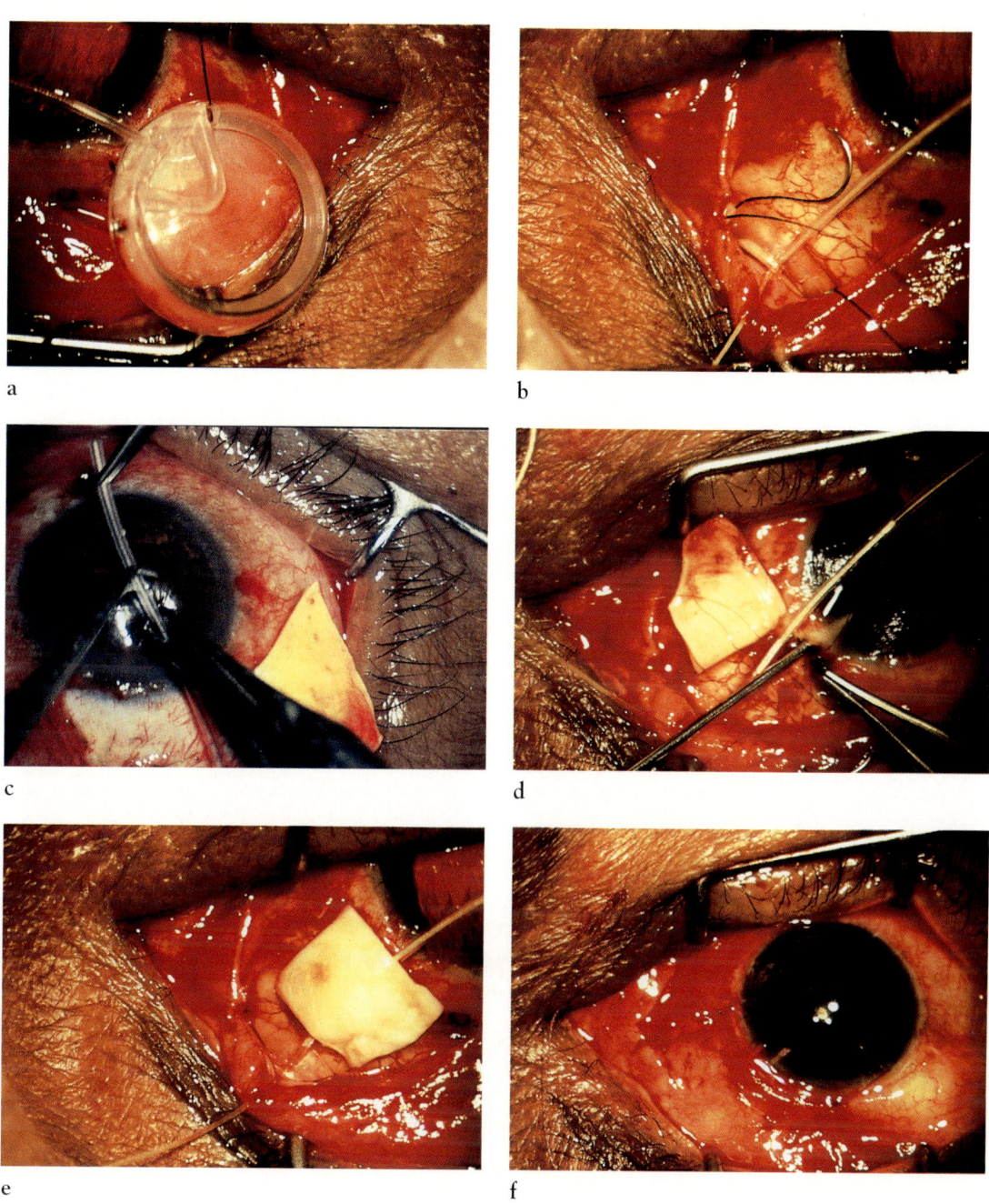

DRAINAGE IMPLANT SURGERY

Technique of Ahmed Implantation

III39a.   The plate of the Ahmed glaucoma valve is shown in this photograph just before implantation. With any drainage implant device that contains a pressure-regulating valve, the tube should be flushed with balanced salt solution to confirm that the valve is functioning properly.

III39b.   The plate of the Ahmed valve has now been inserted into sub-Tenon's space between the superior and lateral rectus muscles. The plate is sutured to the sclera with the anterior border measured 9 to 10 mm behind the limbus.

III39c.   A 23-gauge needle is used to create a track into the anterior chamber at the limbus for insertion of the tube.

III39d.   The tube is then placed over the cornea and cut with the bevel up. When inserting the tube into the vitreous cavity at the pars plana, the tube should be cut bevel down.

III39e.   A rectangular piece of donor scleral, measuring approximately 5 × 7 mm, is sutured over the exposed tube adjacent to the limbus.

III39f.   The conjunctival flap is pulled over the donor sclera and secured at the limbus with wing sutures. The tube can now be seen extending well into the anterior chamber.

(All figures on this page were provided courtesy of R. Rand Allingham, M.D.)

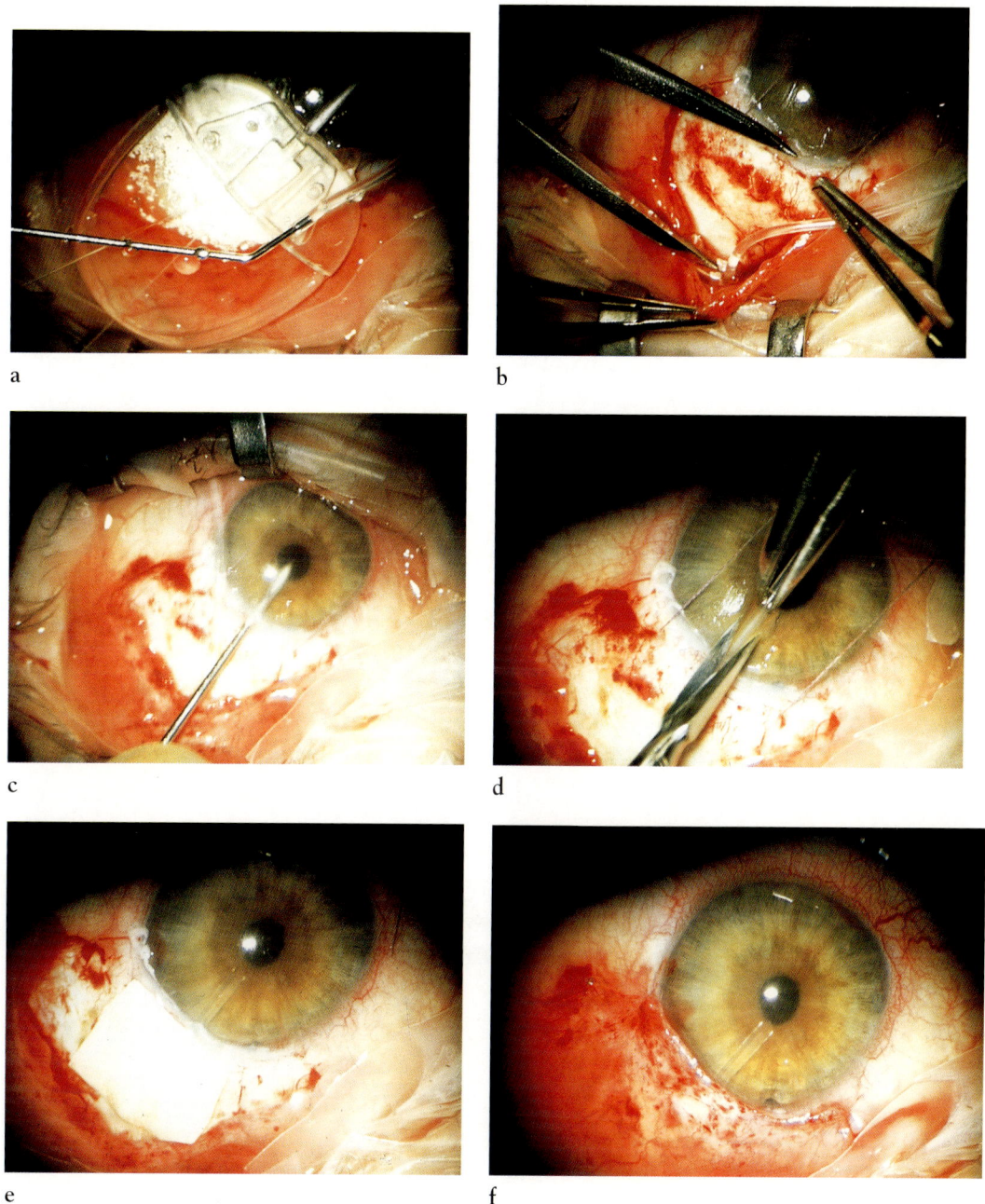

a

b

c

d

e

f

DRAINAGE IMPLANT SURGERY

Technique of Krupin Implantation

III40a.   The plate of the Krupin eye valve with disc is shown just before implantation.

III40b.   After the plate is inserted into the sub-Tenon's space, sutures are passed through the perforations at the anterior ridge of the plate, which is then secured to the sclera, 9 to 10 mm behind the limbus.

III40c.   A partial-thickness, limbus-based scleral flap has been developed, similar to that used with a trabeculectomy. A needle is then used to create a track into the anterior chamber beneath the scleral flap for insertion of the drainage tube.

III40d.   The desired length of the tube is estimated by holding it over the cornea, and the excess is cut off with the bevel up.

III40e.   The drainage tube is inserted into the anterior chamber through the needle track beneath the scleral flap. Special forceps are available with concave platforms for grasping the drainage tube. With most drainage implant techniques, the tube is secured to the sclera (in this case, just behind the scleral flap).

III40f.   After the drainage tube is properly positioned and attached to the sclera, the posterior corners of the scleral flap are approximated. A section of donor sclera is then secured to the sclera over the scleral flap. Processed pericardium is also available commercially for use in place of the donor sclera.

(All figures on this page were provided courtesy of Theodore Krupin, M.D.)

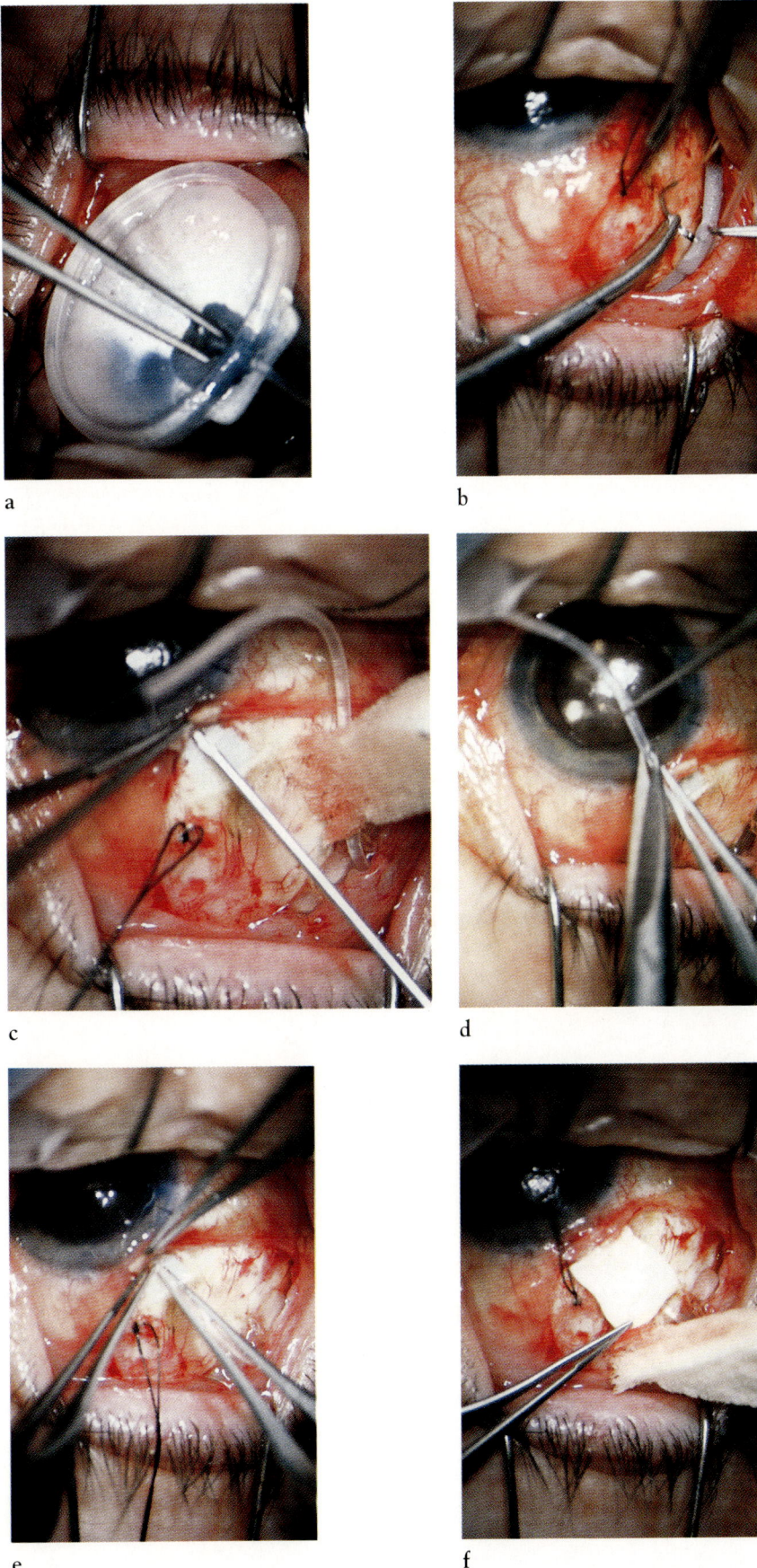

a

b

c

d

e

f

DRAINAGE IMPLANT SURGERY

Joseph Tube and Postoperative States

III41a.   Another example of a valved drainage implant device is the Joseph tube, which is composed of a silicone tube with slit valves in the side that are calibrated to open between 4 and 20 mm Hg. The tube is attached to a 9-mm-wide silicone rubber strap. This photo shows the strap and the attached tube before implantation.

III41b.   After a large fornix-based conjunctival flap is created, the silicone strap is inserted beneath a rectus muscle and secured against the globe near the equator. The remainder of the procedure is as described on the previous pages for implant devices.

III41c.   Glaucoma drainage implant devices are especially useful for cases in which a high risk is present of failure of long-term filtration with standard techniques. In this patient with neovascular glaucoma, a Molteno tube is clear and well positioned.

III41d.   A relatively common complication of drainage implant surgery, in addition to the previously mentioned early hypotony, is obstruction of the internal portion of the tube. In this photograph, a Molteno tube is seen overlying an anterior chamber intraocular lens, with a fibrin plug in the opening of the tube.

III41e.   This postoperative photograph shows a properly positioned drainage tube (*arrow*) in the anterior chamber, well away from both the cornea and iris.

III41f.   In this postoperative photo, the internal portion of the drainage tube is seen through a peripheral iridectomy in the vitreous cavity. In eyes that have had a complete vitrectomy and are aphakic or pseudophakic, inserting the drainage tube into the vitreous cavity through the pars plana helps to reduce the risk of certain postoperative complications, such as corneal damage, obstruction of the tube by iris, and epithelial downgrowth.

(Figures III41a and III41b were provided courtesy of Fathi El Sayyad, FRCS, George L. Spaeth, MD, and M. Bruce Shields, MD from the book THE REFRACTORY GLAUCO-MAS, Igaku-Shoin Medical Publishers, New York, NY; 1995. Figures III41c and III41d were provided courtesy of Jeffrey Freedman, M.D., Ph.D.)

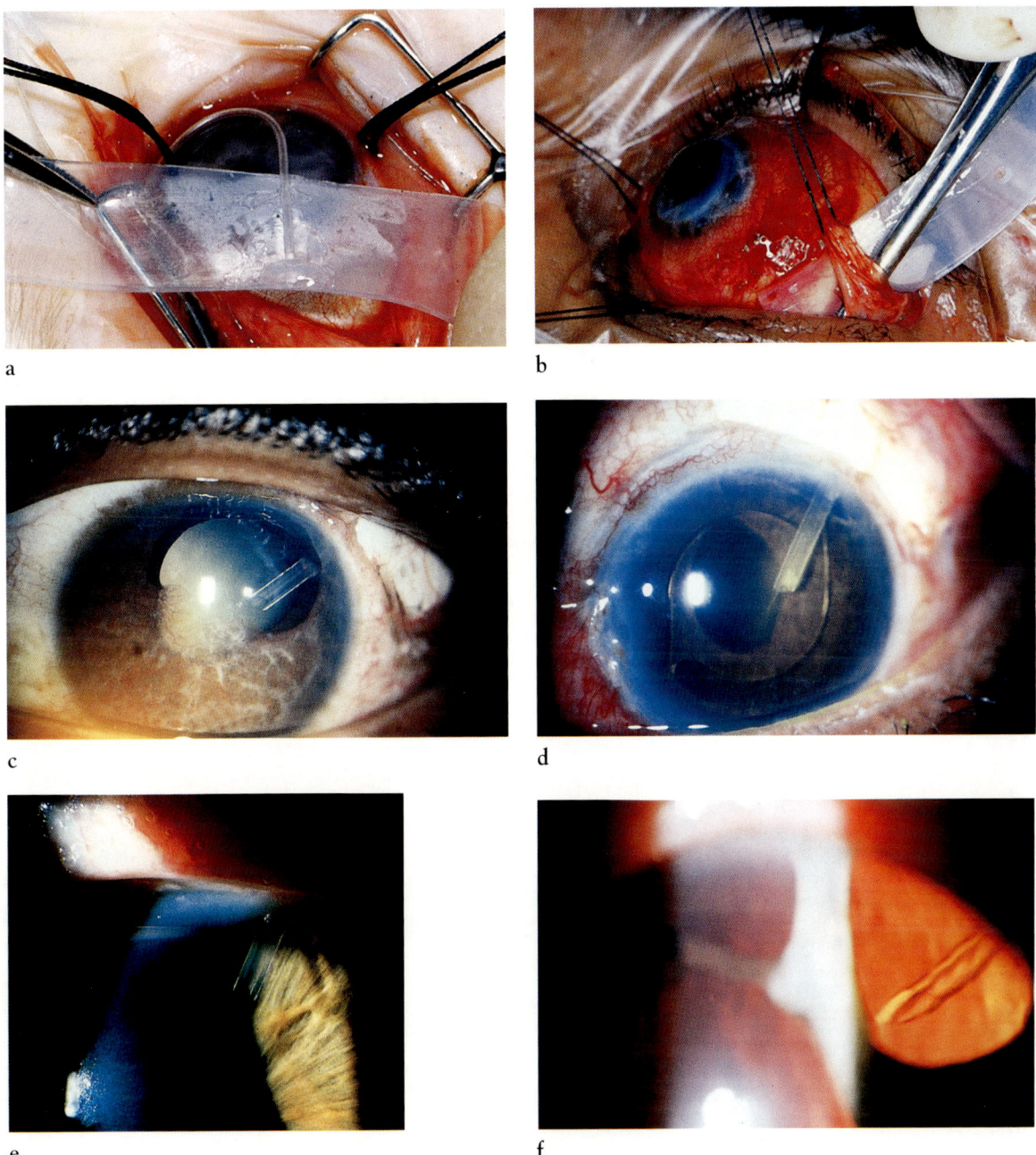

a

b

c

d

e

f

CYCLODESTRUCTIVE SURGERY

Cyclocryotherapy

When surgical procedures that improve aqueous outflow have repeatedly failed or are felt to be contraindicated, an alternative approach is to reduce the rate of aqueous production by partially eliminating the function of the ciliary processes. These operations have been collectively referred to as cyclodestructive procedures. Several cyclodestructive techniques have been used in the past, with cyclocryotherapy being the most popular since it was introduced in the 1950s. Subsequent experience with laser cyclophotocoagulation, however, has shown clear advantages over cyclocryotherapy, and it is today the preferred cyclodestructive operation. Another of the newer cyclodestructive techniques is therapeutic ultrasound. We will consider cyclocryotherapy on this page and then look at the newer techniques with laser and ultrasound on the following pages.

III42a. This photograph shows the cross-section of a human autopsy eye with the cryoprobe on the sclera adjacent to the pars plicata, in the proper position for performing cyclocryotherapy. As with all transscleral cyclodestructive procedures, the destructive element must pass through conjunctiva, sclera, and ciliary muscle before reaching the target tissue, which is the epithelial layers of the ciliary processes.

III42b. The tip of a 4 mm cryoprobe is shown in this photograph.

III42c–e. The technique of cyclocryotherapy is shown in these three photographs. The tip of the probe is placed approximately 2.5 mm from the limbus (III42c). The temperature at the probe tip is reduced to approximately −80° C and maintained for 60 seconds. III42d shows the typical ice ball 30 seconds after initiating freezing. After the 60-second freeze, the probe is irrigated with saline solution, as shown in Figure III42e before removing the probe from the conjunctiva. Note the area of hyperemia around the probe tip.

III42f. Cyclocryotherapy can also be performed on infants under general anesthesia. Because infants and young children tend to do poorly with filtering surgery because of excessive conjunctival scarring, cyclodestructive procedures are frequently useful in the management of childhood glaucomas.

(Figures III42b–e were provided courtesy of A. Robert Bellows, M.D.; Figure III42f was provided courtesy of Irvin P. Pollack, M.D.)

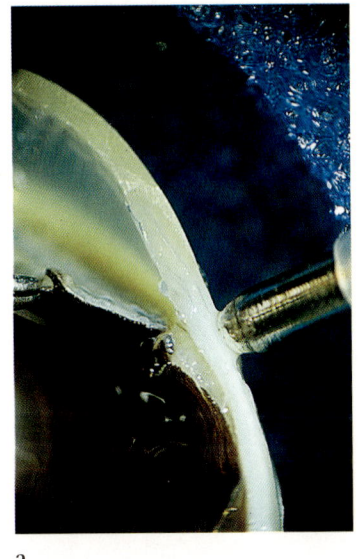

a

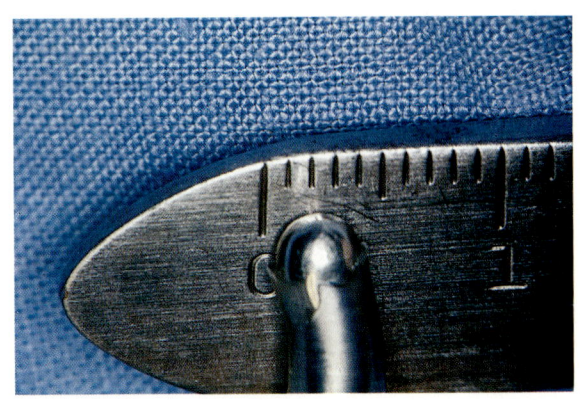

b

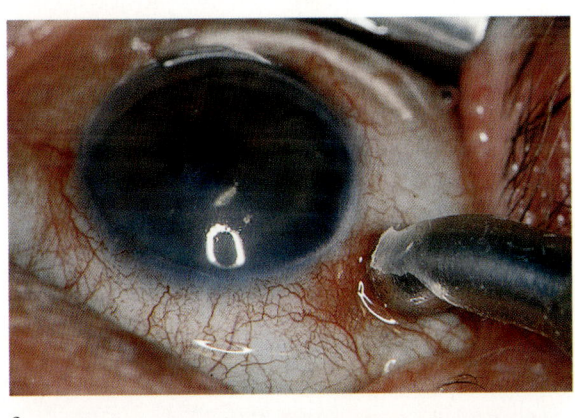

c

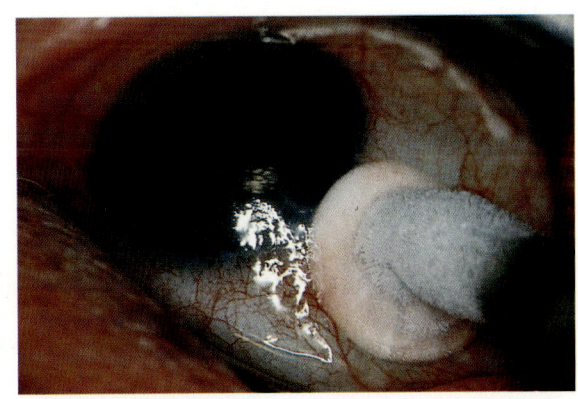

d

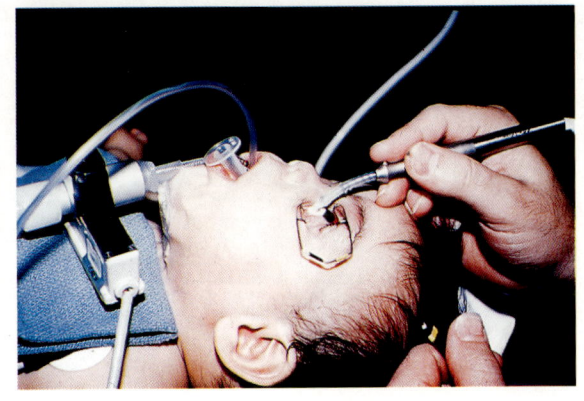

e

f

CYCLODESTRUCTIVE SURGERY

Cyclophotocoagulation

The lasers most commonly used for cyclophotocoagulation are neodymium:YAG (Nd:YAG) and semiconductor diode lasers. Some of the more commonly used laser units for cyclophotocoagulation are shown on this page.

III43a. The Microruptor II (MR II) is a Nd:YAG laser, which provides slit-lamp delivery in the free-running thermal mode with 20 millisecond pulses. It has an adjustable offset between the focal points of the aiming beam and therapeutic beam and is capable of energy levels up to 8 to 9 joules.

III43b. Surgical Laser Technologies (SLT) CL60 provides contact probe delivery of Nd:YAG laser in a continuous-wave mode of 0.12 to 10 seconds. A 2.2 mm sapphire-tipped, hand-held probe is coupled to the fiberoptic delivery system and focuses the laser at 1.5 to 2 mm in air.

III43c–d. The Microruptor III (MR III) also provides continuous-wave Nd:YAG laser energy, which can be delivered by either a slit lamp or a fiberoptic probe. The slit lamp can be operated with the patient sitting in the usual manner, or it can be rotated down, as shown in III43c, for use with the patient in the supine position. The console with the fiberoptic hand probe is shown in III43d.

III43e. One example of the semiconductor diode laser is the Oculight SLx, which provides continuous-wave, contact delivery of the diode laser at a wavelength of 810nm, with a maximum power out of 2.5 to 3.0 W and a maximum duration of 9.9 seconds. Advantages of semiconductor diode lasers include the solid-state construction with compact size (complete unit, as shown in this figure, is approximately the size of a briefcase), low maintenance requirements and no special requirement for electrical outlet or water cooling.

III43f. The Oculight SLx probe (G-Probe) consists of a 600 micron quartz fiberoptic, protruding 0.7 mm from a handpiece designed to center the fiberoptic 1.2 mm behind the surgical limbus and parallel to the visual axis.

(Figure III43b was provided courtesy of R. Rand Allingham, M.D.: Figure III43f was provided courtesy of Theodore A. Boutacoff.)

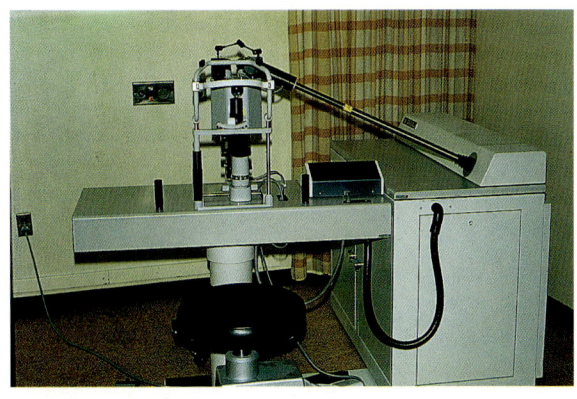

a

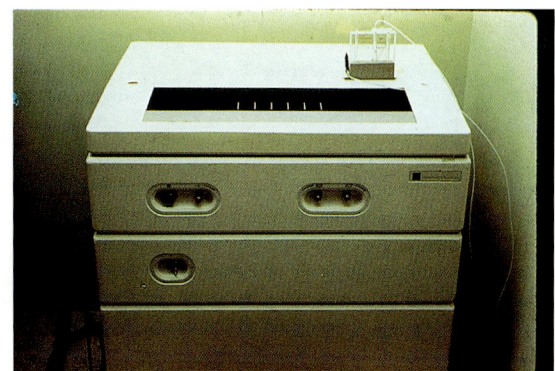

b

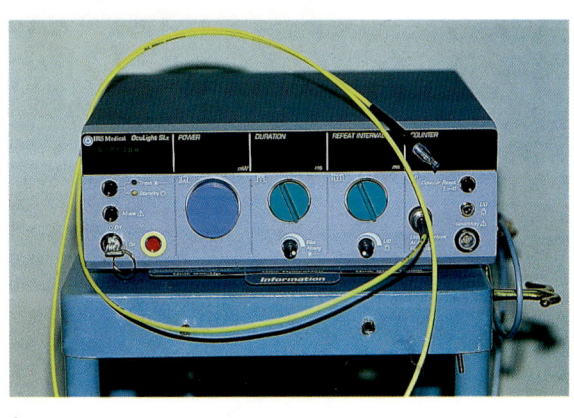

c

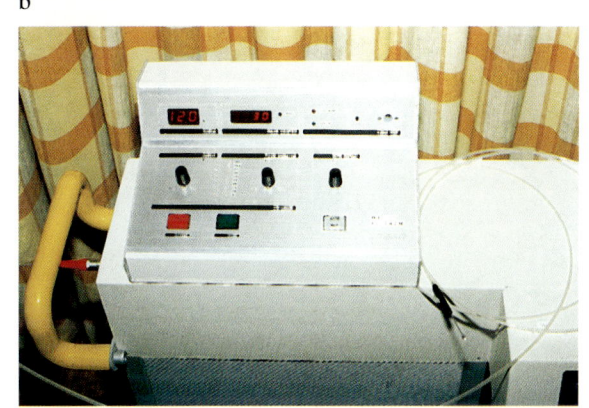

d

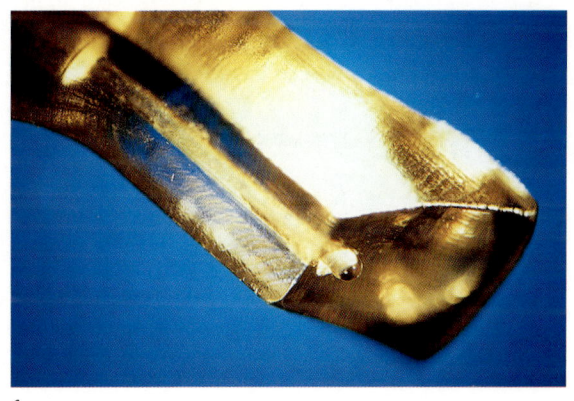

e

f

CYCLODESTRUCTIVE SURGERY

Transscleral Cyclophotocoagulation

III44a.   This cross-section of a human autopsy eye shows the relationship of the ciliary body (the target of cyclophotocoagulation) to the sclera, anterior chamber angle, and iris. With laser energy, the route of delivery in cyclophotocoagulation can be either transscleral (*small arrow*), transpupillary (*large arrow*) or intraocular with the probe entering the eye through either the pars plana or limbus. Note that the angle of approach with transpupillary cyclophotocoagulation allows view and treatment only of the anterior portion of the ciliary body ridge, a limitation with this technique.

III44b.   With transscleral cyclophotocoagulation, the focus of laser energy on the conjunctiva and sclera must be such that the energy will enter the eye at the level of the pars plicata. In this cross-section of a human autopsy eye, a needle has been inserted through the sclera 3 mm behind the limbus. This results in entry into the vitreous cavity at the level of the pars plana. With cyclophotocoagulation, therefore, the laser placement must be more anterior, at a distance of 1.0 to 1.5 mm posterior to the limbus.

III44c.   This light microscopic section of a human autopsy eye was treated with transscleral thermal, pulsed neodymium:YAG cyclophotocoagulation. Note the minimal damage in the sclera (the external defect is an artifact, created with India ink on a needle to identify the center of the laser path for histologic purposes) and the almost imperceptible damage in the adjacent ciliary muscle. When the laser energy reaches the more pigmented ciliary epithelium, however, a broad, blisterlike lesion is created (*arrows*).

III44d.   This light microscopic view shows the ciliary body of a human autopsy eye after treatment with transscleral continuous-wave Nd:YAG cyclophotocoagulation. The longer duration of exposure (700 to 1000 milliseconds) produces a more gradual contraction and coagulation of the uveal tissue, compared with the more explosive, blisterlike lesion with the thermal, pulsed mode (20 milliseconds) in the previous figure.

III44e.   This section of a porcine enucleated eye shows three ciliary body lesions created by contact, continuous-wave, Nd:YAG transscleral cyclophotocoagulation. Although the settings (power and exposure) were the same for all three treatment sites, considerably more damage is seen in the lesion to the far right of the view. This illustrates one disadvantage of contact transscleral cyclophotocoagulation, which is variability of tissue reaction related to the amount of pressure applied by the probe and the length of time the probe remains in contact with the eye before delivering the laser energy.

III44f.   This light microscopic view of a human autopsy eye shows the effect of transscleral diode cyclophotocoagulation. Note the increased amount of coagulation in the ciliary muscle (*arrows*), compared with that in III44c. This is related to the greater absorption of diode wavelength by melanin, compared with Nd:YAG wavelength.

(Figure III44b was provided courtesy of A. Robert Bellows, M.D.)

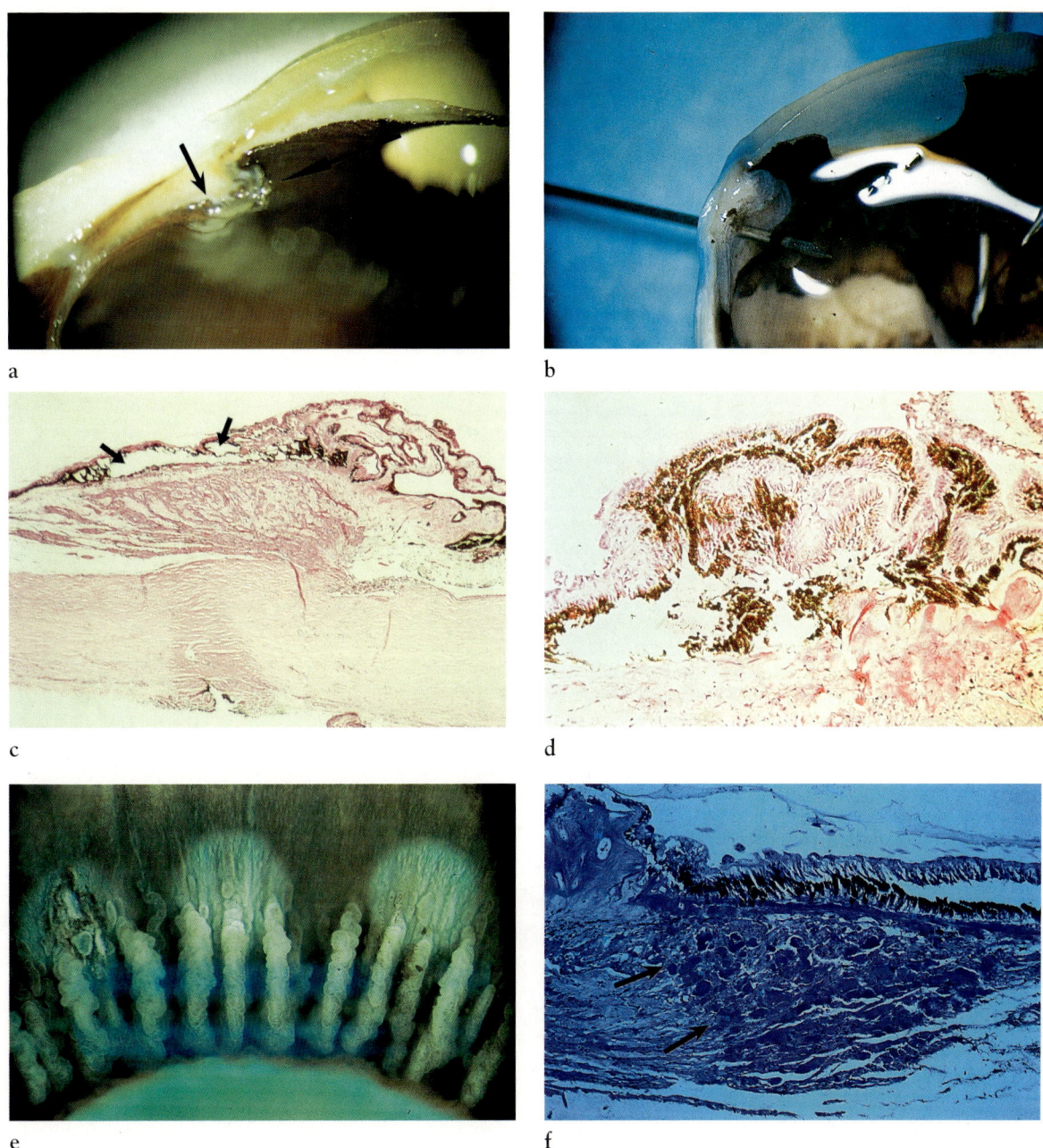

CYCLODESTRUCTIVE SURGERY

Technique of Non-Contact, Transscleral Cyclophotocoagulation

III45a.   Non-contact, transscleral Nd:YAG cyclophotocoagulation, which utilizes the MR II, can be performed with or without a contact lens. This photo shows a lens that has been developed for this operation, which provides the advantages of compressing and blanching the conjunctiva, maintaining lid separation and providing measurements from the limbus.

III45b.   After administering retrobulbar anesthesia, the patient is positioned at the laser slit lamp, and the contact lens is positioned on the eye. The cut portion in the periphery of the contact lens is designed to facilitate proper placement of the lens in an individual with a prominent brow.

III45c.   This slit-lamp view shows the appearance of the eye with the contact lens in position. Note the blanching of the conjunctiva in the superior quadrant, created by the pressure of the contact lens. A standard protocol for non-contact, transscleral Nd:YAG cyclophotocoagulation is 30 to 40 applications for 360°, spaced 1.0 to 1.5 mm behind the limbus, with energy levels between 4 and 8 joules.

III45d.   This photograph was taken immediately after non-contact, transscleral Nd:YAG cyclophotocoagulation, in which the contact lens was used to treat the 180° to the right of the view, but was not used in the 180° to the left. Note the greater degree of conjunctival burn that occurred without the conjunctival blanching produced by the contact lens.

III45e–f.   Even without the contact lens, the conjunctival burns heal quickly. III45e was obtained one day after non-contact, transscleral cyclophotocoagulation without a contact lens. Although the burns were prominent immediately after the procedure (as in III45d), they are barely seen at this time. III45f shows the same eye one week after surgery, at which time only minimal conjunctival hyperemia is seen at the treatment sites. Note also the clearing of the cornea with the reduction in intraocular pressure.

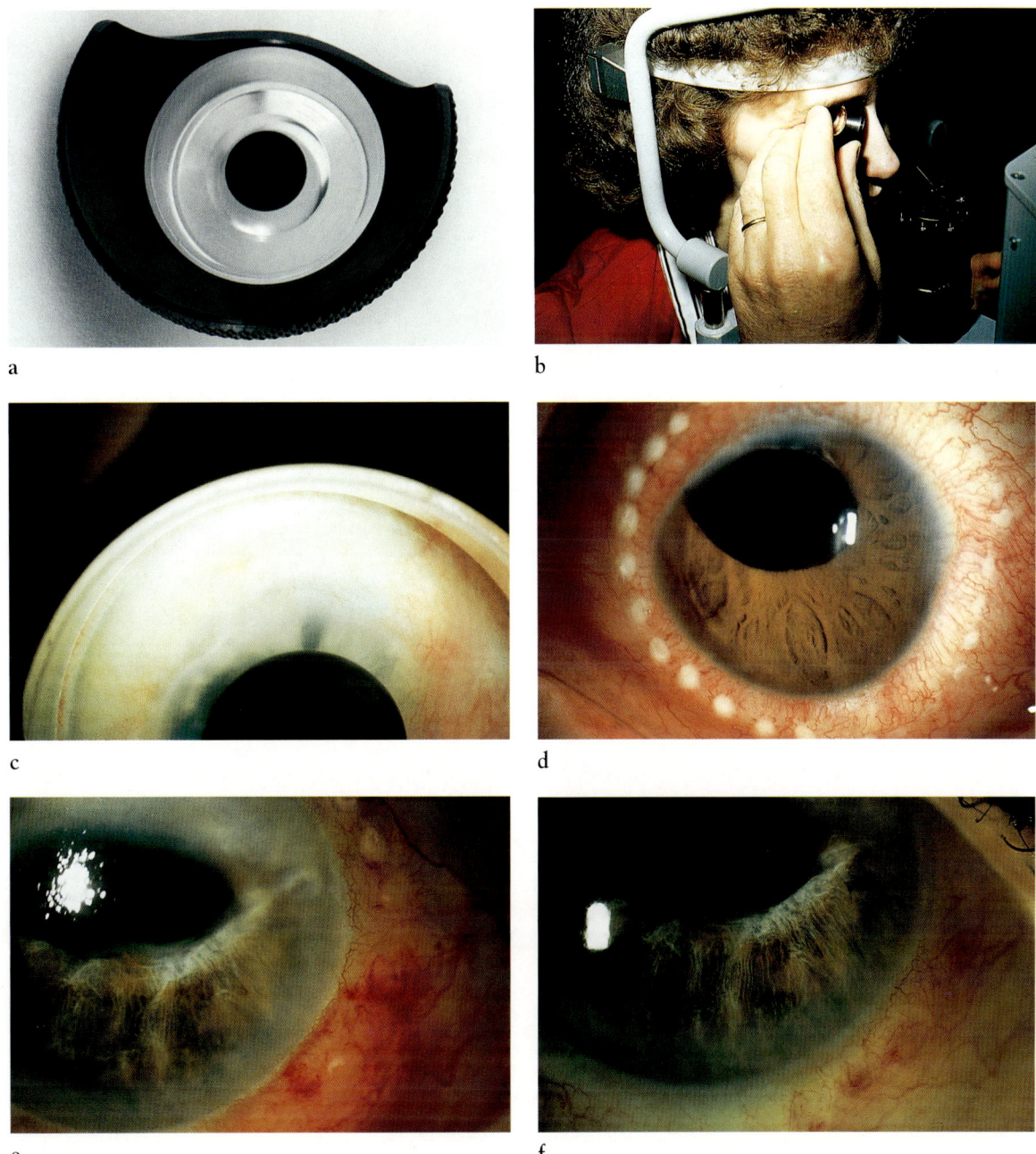

a

b

c

d

e

f

CYCLODESTRUCTIVE SURGERY

Techniques of Contact, Transscleral Cyclophotocoagulation

III46a. Contact, transscleral Nd:YAG cyclophotocoagulation is being performed in this photograph with the SLT CL60. The lids are separated with a lid speculum, and calipers are used to measure a distance of 0.5 to 1.5 mm behind the limbus. The tip of the fiberoptic probe is applied perpendicular to the surface of the conjunctiva with the tip of the probe at the measured site. Treatment protocols vary among surgeons, although that most commonly used involves 30 to 60 applications for 360° with a power in the range of 4 to 9 W.

III46b. This schematic shows the placement of the G-Probe (trapezoidal outline) when performing contact, transscleral diode cyclophotocoagulation with the Oculight SLx. With the footplate adjacent to the limbus, the fiberoptic is positioned 1.2 mm from the limbus. The footplate can also be used to standardize spacing between laser applications, by placing the next application at the margin of the indentation created by the footplate in the previous application.

III46c. The G-Probe is shown in position during transscleral diode cyclophotocoagulation. This procedure can be performed with the patient sitting or supine.

III46d–f. Transscleral diode cyclophotocoagulation with the G-Probe can also be performed at the slit lamp. III46d shows the length of the standard G-Probe in the lower field of view. The shorter probe was designed for use at the slit lamp. III46e and III46f show the use of the short G-Probe at the slit lamp.

(Figure III46a was provided courtesy of Joel S. Schuman, M.D., and used with permission of Lippincott-Raven Publishers. Figure III46b was provided courtesy of Douglas E. Gaasterland, M.D.; Figure III46c was provided courtesy of Irvin P. Pollack, M.D.)

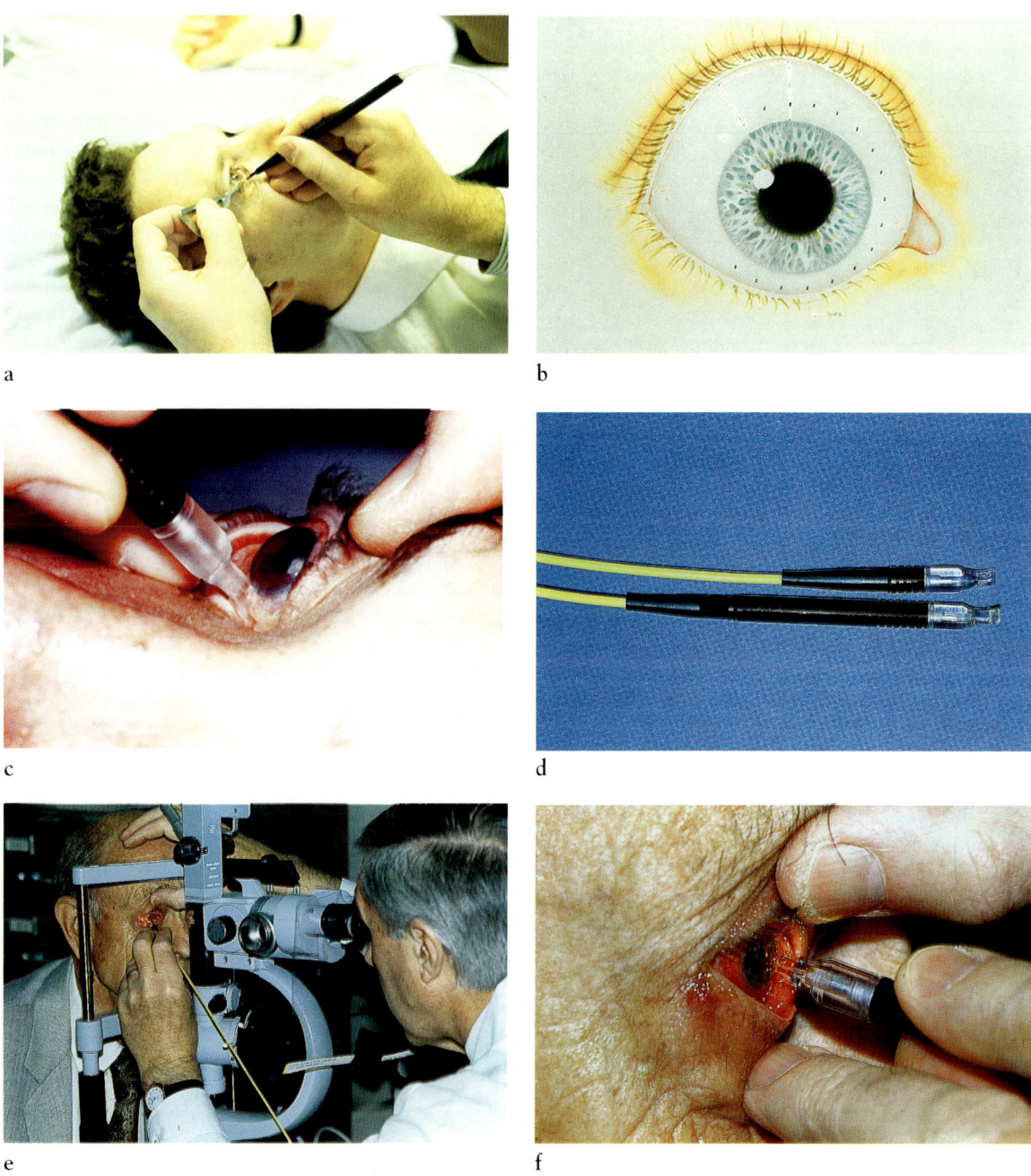

a

b

c

d

e

f

CYCLODESTRUCTIVE SURGERY

Endoscopic Cyclophotocoagulation and Therapeutic Ultrasound

III49a.   Intraocular cyclophotocoagulation is being performed in this photograph under endoscopic visualization. The television monitor for the microendoscope is seen to the left of the picture. This position allows the surgeon to quickly change observation between the operating microscope and the television monitor.

III49b.   Although endoscopic cyclophotocoagulation is commonly performed through the pars plana, it can also be performed through a limbal tunnel incision, as in this photograph. The eye is aphakic and has had an anterior vitrectomy. An irrigation cannula is positioned through a clear corneal incision to maintain anterior chamber depth, and three flexible iris retractors are used to pull the iris anteriorly. The probe of the microendoscope has been inserted through a scleral tunnel incision 180° from the iris retractors, and intraocular cyclophotocoagulation can be performed for approximately 180°.

III49c–d.   These two photographs show laser lesions in a monkey eye that were produced with an early, prototype endophotocoagulator, in which an argon laser fiberoptic was attached to a direct-viewing endoscope. III49c shows a cluster of five ciliary processes treated with the endoscopic argon cyclophotocoagulation. III49d shows the light microscopic appearance of a treated ciliary process to the left, with an adjacent, normal-appearing, untreated ciliary process to the right. This demonstrates the precision that can be achieved with endoscopic cyclophotocoagulation.

III49e–f.   These two photographs show the use of therapeutic ultrasound as a cyclodestructive procedure. The basic technique involves an emersion applicator (III49e) with which an average of 6 to 7 exposures of ultrasound are delivered at an intensity of 10 kW/cm^2 for 5 seconds each to scleral sites near the limbus. III49f shows the light microscopic appearance in a porcine eye after therapeutic ultrasound. Note the extensive scleral damage, in addition to the destruction of ciliary processes. It has been postulated that the selective thinning of scleral collagen and separation of the ciliary body from the sclera may improve aqueous outflow, in addition to the reduced inflow produced by the cyclodestruction.

(Figures III49e–f provided courtesy of D. Jackson Coleman, M.D., and Barrett G. Haik, M.D.)

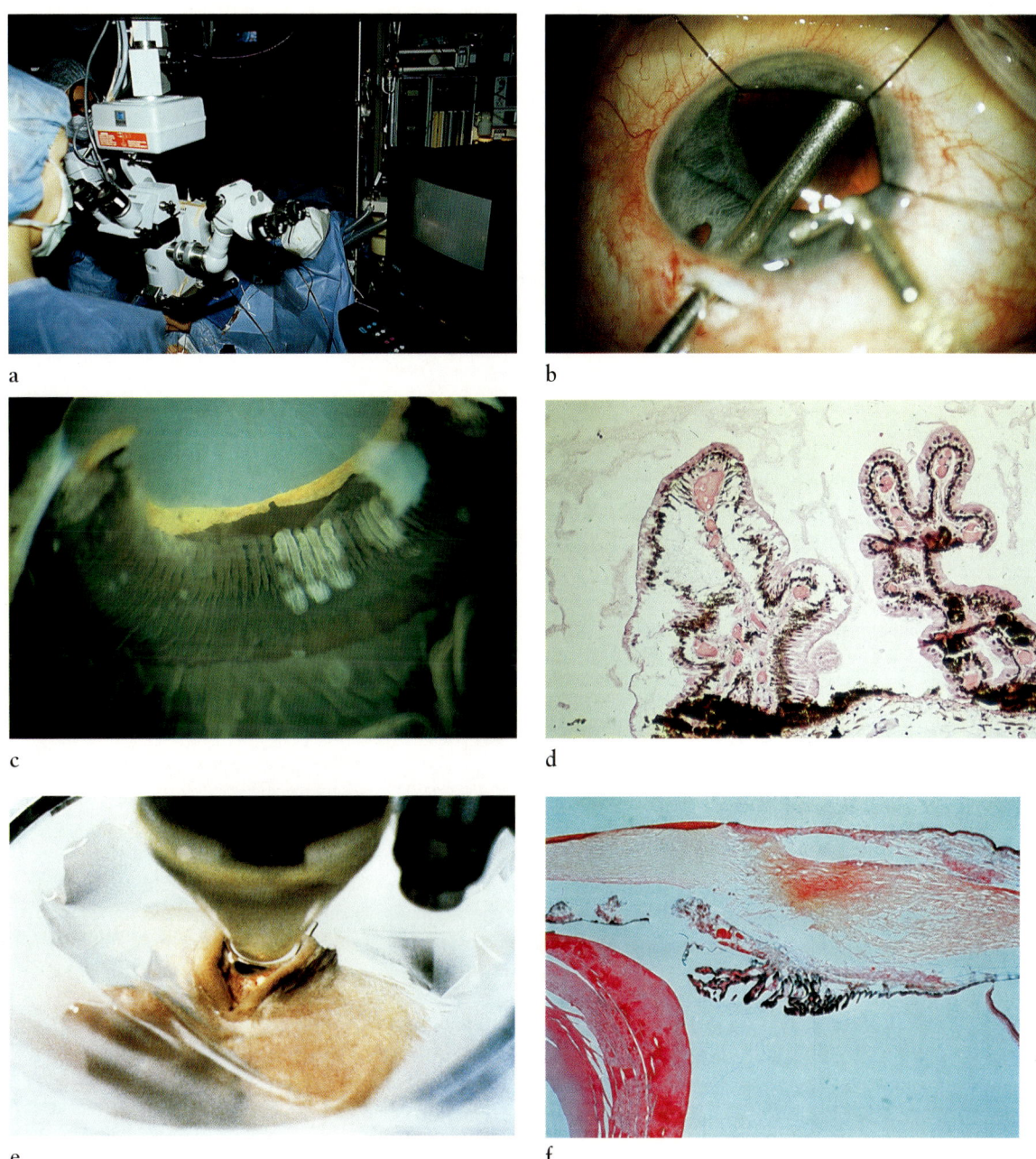

SURGICAL APPROACHES FOR CO-EXISTING GLAUCOMA AND CATARACT

Management of the Small Pupil

A common problem in performing cataract surgery on patients with glaucoma is the irreversible miosis from chronic miotic therapy. A wide variety of techniques have been described to surgically enlarge the pupil. In the era of extracapsular cataract extraction, various combinations of iridotomies and sphincterotomies proved to be effective. With the popularity of small incision phacoemulsification, however, newer techniques, such as iris retractors and stretching techniques, have been successfully employed. We will consider one of the former techniques with extracapsular surgery on this page, and then review approaches to mechanical pupillary dilation with phacoemulsification on the next page.

III50a.   This eye is being prepared for combined extracapsular cataract extraction and glaucoma filtering surgery. The size of the pupil represents the maximum dilation that could be achieved with mydriatics, and is not that uncommon in patients on long-term miotic therapy.

III50b.   After creating the cataract incision with a chord arc of approximately 10 mm and deepening the anterior chamber with a viscoelastic, iris scissors are introduced into the anterior chamber, with one blade in the posterior chamber to create an inferior sphincterotomy.

III50c.   Two inferior sphincterotomies have now been created. It is important to extend the incision of each sphincterotomy just beyond the sphincter muscle to allow adequate dilation, but not beyond that point.

III50d.   The next step is to create a superior sector iridotomy, as shown in this photo. One technique for creating the sector iridotomy is to first create a small, peripheral iridotomy, then extend one blade of the iris scissors through the iridotomy until the tips are beyond the margin of the pupil and then complete the sector iridotomy with a single cut.

III50e.   After the two inferior sphincterotomies and the superior sector iridotomy are completed, additional viscoelastic is injected into the anterior chamber, which mechanically expands the pupil, as shown in this photo. Such a pupillary opening is usually sufficient for extracapsular cataract extraction.

III50f.   This slit-lamp view shows the postoperative appearance of a patient who has had the two inferior sphincterotomies and superior sector iridotomy. Some surgeons prefer to close the sector iridotomy with an iris suture. This can be technically difficult, however, and patients generally tolerate the sector iridotomy, most of which is covered by the upper lid. Leaving the iridotomy open also facilitates future fundus examination. It is advisable with this technique, however, to rotate the haptics of the intraocular lens horizontally, especially with sulcus fixation.

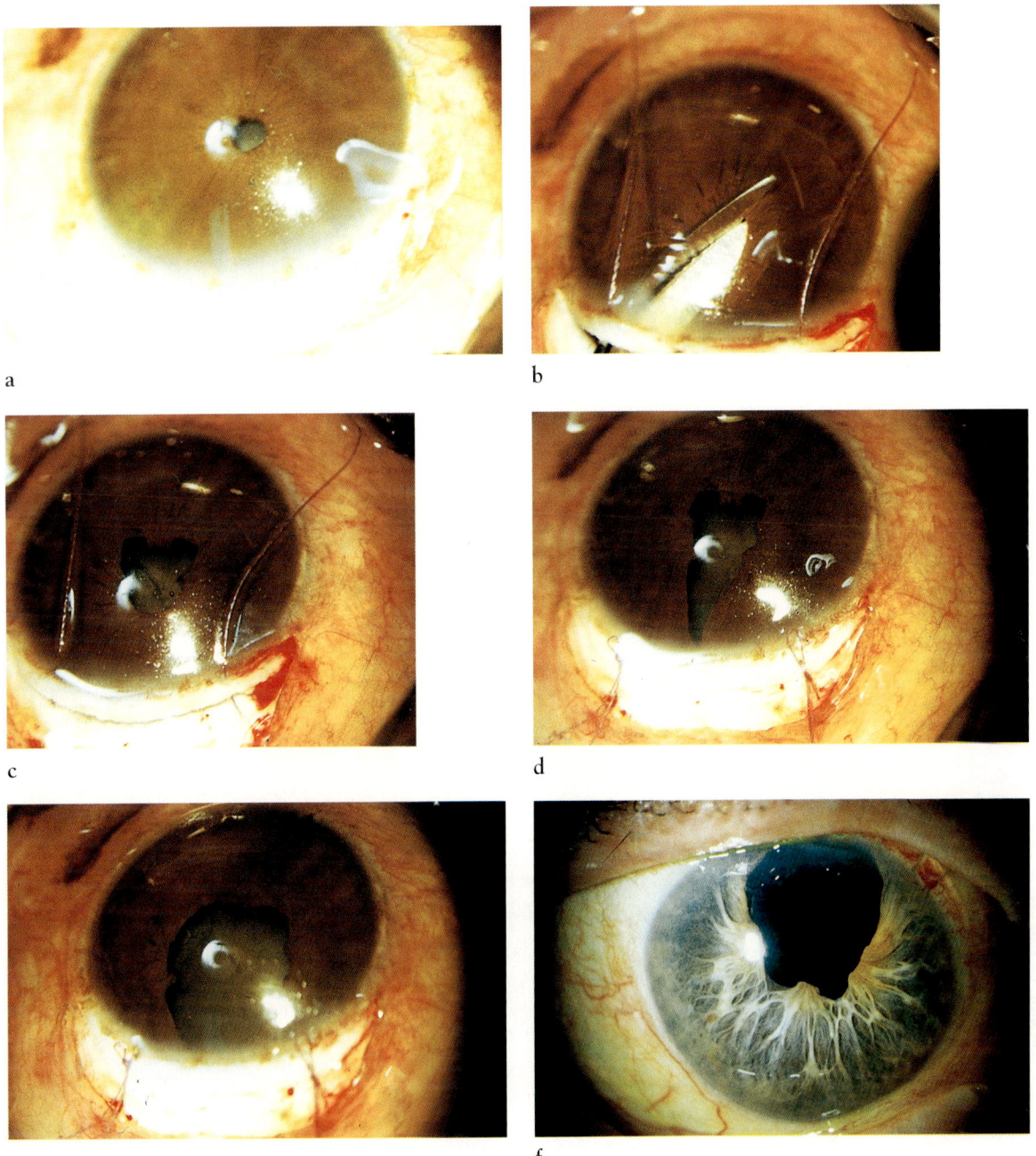

a

b

c

d

e

f

SURGICAL APPROACHES FOR CO-EXISTING GLAUCOMA AND CATARACT

Management of the Small Pupil

III51a.   A technique that has proved to be especially useful in conjunction with small-pupil phacoemulsification is the use of the flexible iris retractor, as shown in this photo. The retractor is fashioned from nylon suture material, and the hook at one end is sufficiently rigid to maintain iris retraction, but also flexible enough to facilitate removal of the retractor through the corneal incision. A Silastic sleeve on the retractor can be positioned to help maintain tension on the iris.

III51b.   Before inserting the retractors, the anterior chamber is deepened with viscoelastic (although not too deep, because that makes it more difficult to engage the hook around the pupillary margin) and four stab incisions are made at the limbus. Two incisions should be to either side of the cataract incision, and the other two are equally spaced in the inferior quadrants. In this photo, a diamond blade is being used to create the stab incisions, although any sharp, pointed blade will suffice.

III51c.   After the four stab incisions are made, the iris retractor is now inserted through the incision, into the anterior chamber, and the hook is engaged around the pupillary margin.

III51d.   In this photo, the hook has been engaged around the pupillary margin, and slight tension is put on the iris sphincter by advancing the Silastic sleeve to the limbus. The pupil should be dilated only minimally at this time, because that will help the placement of the other retractors.

III51e.   All four retractors have now been positioned, with partial tension on the iris sphincter.

III51f.   After all four iris retractors are in position, the tension on each retractor can be increased to achieve maximal dilation, as shown in this photograph. The pupil will now remain reliably dilated throughout the phacoemulsification procedure. One note of caution, however, is that the retractors lift the pupillary margin, and care must be taken in going over this elevated margin with the phacoemulsification tip and other instruments. After completion of the cataract extraction (but before insertion of the intraocular lens) the tension on the iris sphincter is released, and the retractors are easily removed through the corneal incisions.

Other techniques for mechanically enlarging a miotic pupil in conjunction with phacoemulsification include mechanically stretching the pupil and a variety of iris suture techniques.

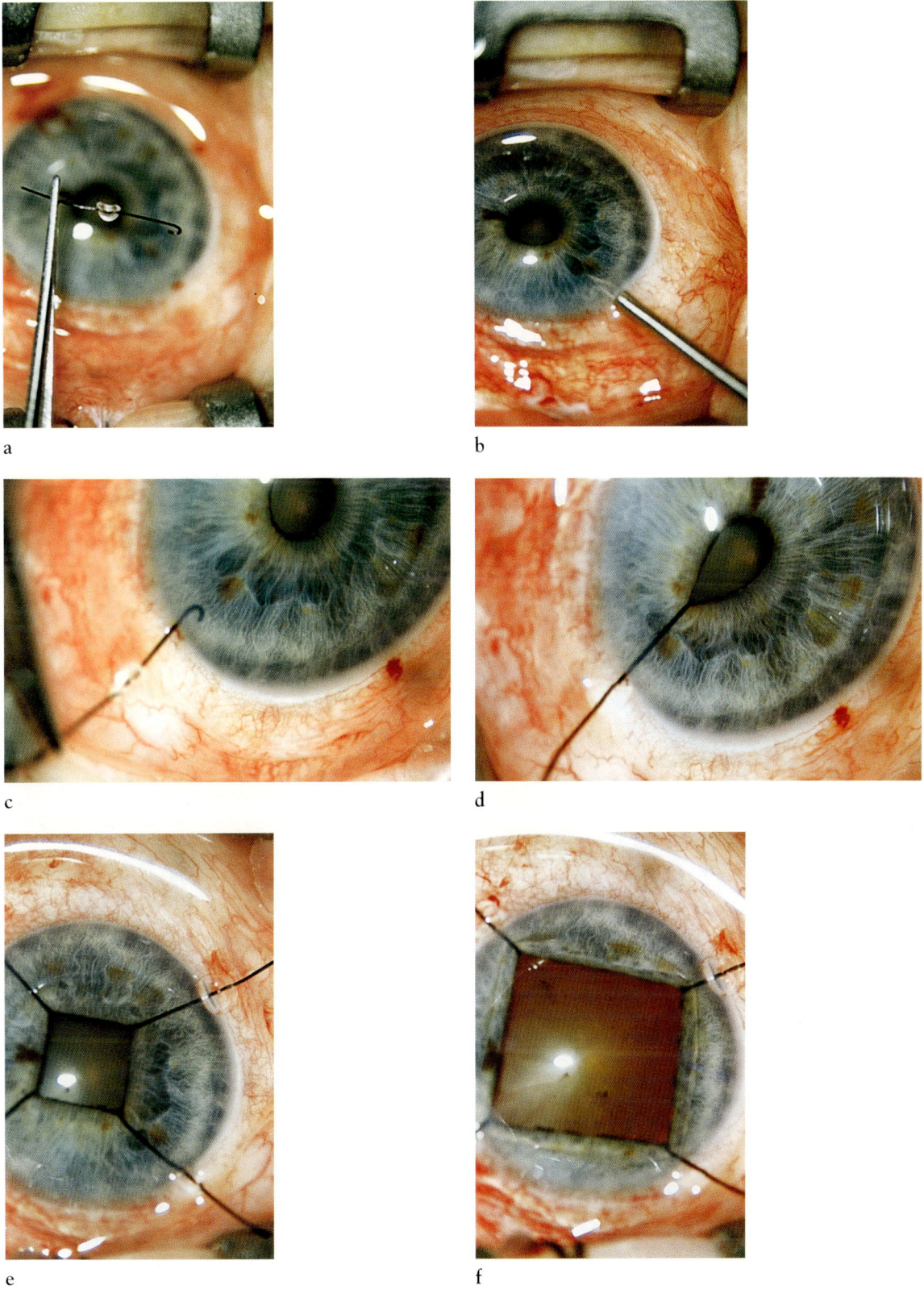

a

b

c

d

e

f

SURGICAL APPROACHES FOR CO-EXISTING
GLAUCOMA AND CATARACT

Combined Phacoemulsification and Glaucoma Filtering Surgery

III52a.   A conjunctival-Tenon's capsule flap is first prepared in the same manner as previously described for a trabeculectomy. In this case, a limbus-based flap is being used. Many surgeons prefer a fornix-based flap for the combined surgery, and postoperative results appear to be similar with the two techniques.

III52b.   The conjunctival-Tenon's capsule flap is dissected to the limbus, using blunt dissection whenever possible, and clipping tissue strands only when necessary. As noted with the trabeculectomy technique, it is advisable to leave Tenon's capsule inserted at the limbus to provide a thicker filtering bleb postoperatively.

III52c.   Most surgeons choose to use an antimetabolite, since combining the glaucoma filtering procedure with cataract extraction is felt to increase the risk of late failure of the filtering bleb. Postoperative 5-fluorouracil has not been found to be helpful in these cases, but there is an impression that intraoperative mitomycin-C is beneficial. In this photo, a Merocel sponge, saturated with mitomycin-C, is being placed under the conjunctival-Tenon's flap. The details of this procedure were discussed under Trabeculectomy.

III52d.   After applying the mitomycin-C and irrigating the site with balanced salt solution, the scleral tunnel incision is created in the usual manner. The width of the tunnel will depend upon the intraocular lens that is to be used.

III52e.   This photo shows the use of the flexible iris retractors, as discussed on the previous page, in conjunction with the standard phacoemulsification procedure.

III52f.   After completing the cataract extraction, but before inserting the intraocular lens, it is advisable to remove the flexible iris retractors. The iris will remain sufficiently dilated at this point, and it is easier to insert the intraocular lens without the elevation of the pupillary margin created by the iris retractors. In this photo, a rigid intraocular lens is being inserted into the capsular bag through a 6 mm tunnel incision. Foldable lenses can also be used in the combined procedure and have the obvious advantage of a smaller incision.

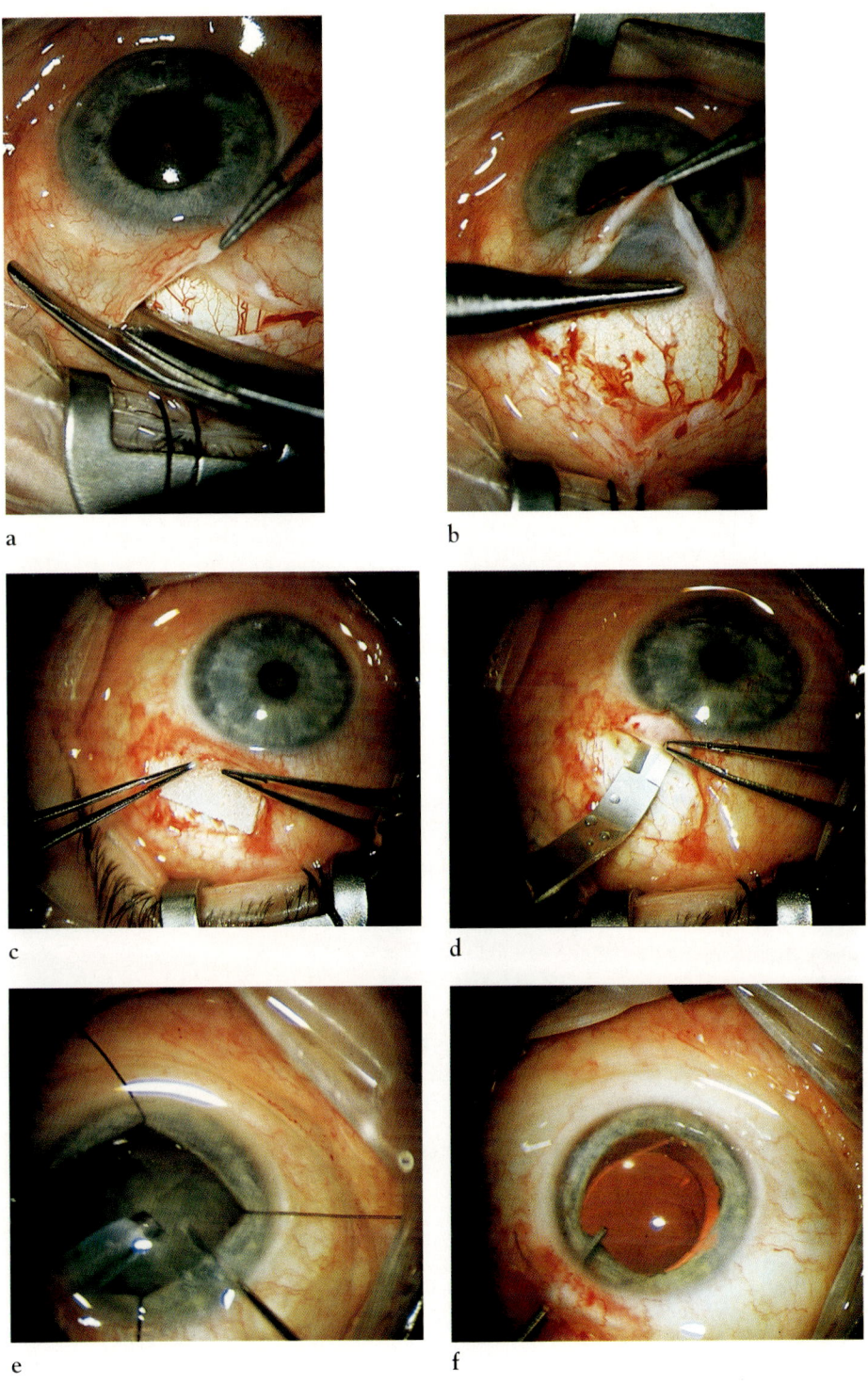

a

b

c

d

e

f

SURGICAL APPROACHES FOR CO-EXISTING GLAUCOMA AND CATARACT

Combined Phacoemulsification and Glaucoma Filtering Surgery

III53a. Having completed the phacoemulsification and posterior chamber intraocular lens implantation, as described on the previous page, it is now time to perform the glaucoma filtering portion of the operation. In the technique shown here, the guarded filtering procedure is incorporated into the standard scleral tunnel incision. Two radial incisions are first made in the posterior lip of the tunnel incision. The two incisions are approximately 2 to 3 mm apart and are extended to within less than 1 mm of the entry site for the tunnel incision. With a 6 mm incision, adequate exposure for this step of the operation can usually be achieved by lifting up the anterior lip of the tunnel incision. For smaller incisions, it may be necessary to make a radial incision at one end of the anterior lip in order to provide adequate exposure for creation of the fistula.

III53b. Having made the two radial incisions, the flap of deep limbal tissue is reflected, exposing the anterior chamber angle structures, and the fistula is completed by cutting along scleral spur. This photo shows the completed fistula in the posterior lip of the scleral tunnel incision.

III53c. After the fistula is created in the posterior lip of the scleral tunnel incision, the incision is then closed with one 10-0 nylon suture on either side of the fistula. In this way, the anterior lip of the scleral tunnel incision serves as the guard over the fistula in the internal lip, creating a situation similar to that in a standard trabeculectomy.

III53d. Before closing the conjunctival-Tenon's capsule flap, it is advisable to test the integrity of the scleral tunnel incision by injecting balanced salt solution into the anterior chamber through one of the corneal stab incisions used during the phacoemulsification procedure. This maneuver should be associated with a deepening of the anterior chamber before fluid is seen to flow slowly through the incision site. If the flow is too brisk, and the anterior chamber shallows, additional sutures should be placed in the scleral tunnel incision.

III53e. The conjunctival-Tenon's capsule flap is closed in the same manner as previously described for a trabeculectomy, using a double, running closure of 10-0 absorbable suture on a fine, non-cutting needle. After the closure is complete, balanced salt solution should again be injected into the anterior chamber. This step should be associated with a further deepening of the anterior chamber and an elevation of the conjunctival flap, with no evidence of wound leakage.

III53f. This slit-lamp view shows the postoperative appearance after phacoemulsification, posterior chamber intraocular lens implantation, and guarded filtering surgery with adjunctive mitomycin-C. The postoperative management of these patients is essentially the same as previously described for trabeculectomy, including the use of digital pressure and laser suture lysis, as required to promote a successful filtering bleb.

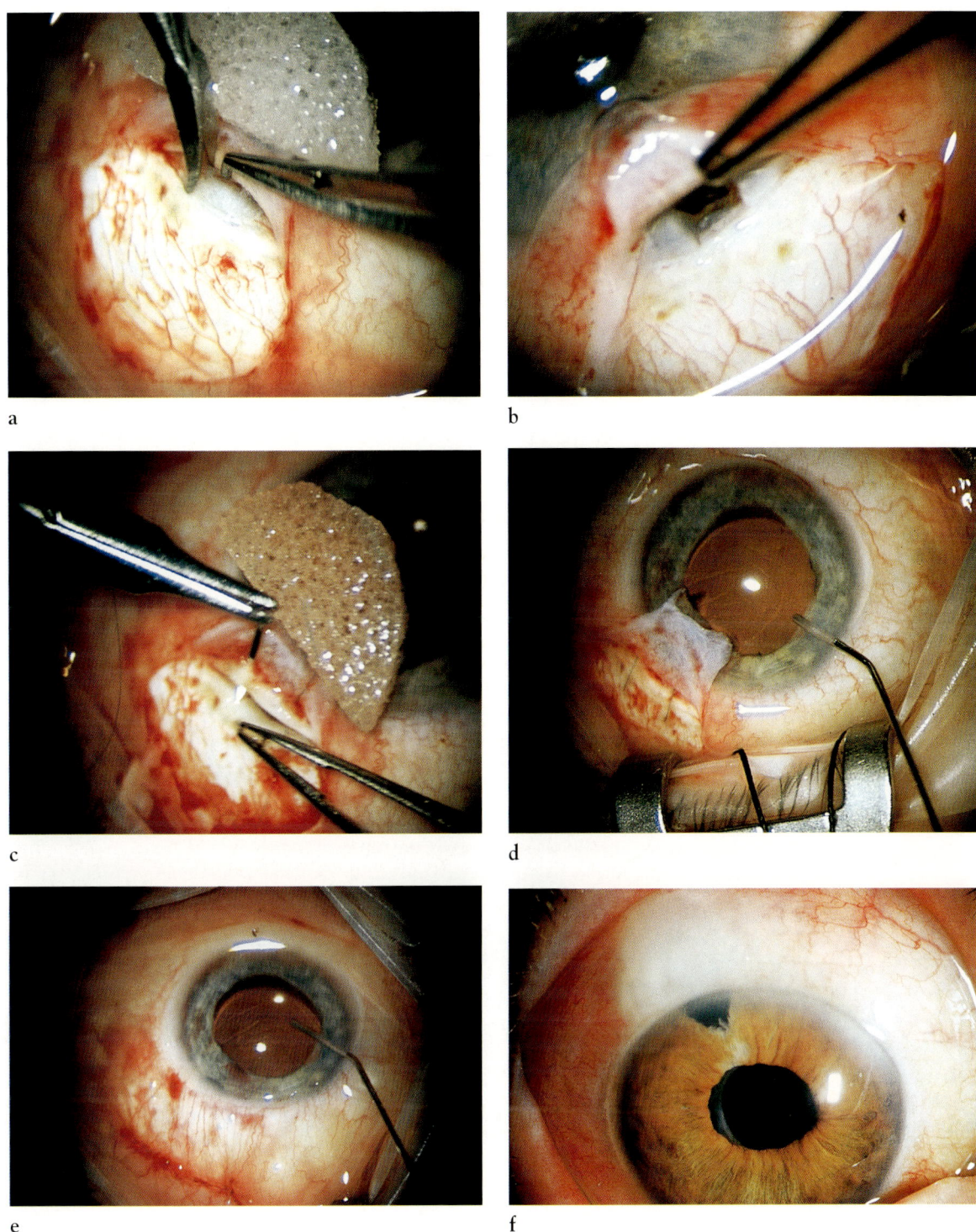

a

b

c

d

e

f

SURGICAL APPROACHES FOR CO-EXISTING GLAUCOMA AND CATARACT

Phacoemulsification After Filtering Surgery

III54a.   Cataract surgery is occasionally required in an eye with a functioning glaucoma filtering bleb. In some cases, the filtering surgery may have been performed years earlier, and the eye has subsequently developed a cataract. In other cases, the cataract surgery may be the second part of a two-stage approach to co-existing cataract and glaucoma. The latter approach is often used when the glaucoma is uncontrolled despite maximum medical therapy and trabeculoplasty and poses an immediate threat to the patient's vision.

III54b.   Small-incision, clear-cornea phacoemulsification has become the ideal technique for cataract extraction in an eye with a functioning filtering bleb. Some surgeons prefer to use a temporal incision. A supero-temporal or infero-temporal incision can also be used, however, and has the advantage of allowing the surgeon to operate from the customary position. In this photo, the anterior chamber is being entered through clear cornea with a 2.5 mm diamond keratome.

III54c.   The phacoemulsification procedure is next performed in the usual manner. Flexible iris retractors or other techniques of mechanical pupillary dilation can be used, when necessary. In many of these patients, however, who are no longer on miotic therapy, adequate dilation can be achieved with mydriatic drops.

III54d.   After the cataract extraction is complete, the corneal incision is enlarged to 3.5 to 4.0 mm with a keratome, and a foldable lens is implanted in the capsular bag.

III54e.   In some cases, wound closure may be adequate to preclude the need for a suture. When in doubt, however, it is advisable to use a single 10-0 nylon suture across the corneal incision, which can be removed in the early postoperative course. This technique of clear-cornea phacoemulsification, with posterior chamber lens implantation, is usually well tolerated by the filtering bleb. It is not uncommon, however, to see a slight rise in the long-term intraocular pressure, and some patients will require resumption of glaucoma medication.

III54f.   With modern phacoemulsification techniques, extracapsular cataract surgery is rarely required. If extracapsular extraction is felt to be indicated (e.g., in an eye with an unsually hard nucleus or a hypermature cataract) in an eye with a functioning filtering bleb, the clear cornea approach can again be used. In this case, a large incision in the peripheral cornea with a chord arc of 10 mm is created to express the nucleus. Multiple, individual sutures or a running suture can then be used to close the wound at the completion of the procedure, as shown in this photo.

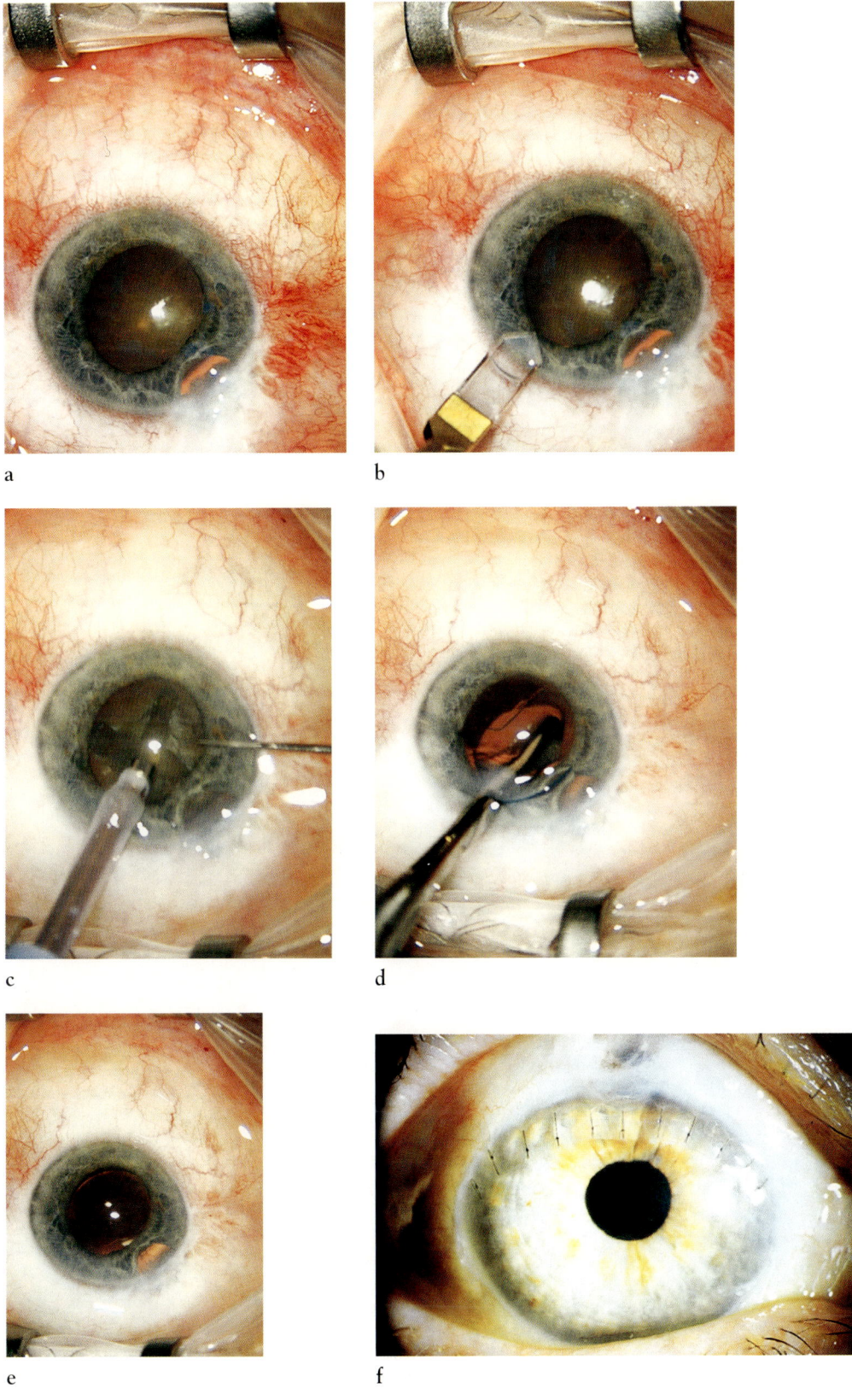

a

b

c

d

e

f

INDEX

LIBRARY
POST GRADUATE CENTRE
KETTERING GENERAL HOSPITAL